11th CONGRESS OF
THE INTERNATIONAL
FEDERATION OF HOSPITAL
ENGINEERING

11e CONGRÈS DU
FEDERATION
INTERNATIONALE
D'INGENIERIE HOSPITALIERE

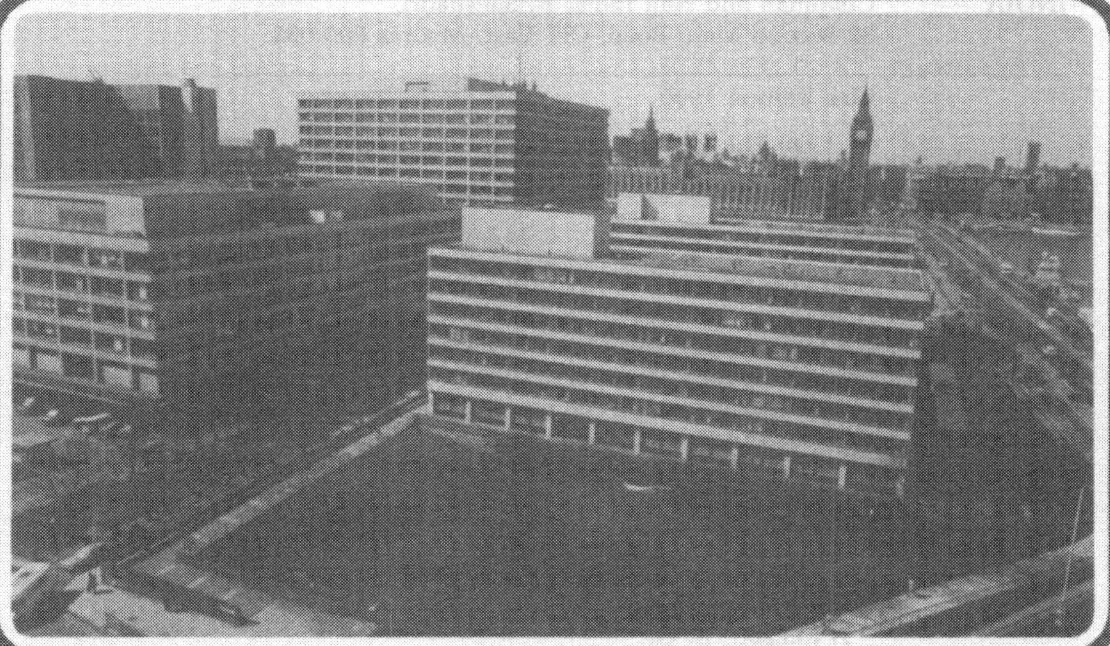

Photograph of St Thomas' Hospital, London by courtesy of Landis & Gyr.

The Changing Scene of Health Care and Technology
Evolution Des Soins et Technologie

at THE QUEEN ELIZABETH II CONFERENCE CENTRE, LONDON, 4-8 JUNE 1990

Editor in Chief:
R. G. Kensett
BA(Hons), CEng, MIMechE, MCIBSE, MInstE, MBIM, FIHospE

Routledge
Taylor & Francis Group
LONDON AND NEW YORK

First edition 1990
By Chapman & Hall.
Published 2004
by Spon Press,
2 Park Square, Milton Park, Abingdon, Oxon OX14 4RN
711 Third Avenue, New York, NY 10017, USA

First issued in hardback 2017

Routledge is an imprint of the Taylor & Francis Group, an informa business

British Library Cataloguing in Publication Data

The changing scene of health care and technology
1. Health services
1. Kensett, R. G.
362.1

ISBN 13: 978-1-138-40234-8 (hbk)
ISBN 13: 978-0-419-16740-2 (pbk)

INTERNATIONAL FEDERATION OF HOSPITAL ENGINEERING
FEDERATION INTERNATIONALE D'INGENIERIE HOSPITALIERE

The First Twenty Years

In May 1970 the Federazione Nazionale Tecnici Ospedalieri (FeNATO) organised an International Congress of Hospital Engineering in Rome. It was during this Congress the need was recognised for an organisation which would encourage international communication between hospital engineers and to ensure that congresses of this type would be held at least every two years. A working party, drawn from the six nations expressing an interest, considered how this might be achieved and proposed at the Congress that an International Federation of Hospital Engineering be set up. This was accepted and a Deed of Partnership was signed by:-

George Rooley — Institute of Hospital Engineering — United Kingdom
Osvaldo Amato — Federazione Nazionale Tecnici Ospedalieri — Italy
Jean Aloy — Association Nationale des Ingeniers Hospitaliers — France
Zissimos Tzartzanos — Technikon Epilmelitirion tis Ellardos — Greece
Eduardo Caetano — Portugal
Jan Thorp — Sweden
Bruno Massara — FeNATO — Italy who became the first General Secretary.

The objectives of the IFHE are:- to promote, develop and disseminate hospital engineering technology; to compare international experience; to promote the principle of integrated planning, design and evaluation by improved collaboration between professions; to promote more efficient management of operation, maintenance and safety of hospitals, their engineering installations, equipment and buildings; and to offer collaboration with other international organisations.

Initially the membership was drawn from Institutions/Associations of Hospital Engineering as Full Members, and Associates from countries where such organisations did not exist. As the objectives of the Federation became more widely known, mainly through the bi-annual congresses, more individuals and organisations associated with hospital engineering wished to subscribe and help to increase its activities.

In 1983 the Statute was amended to widen the membership to include individuals ('B' Members), public authorities ('C' Members), industry and professional consultants ('D' Members). The Institutions/Associations are the 'A' Members and form the Council which controls the affairs to the Federation. Now, in 1990 there are 26 'A' Members from 24 countries and 57 members in the other categories.

In 1987 the IFHE was recognised by the World Health Organisation as a 'Non-Governmental Organisation in Official Relationship with WHO'. IFHE is collaborating with WHO, as far as its limited resources will permit, to improve standards of engineering management in the developing countries.

Since 1973 the Institute of Hospital Engineering has produced for IFHE quarterly International Issues of 'Hospital Engineering' which has recently been re-named 'Health Estate Journal' to reflect the wider interest of its readers. The Editor would be pleased to receive as many articles as possible especially from countries outside of the United Kingdom.

Congresses have been held every two years in Rome, London, Athens, Paris, Lisbon, Washington, Amsterdam, Melbourne, Barcelona and Edmonton. The 12th Congress will be in Bologna, Italy in 1992.

The Presidents of IFHE:-

Osvaldo Amato	—	Italy	**Vinson Oviatt**	—	USA
George Rooley	—	United Kingdom	**Cor Sonius**	—	The Netherlands
Zissimos Tzartzanos	—	Greece	**Robert Cottrill**	—	Australia
Jaques Ponthieux	—	France	**Antonio Bonnin**	—	Spain
Eduardo Caetano	—	Portugal	**Steven Morawski**	—	Canada

The President Elect for June 1990-1992 **Basil Hermon** — United Kingdom

General Secretaries have been:-

Bruno Massara	—	Italy	—	1970-1980
Joao Galvao	—	Portugal	—	1980-1984
Basil Hermon	—	United Kingdom	—	1984-1988
Duncan MacMillan	—	United Kingdom	—	1988-1989
Michael Franck	—	United Kingdom	—	takes over in June 1990

The IFHE is grateful to the Institute of Hospital Engineering for organising the 11th Congress in London 4-8 June 1990 and to the generosity of the following sponsors for their support of this event:-

British Coal
Department of Health
RW Gregory and Partners
Haden Young
Hospital Engineering and Estate Management Centre
IFHE
John Laing Construction
Landis & Gyr
Ohmeda
SISealy & Associates
Donald Smith Seymour & Rooley
Static Systems
Widnells

INTERNATIONAL FEDERATION
OF
HOSPITAL ENGINEERING 11TH CONGRESS

The Changing Scene of Health Care and Technology

CONTENTS

Foreword

It is my privilege and pleasure to introduce the Proceedings of the 1990 International Congress on hospital engineering and estate management.

The task of selecting the papers which are to be given at the Congress and which form these Proceedings was both difficult and complex. This was not because of a lack of choice but rather because of the number and quality of the papers offered. To the unsuccessful the Programme Committee offer their grateful thanks and only regret that time did not allow us to take advantage of the depth of knowledge and experience you were willing to share with those engaged in the Health Care field.

When reviewing the papers offered the complexity of hospital engineering in all its facets and the advances which have taken place since the UK last hosted the Congress in 1972 were readily apparent. The Programme Committee trust that their selection will offer a range of experience and information which will be of assistance to you all.

I hope our many delegates from so many countries will enjoy their stay in the UK and will find the Congress informative. It is to be hoped that the informal contacts, which always form such a valued part of the Congress, will endure and perhaps enable the interchange of views and experiences to continue long into the future.

Ray Kensett
Chairman
Congress Technical Programme Committee

Energy Strategy in English Hospitals

by

Brian Oliver
CEng, MIMechE, MInstR, FIHospE
Head of Energy Efficiency,
Department of Health, London

This paper sets out to address the need for a co-ordinated energy strategy for the National Health Service. But first, in order to put this into context, especially for delegates from abroad, it will be necessary to give some background to the NHS and to its record in respect of energy management.

The National Health Service in England has an estate consisting of some 2,000 hospitals and 10,000 other buildings with a current replacement value of about £70B. Over 50% of this estate is comprised of buildings built before 1919. On the whole this group have a good energy performance especially when upgraded or refurbished.

Of the remainder about half consist of buildings completed between the two world wars, many of which include temporary buildings with considerable variability of construction, often on the same site.

The final 20% or so, is made up of relatively new buildings, which vary from the tower block and deep planned constructions of the 60's and 70's to the modern Nucleus and Low Energy designs. Unfortunately buildings erected during the early part of this period are among our worst energy performers.

It was in the early part of the 1960's that work commenced on a range of guidance to assist in the design and operation of the hospitals built and used in the NHS. This guidance consisted of Hospital Building Notes, Technical Memoranda and Equipment Notes. For the first time medical planners, nurses, architects and engineers were brought together so as to optimise design and operation. This guidance is now renowned throughout the world.

At this time energy was recognised as a significant factor within the design process and a good deal of expertise was gained and incorporated, both within the Building Notes and the associated Design Guides and within the operation and estate management modules that were produced.

Because of the low price of energy, the design of a UK hospital in the 60's was not, by todays standard, energy efficient. Nevertheless it was energy conscious and included a high degree of sophistication. Cost effectiveness played an important part of design and discounted cash flow techniques were recommended for the option appraisal of design. It was also considered imperative that adequate security of service should be provided with backup supplies of fossil fuel and electricity. This is a subject somewhat forgotten with today's emphasis on efficiency and is a matter I shall return to later.

It was not until the OPEC energy crisis in 1972 that we had to take more concerted steps to limit the use of energy. This involved the injection of £13.3M of capital for local initiatives in the UK NHS and the employment of a small section of staff at the Department of Health in London. Initially the team worked on the analysis of energy consumption and the selective improvement of hospital engineering plant. Particular attention being paid to energy conversion equipment. Co-ordinated effort was also made to improve energy management but this was not drawn together into a comprehensive energy code (Encode) until 1983.

In the design field, our examples on the Isle of Wight and in Northumberland have given a clear lead for new build. These are based on the Nucleus concept which in itself is an energy efficient hospital design making the most of natural light and ventilation and thereby minimising the need for additional energy systems. Added to this are a range of engineering provisions to minimise and recover energy. The features used are much the same as recommended in Encode, differences of emphasis only occurring because the energy code relates to the wide variety of old and new buildings in use in the UK NHS.

The strategy adopted for the energy code defined a need to stimulate, in concert with both new health building and the estate management processes, the public sector and private enterprise, in the provision of tools and services to reduce the energy consumption and cost within the health service. This was seen to involve the provision of improved management services, better and more efficient technical equipment and more energy efficient building design standards. Data collection and management was identified as an area needing particular attention.

In order to meet the strategy the Department has concentrated on the following:-

(1) Continuing research and development in discrete areas, especially on new build.
(2) Compilation of case studies.
(3) Comprehensive guidance.
(4) Application of computer technology for better management.
(5) Promotion of energy awareness.

Whilst we are aware that much still needs to be done the 20 year programme to date has saved an impressive amount of money estimated to be running currently, at today's prices, at over £70M/year. Looked at in another way this amounts in total over the period to the cash equivalent of over 20 new district general hospitals.

Despite this impressive record there is no room for complacency and the main purpose of my paper is to review the operational strategy which is presented in the new Encode Strategic Guide and to look at the lessons learned over the last 20 years of energy management. Before doing this let me outline the achievements and lessons we have learnt in these five areas of initiative as it relates to the existing estate.

STRATEGIES ENERGETIQUES EN MILIEU HOSPITALIER (GRANDE-BRETAGNE)

Cet article établit la nécessité d'une nouvelle stratégie énergétique bien coordonnée pour le National Health Service. Une historique est esquissée et un résumé de la situation est donné dans le domaine de la gestion de l'énergie pas le NHS.

En Grande- Bretagne, le NHS a un parc de quelque 2000 hôpitaux et 10,000 autres bâtiments (prix de 'remplacement' actuel: 70 milliards de £). Plus de la moitié de ce parc consiste en des bâtiments construits avant 1919. Dans l'ensemble, ce groupe, une fois rénové et réhabilité, est assez performant du point de vue énergétique.

Quant au reste, la moitié consiste en des bâtiments de l'entre-deux -guerres, comprenant souvent des annexes temporaires, de qualité de construction très variable. Souvent, les styles et les époques varient pour un même hôpital.

Les quelque 20% qui restent sont des bâtiments relativement modernes, parfois des multi-étages remontant aux années 60 ou 70, et parfois des bâtiments sur plans Nucleus ou Faible Energie. Les premiers de cette catégorie sont de loin les moins performants.

C'est au début des années 60 que les travaux ont commecé sur une série de recommendations visant à améliorer le design et le fonctionnement des hôpitaux du NHS. Cet article décrit le développement de la stratégie énergétique depuis le début de cette période, en passant par la crise de 1972, jusqu'à l'heure actuelle.

1. R&D

In this area technical performance is very good and my Department now find it to be most cost effective to assist and encourage those delivering health care to carry out research projects at a local level. Good examples are to be found nationwide and include a range of innovative projects including combined heat and power (CHP), waste burning boilers, lighting control and variable speed drives for ventilation systems. Whilst most of these have general applicability it is worth commenting initially on the ventilation and air conditioning scenario in the UK, which has a more limited scope.

1.1 Ventilation: Generally both modern hospitals, and their older counterparts are designed for natural ventilation, so cost savings on plant are limited and mostly related to intense areas of medical care. As a result the potential for large energy saving is limited to the large hospitals built in the 60's and 70's which are deep planned and have extensive ventilation systems. Case histories on these have shown that very significant savings, up to as much as 80%, can be made in the fan electricity bill. It must be stressed however that reductions are usually limited to general wards and office accommodation and that modifications can only be carried out with the full co-operation of medical staff, patients and particularly the virologists and bacteriologists.

1.2 Lighting: This is another, and more general, area of high electricity use, which is attracting research and development. At the top of these in retrofit projects, is control using mains borne signalling techniques. Because of interference problems however such systems are not currently recommended by the Department although new guidance is expected shortly allowing the use of low frequency band width systems. Lighting normally represents over 10% of a hospitals energy consumption, which can account for more than 30% of the fuel cost, so this area is of particular importance.

1.3 CHP: This is particularly fashionable at the current time and has considerable potential as electricity consumption and price continues to rise. CHP application and installation is however extremely complex and properly constituted option appraisals are essential.

There are a number of key elements in this:-

1.3.1 The final selection of a CHP scheme can only be justified following a proper comparison of a whole range of measures set against a properly constituted programme of work. There are still very many value for money schemes with potential investment returns higher than 20% (IRR). It should be noted that the use of simple payback criteria is an unacceptable method of selection, except where very short paybacks of less then two to three years can be proven.

1.3.2 Schemes must take full account of the strategic needs of the hospital with particular attention being paid to fossil fuel reserves and emergency electrical supplies. In practise this will normally require the total integration of the CHP plant with the essential electrical services, and the standby boiler plant. In general this will mean reciprocating oil engines driving synchronised generators.

1.3.3 In taking account of the emergency electrical service it is acceptable to discount a very large proportion of the CHP plant in respect of the replacement value of the emergency generator capacity. In the UK it is common to have an installed emergency capacity equal to the hospital's maximum demand. This size of plant, made up of three or four engines, gives the flexibility of heat output required by a hospital.

1.4 Waste Heat Boilers: Due to impending UK and EEC environmental legislation, the waste disposal policy in UK hospitals is under review. This is a wide subject on which we could spend the whole day in debate, but its net effect in the UK NHS will mean the provision of alternative services and the renewal or upgrade of hospital incinerators. Additionally, against this background we have not generally found it cost effective to recover energy from incinerators. This situation has therefore opened up considerable potential for waste burning boilers which, whilst they are not cost effective in the energy sense alone, can go a large way toward offsetting the cost of the disposal of both clinical and domestic hospital wastes. Typically the cost of disposing of clinical waste can be reduced from some £300/tonne to less than £50.

2. Case Studies

Based on the results of discrete NHS R&D projects we publish a range of case histories. Much of these results are embodied in the revised Encode guidance whilst day to day studies are reported in the DH/NHS estate house journal Health Service Estate (HSE). Many with general appeal are also sponsored and publicised by the Energy Efficiency Office of Department of Energy.

3. Guidance

Comprehensive guidance is given to the UK NHS and to private purchasers through the energy code ENCODE. This consists of a wide range of guidance in two basic volumes. The first deals with the process of Survey and Audit and provides a basic guide for the setting up of monitoring and targeting systems within an organisation. The second volume gives technical support on a wide range of management, building, engineering and financial aspects as appropriate to the improvement of energy consumption and cost. Additionally the 'Strategic Guide' provides help to hospital executives. It references the need for financial appraisal, staff training and promotion, information technology and fuel procurement and conversion. The primary objective of the guide is to convey the importance of a revenue saving strategy to general managers, treasurers and administrators so that estate staff can receive support for cost effective measures.

4. Computer Technology

This area is considered to be the key to better management. If we are honest we will admit that even the best written management books and guides remain on executives bookshelves. Software on the other hand is more readily used and what is more, can guide the user in an instructional way through the maze of decision making processes.

To support ENCODE we have devised a range of programs to assist the energy manager.

4.1 Firstly there is a suite of programs to complement ENCODE1 and assist in the survey and audit process. This includes programs for assessing the building and engineering attributes (ENBUILD and ENPLANT), for producing an audit (ENAUDIT), and then ranking energy improvement measures into a programme of work (ENCOST) using discounted cash flow techniques.

4.2 Two separate programs assist the site manager in his day to day energy management. ENCAP, which operates on a hand held device, supplements any data collected by an installed building energy management system (BEMS), by facilitating easy data capture of outlying energy meters. This data and that provided by the WIMS can then be fed into the monitoring and targeting program (ENMATS) which provides a comprehensive range of analysis and reporting facilities.

4.3 We have also established a program to deal with the central analysis of data (ENDATA) for establishing and maintaining a national or regional data base of energy statistics with a corresponding range of analyses and reports.

4.4 Finally there are two research exercises for which prototype software has been written. They both address the need for a more co-ordinated approach to the procurement and operation of BEMS, which is an increasingly essential requirement of a corporate organisation. ENSEVEN is a software/operational requirement package in support of a standard approach to low cost building management systems for operation on a personal computer (PC). ENACT is an ambitious real time package designed to supervise a range of proprietary BEMS. This can consist of either complete systems or individual outstations. Manufacturers full collaboration is encouraged and software licences are offered to help them establish their systems in the health market.

5. Energy Awareness

This has been found to be one of the most difficult areas to address centrally. Much can however be done locally if an energy management officer has the freedom to transgress professional boundaries and promote energy awareness to all staff and patients. Much though is down to basic education and experience. No doubt the 'green' lobby will do much to improve the public's perception.

The new Strategic Guide to hospital executives will encourage managers to take energy management more seriously and set aside resources for both capital work and good day to day management. This will need designated energy officers with adequate time and resource to promote energy awareness. There are already some good examples of this in the UK NHS and a number of health authorities publish house magazines on energy efficiency. The Department, with the help of the Great Ormond Street Hospital, has produced a Video film entilted 'A Matter of Conscience'. Copies of this VHS Video are available through the Department.

Outstanding Potential

As I said earlier the potential for saving is still good and in the UK this has been estimated, and confirmed by an ongoing review of the Audit Commission, to be in excess of 25%. Which in England is about £60M of the current £250M bill.

Based on our experience then, what are the shortcomings and the potential remedies?

Firstly, it must be said that there are few easy solutions left. It is true that some low cost measures can still be identified on many sites, typically items like valve insulation, but these are relatively insignificant. It is also generally true in the UK that engineering solutions will not have a great effect as most plant is already very efficient. The next steps require major strategic decisions backed with the necessary cash and human resource.

Primarily it is up to management to recognise the need for a proper management infrastructure with good communications and reporting services. In practice this means the appointment of a manager with complete responsibility for both day to day energy management and an associated programme of capital works. It will not be possible to justify a full time manager in smaller organisations but a properly designated part of an officer's time is essential. Alternatively the part time services of an external professional can be employed under contract. A good guide to the required budget can be related to the fuel bill and a simple payback of less than three years.

Once established an energy manager should have access to top management and be allocated a budget for energy and environmental improvement work. As a guide the Audit Commission and Department of Energy recommend an initial budget of 10% of the fuel bill, but the final one should be based on a viable programme of measures selected on a call off basis. These measures will of course need to be fully related to other estate building and engineering projects and supported by competent option appraisals for each scheme. The use of the ENCOST computer program is ideal for this purpose.

In order to determine potential work, select appropriate fuel procurement contracts and manage daily operations the manager will be well served by good support services. In efficiently run hospital estates this will include the Works Information System (WIMS) and a Building Management System supported by a range of reporting and accounting systems. A key element in this is the data collection transducer which is all too often absent in today's systems. It is a valid criticism of current UK BMS or BEMS that they pay too much attention to control systems and far too little to information gathering. Some transducers are inherently expensive, particularly those for measuring heat flows, but technology is advancing and there is no excuse for not providing an adequate range of temperature sensors throughout a building, nor for not installing cheap secondary electrical meters. Without such provision it is difficult to see how proper general or energy management can take place.

Strategic Influences

Having laid these foundations, what then are the main aspects affecting the strategic criteria to be considered. These I will necessarily look at from an English point of view, but many will be applicable to the international scene. These influences include the introduction of capital charges, the loss of Crown Immunity, the current and forthcoming reviews by the Audit Commission, the new environmental legislation 'Green Bill' and not least the problems with computer policy.

1. Capital Charging of Assets

Accountability, or the lack of it, has inhibited proper investment and option appraisals on value for money schemes, and thereby made it difficult for estate staff to acquire adequate funding for many viable estate saving measures. It has also limited the proper staffing of energy management posts. These changes are therefore most welcome and can only work towards improving our energy performance.

2. Crown Immunity

It is not appropriate for me to deal with the subject of Crown Immunity, but it is an issue which needs reinforcing in your minds as it will have important ramifications for the Estate Manager. It is not perhaps the more obvious factors like clean air and the control of pollution that will have the most significant impact; these are in principal adequately covered already by the existing protocols, whereby we act within the legislation even if not bound by it. It is other more obscure issues of Building Regulations and Local Authority Planning that are more likely to need attention.

3. Audit Commission Energy Review

This review follows the one started in 1985 in respect of local authorities and is based on the experience gained by the Audit Commission, and on the work already done within the NHS. The auditors have sensibly drawn together a team of advisors with experience in the health service and the Audit Guide for the NHS audit reflects this in its compilation. The guide refers to ENCODE and draws upon its text for much of its content.

It is too early to draw firm conclusions but its effect on the NHS is likely to be profound. Our main weakness within the NHS and at the Department has been our inability to direct top management to apply adequate resource to energy management. The NHS in general has also been slow in some areas of technology, particularly where it is of strategic importance affecting security and fuel purchase flexibility. This will change with the external influence of the Audit Commission and its report.

4. The Green Bill

This will also have significant effect on the Health Service Estate. Initially it is leading to changes in the disposal of hospital waste and in particular the operation and staffing of hospital incinerators, which themselves will be the subject of new and stringent regulations covering dangerous emissions into the air. In the medium and long term we will also see considerable improvement in the way we classify and handle waste. Segregation will no longer be a satisfactory management tool for the separate disposal of domestic and clinical waste, and all wastes will have to be disposed of by incineration. These changes will include some expensive but necessary improvements in both the handling and storage of hospital waste.

The concern for the environment will also lead to improvements in boiler plant and a more efficient use of resources. The ENCODE energy strategy, to be published later this year, puts forward an 'ideal boiler house' concept where waste burning boilers and CHP form a co-ordinated approach to energy conversion, with secondary and emergency provision supplied by conventional heating plant. It is also foreseeable that it will be necessary to provide tighter emission control to conventional boilers, especially those burning heavy oil and coal.

The effect on energy policy will be substantial, as to be most cost effective the energy in the waste material will need to be fully recovered. It is a fact that the waste generated by the NHS has a calorific value equivalent to about 15% of current fossil fuel energy consumption. This exceeds both that of the coal and electricity we currently use.

5. Computer Policy

The NHS in the UK has been at the forefront of computer application. It was some 20 years ago that the Ministry of Health, as it was then, pioneered computer aided design applications, and this research is embedded in many of the modern systems used for building and engineering design within the NHS. On the operations side the Works Information Management System (WIMS) is now used in over 30 countries world wide and within almost all of the NHS districts. Subsequent to these early developments much has been done to rationalise the data to the point where we now have a national minimum data set of which the Estate Data Base forms an integral part.

Against this background however there are immense hardware co-ordination problems, which grow with every new procurement of computer system or solid state controller. Initially the smaller systems standardised on the CP/M operating system which has since been superseded by MSDOS and its derivatives. With larger scale computing, which is increasingly necessary for data analysis, there has been a diverse array of equipment and systems. Here we see the emergence of UNIX as a standard operating system, with the language 'C' providing portability. Added to the hardware problem is the diversity of software and communication protocols that exist, even on PC's. It is to be hoped that the 'Open Systems' initiative will clear the way to a more co-ordinated future, but at the current time a quick solution seems unlikely. Fortunately much of our estate operations are still based on the WIMS and our best policy for the future is to retain and build on the framework it provides.

There is however chaos in the world of computing, and much of this affects computing in our hospital service. The principal blame for this must fall to the computer industry, particularly those in software development, who seem to profit from confusion. In addition the hardware developments are hard to keep abreast of, and in pace with. I have an interest in home computers and it is still a fact, as it was 15 years ago, that personal machines lead the way in low cost computing. I have a 25MHz 386 in my office, but my home computer is faster and better structured and at a lower price.

Strategic Criteria

Having laid these foundations what are the main strategic criteria to be considered. Again I can only look at these from an English point of view, but all are applicable to the international scene. I shall not dwell on them as they are embodied in the new DH Strategic Guide and you can equally well derive your own conclusions from my paper. In essence they can be summarised in priority order as:-

(1) Hospital Strategic Needs;
(2) Cost Effectiveness;
(3) Energy Efficiency, and not least
(4) Energy Conservation.

1. Hospital Strategic Needs

These are reasonably straightforward but not always appreciated in today's effort to cut costs. There is however long standing guidance in respect of the need to provide an adequate level of security of service in all hospitals and in particular those providing an acute or emergency service. The UK Government through its Building Notes and Technical Memoranda provide details of these essential services, which in the energy field can be summarised as follows:-

1.1 On site storage of heating fuel. Normally this should be a minimum of 10 days at peak load. This requirement demands that appropriate plant is installed to burn the fuel stored.

1.2 Proper segregation of essential electricity supplies in accordance with HTM11 and/or the provision of adequate emergency electrical generation capacity to meet the essential needs of the hospital at peak periods.

1.3 Both of these requirements demand the provision of adequate back up in a time of emergency. This means that the emergency service has to be provided as a multiple of units.

1.3.1 With the heating and hot water plant it is normally adequate to add one boiler to the normal provision so that another is available if one fails or is down for overhaul. It is generally better to have more than three units but the full capacity must be operable with the stored emergency fuel, which is normally coal or oil.

1.3.2 On the electrical side it depends to some extent upon the nature of the hospital, but in large acute units plant should consist of at least three engines capable of full operation on a stored fuel (normally oil), and of reaching their operating speed within 15 seconds. Each engine should be able to meet the essential supply, with load shedding where obtainable, and with full automation. The equipment will also need to meet the Electricity Council's G59 Regulations.

2. Cost Effectiveness

Whilst it is desirable to install the most efficient systems, these must be consistent with lowest cost which is often an overriding factor. Commonly a less expensive fuel will be less efficient but incur more capital outlay. Only by carrying out proper option appraisals using discounted cash flow can the most cost effective solution be selected. All factors must be considered including those related to security of service and staffing. The sensitivity adjustment to allow the fuel price changes, which is usually the most difficult aspect, is helped by the security provision of multi-fuel plant.

3. Energy Efficiency

This aspect takes third place behind the strategic and value for money needs. Caution is required when comparing systems using a different fuel, particularly when high electrical consumption is involved. Efficiency really only comes into play when comparing two similar pieces of equipment.

4. Energy Conservation

Last but not least. This is the most important aspect and will always have the greatest potential for saving. The cliche that 'a room can be heated by a 40w lamp' may not often be cost effective but it is nonetheless true. All energy is eventually wasted as heat and at the end of the day we need better building design using better materials, and, not least, users that are aware of both the cost of wasting energy and its damage to the environment.

Steam Raising Solar Array

by

Alan Moore
CEng, MIHE(Aust), FIMechE, FCIBSE
Hosplan, Private Bag 5
Rozelle, NSW 2039
Australia

The Campbelltown District Hospital installation is a pilot development solar steam plant and as such should not be taken as representative of a normal steam production plant.

The purpose of developing a pilot plant on this scale was not only to demonstrate a new technology, but to measure performance and check design parameters, before any large solar projects of this type are undertaken.

The array is simple in concept and Figure 1 will show basically how it works.

As a pilot scheme it was therefore expected that various features of design and material use would be revised during the construction, installation and commissioning period. These expectations were met and the revisions continue to be of great value in this regard. Some of the revisions will indeed effect the directions of future design of solar plants producing steam.

Although this is a pilot scheme, it will be accepted by the Hospital as a useful energy source to decrease their electrical energy consumption. The array will be monitored for some years to record the array performance and any necessary maintenance.

One of the largest potential markets for renewable energy is that of heat supply. In Australia, more than half of all end use energy is thermal, and most of this energy lies outside the operating range of conventional flat plate solar water heaters. However, much of it lies in the temperature range (100-500°C) which is, in principle, able to be supplied by relatively simple evacuated tube solar collector technology.

Relatively few attempts have been made to exploit this large potential market. There were valid reasons for this. First and foremost, the cost of competing conventional energy supplied to industrial markets, where much energy above 100°C is used, as in Australia, bulk industrial fuel is often available for 2 to 3 cents Australian per kWh.

The new technology is extremely simple, having no moving parts in the collector field except for a seasonally adjusted mirror and passive valves and vents. It requires relatively little maintenance (although it was found that, with the concentration level used in the project, careful initial array alignment to within 5° of true north is necessary to reduce the frequency of mirror adjustment to acceptable levels). Replacement of tubes or mirrors does not require array shut down. Components are also very light and have a small unit size to allow relatively easy assembly.

In all, the technology allowed, represents a plausible extension of simple and cost effective solar collector technology into a relatively larger potential market. It is a young technology, but the present performance of the technology in the range of applications below 250°C is unlikely to improve markedly, as peak efficiencies are already high.

The solar collector uses evacuated tubular absorbers and 1.4m long parabolic through mirrors with an aperture area of 0.6m sq each. These are fabricated from galvanised iron sheet and lined with 0.3mm highly polished anodised aluminium foil. Fourteen such mirrors are attached together in a single module using a planar arrangement of steel heat transfer pipes. The evacuated collector tubes are simply slipped over the steel pipes, and can be very easily replaced if damaged.

The collectors are not tracked, but are instead periodically tilt adjusted about a dozen times a year. All 14 mirrors in a module are linked by inexpensive gavlanised wire, and in this installation, two modules are linked together, so that 28 mirrors can be adjusted in one operation. Adjustment of the entire array takes between 10 and 15 minutes, and is carried out about 12-15 times a year.

Heat transfer takes place as a result of direct boiling of water in the steel tubes which are enveloped by the evacuated tube. The array modules are slightly angled so that vapour flows to the high end of the module, where it is collected by a manifold which leads off to the application. In the case of Campbelltown Hospital, the roof is slightly angled, so the collector modules were installed parallel to the roof.

The entire system was intended to operate in parallel with the existing electric steam boilers, using the same evaporant with corrosion inhibitors from the same reservoir. The existing hospital boilers use a feedwater pump to pump evaporant into the boiler against boiler pressure. In the case of the solar boiler, hospital staff adapted one of the existing feedwater pumps to pump feedwater to a rooftop reservoir connected to the solar boiler. This reservoir contains a float valve which shuts the pump off when the array water level is acceptably high. The pump is not used during collector operation unless the water level drops too low. Future systems may dispense with pumps and float valves entirely, to improve reliability.

The reflectors for this project are of a cylindrical parabolic design which optimises delivered energy on the absorber tube for a given mirror area. Higher concentration designs would require much more frequent adjustment whilst lower concentration reflectors would use a larger number of evacuated tubes and mirrors. The design chosen has the potential to deliver energy at a price comparable to fossil fuels, but real systems must also include variables such as the likelihood of accurate adjustment and installation by available staff. It may be that the higher cost of more

GROUPE SOLAIRE A PRODUCTION DE VAPEUR

Le projet consiste en un groupe solaire de miroirs paraboliques réfléchissants concentrés sur des tubes de verre vidés d'air recouverts d'une surface émissive et glissant sur d'autres tubes d'acier semi-dur noirs remplis d'eau.

Ce projet a eté financé par le NERDDP (programme national de recherche et d'application dans le domaine énergétique) du Département Fédéral (Minéraux et Energie) australien — qui a depuis été remplacé.

La collaboration de l'Université de Sydney, et plus particulièrement de l'Ecole de Physique a été acquisé pour la mise au point de ce réflecteur parabolique et des tubes à vide. C'est le Dr David Mills qui s'est chargé de diriger la recherche, le développement et la production du groupe solaire. Hosplan a été responsable des détails tecniques du chantier.

A l'origine, avant la prise en charge financière de l'ensemble du projet par le NERDDP, une étude des coûts de mise au point et de production avait été effectuée par une organisation (Wildridge and Sinclair, Sydney, NSW). Le NERDDP avait ensuite donné son accord, autorisant les travaux à commencer.

Le projet a été victime des délais habituels dans ce genre de cas; le site prévu à Cantorbéry (ville satellite de Sydney, NSW) n'a pas fait l'affaire car d'autres bâtiments voisins apportaient de l'ombre sur le toit de l'hôpital de Cantorbéry. Le chantier s'est finalement installé à l'hôpital de district de Campbelltown, ville située à quelque 50 kms au sud-ouest de Sydney.

La construction et l'installation à l'hôpital de Campbelltown ont commencé en avril 1987. L'ouverture officielle a eu lieu, en présence des représentatants du governement du NSW et du gouvernement fédéral d'Australie en novembre 1988.

'forgiving' lower concentration units might be tolerated in the future, particularly in the light of the possibility of Greenhouse Pollution taxes on fossil fuel. It is believed that higher concentration factors than the 4.5 X chosen would be ill-advised without tube redesign, since stagnation temperatures of 517°C have been recorded with these units on days with particularly high insolation. This is close to the softening point of glass.

The mirrors use a thin anodised foil obtained from Germany as a reflector. The foil lines a substrate of galvanised steel which is held in shape by pop-riveted end plates, also of galvanised steel. This method of mirror construction is heavily labour-intensive and this was reflected in the large mirror unit costs faced by the project supervisors, about Australia $85 each for a 0.6m sq reflector. The shortness of the production run prevented any other possibility.

The present reflector foil is considered a temporary measure, and more corrosion resistant material will be installed at Campbelltown District Hospital when available. New mirror liners are being developed with the assistance of DuPont, who have developed a suitable polymer which is completely transparent and unaffected by UV. There is some possibility that the entire mirror may be moulded from this very tough and extremely corrosion resistant material, which has shown no degradation in a decade of desert testing. It is hoped that the mirror foil production can be carried out in Australia.

The mirrors are mounted using a cylindrical length of galvanised pipe welded over a hole in each end plate, the mirror sliding over the tube. In the future, the mirrors will be designed to be stacked and will have only a hole in the end plate, which will fit over a length of pipe attached to the structure.

Differential expansion between the mirror attachment points on the module centreline manifold, and the attachment points on the module edge, was acceptable on the original single module but is a problem on the double modules used at Campbelltown District Hospital. It is suspected of breaking tubes at the module ends and may lead to pipe fatigue if left unattended. This is being corrected at Campbelltown District Hospital with expansion joints between joined modules, but an upcoming revision of the pipework will allow much greater flexibility and tube movement. This will eliminate the need for the above expansion joint.

In large scale production, stamped or moulded mirror substrate (which can be nested for transport) appear to be the preferred option. These would be lined with replaceable mirror film of the type discussed earlier. There seems to be every indication that the mirror costs outlined in the production engineering study of this project can be achieved, but all low cost methods require high initial capital investment with the possible exception of fibreglass construction in countries with very low labour costs.

The module pipework was of all welded construction and was painted with temperature resistant paint before assembly. The assemblies were pressure tested in the factory and taken to the site. There were problems with inaccurate factory welding and a number of pipes needed straightening, but this was successfully done on site.

As the steel manifolds are closed, the extent of corrosion inside them is uncertain. However, a blowdown system has been designed and a very cost-effective solution has been devised which uses main steam line pressure from below to push steam through the array from time to time. It has been decided to take one module and cut up the manifolding to determine the rate of corrosion or scaling. Consideration is being given to replacing the module manifolding with stainless steel. A new, inexpensive stainless steel pipework arrangement is currently under test at the University of Sydney and if its performance is satisfactory, it will then be installed at Campbelltown District Hospital.

Freezing of the array pipes could cause extensive damage. Preliminary discussion before array installation had suggested that freezing was unlikely, but the installers of the array reported ice on the roof. As a result, a system valve is being installed to drain fluid from the array at a trigger temperature just above freezing. The system and reservoir, being empty, will automatically refill with warm water from the boiler reservoir. It is unlikely that the present Campbelltown District Hospital system will be triggered in practice, but this anti-freeze system would be an essential safety feature in many areas.

The array uses a one way valve to prevent reverse steam flow to the array from the main steam line when the array is not sufficiently warm. When the array is up to pressure, the valve allows full passage of steam from the array to the application. Emergency vents are installed on both sides of the valve, and on the upper manifold of each half-array.

A problem that arose during initial tests was that the steam was too wet for the autocalves to accept. A standard steam separator was installed to overcome this problem. Consideration of the installation of steam separating and drying equipment should be covered on all future arrays, as some water will inevitably be carried along with the steam. In future array the pipework will have a small stainless steel separator installed on each module pair.

The reservoir suffered problems of overfilling due to oscillations of the float valve during refilling. Shortage of funds prevented a redesign of the float and reservoir, however the feed water pump was adapted to limit the 'on-time' of the pump, and the problem has not reappeared since. This reservoir would be eliminated in the large storage systems proposed for the future, which operate on a pumpless resyphoning principle.

The evacuated tubes have performed well on the project but a number have been lost for various reasons. The biggest source of loss was during a particularly bad and quite non-typical period of hail in the Spring, during which about 25 tubes were lost. There were three separate storms, and the hail was severe enough to dent the reflectors, although optical collection has been apparently unaffected due to the low concentration factor used. A modification, which involves a shaped, possibly transparent, deflector mounted in front of the tube would not only deflect hailstones, but discourage bird landings. This would not affect performance seriously, as most tube absorption is from below, via the reflector. However, such a solution must be very inexpensive if it is to be cheaper than paying for lost tubes; if such a storm were to happen once every five years, at Australian $30 per tube this represents a cost of Australian $150 per year, or about Australian$0.5 per installed array tube. Over 15 years, each device must cost less than Australian $1.50 to be cost effective. Savings through prevention of bird landings are unlikely with improved inert, non-stick mirror films, which should not be affected by bird droppings.

In all, the installers adapted quickly to the technology and they stated that if the module manifold were threaded where it connects to the main array manifold, the whole array could have been assembled with three spanners. There is possibly some merit in pursuing this philosophy, since corroded pipes could be removed for inspection at any time and little site welding would be needed. On the other hand, the possibility for leakage is increased, an undesirable thing from the point of view of passive downward heat transport systems being contemplated for the future, which rely on partial vacuum in the pipes for refilling. Certainly, decreased module manifold size would allow easy placement during construction by one or two men, and there appears to be some case for restricting the size of all parts according to this criterion, should rooftop module construction become the rule.

Whilst the available data is encouraging the array has produced too much energy for the application. Peak power of the array is about 100kw as measured by an accurate Spirax-Sarco density compensated steam flow meter. This figure exceeds autoclave usage by between 10 and 30kw. Therefore, it has been found necessary to divert excess steam to the hospital's hot water supply, which also supplies space heating to a nearby children's ward. Hospital records of fuel use will be used to monitor the contribution to hot water supply, but overall steam production will be directly measured.

The hospital roof is aligned about 12° from true north. For conventional tracking or flat plate solar collectors, this is close to ideal alignment, since these classes of collector continually accept direct beam radiation and the change in alignment at noon would only amount to a cosine performance loss of about 2% at noon and nearly zero over the day because of compensating collection times before and after noon.

The array was duly aligned with the building, but it became clear that collection times were below what was being achieved by similar collectors in Sydney, which had always faced due north. However, another installation using similar collectors in Sydney was inadvertently misaligned early this year and performance showed that the collectors are quite sensitive to misalignment from true north. The degree of sensitivity has been very surprising in the development of these solar collectors, and is an important finding of the project.

The technology is not threatened by this discovery, but the importance of initial array alignment is clear. At 12° from due north, the Campbelltown District Hospital array must be adjusted twice a day to maintain the performance it would achieve if property aligned and adjusted 15 times a year. This represents a 50 fold increase in adjustment frequency, an unacceptable figure unless labour is very inexpensive. Campbelltown District Hospital has attempted to adopt the twice a day regime, but found it difficult to enforce, particularly in changeable weather conditions, where poor weather not requiring or preventing adjustment can suddenly clear when the staff are otherwise engaged. As a result, it is difficult to say whether the array is or is not properly adjusted when data is being logged, and any estimation of array performance is unreliable unless the project supervisor is continuously present. The modules will be reoriented to true north shortly; this is relatively easy with this technology, but it will be an extra cost for the project.

The data obtained so far has been sufficient to allow modelling of the Campbelltown District Hospital array for an average year. The weather database uses actual hour by hour data from real months so as not to neglect the high frequency interruptions due to clouds. The results indicate that a realigned Campbelltown District Hospital array should deliver about 8MJ per sq m on average throughout the year in Sydney; in inland areas of NSW about 20% higher may be expected.

Future Potential

It is expected that future changes to large system design will reduce rooftop equipment levels and hasten installation. Independent sources have recently evolved a new passive downward heat transport system which would connect the collectors at only one end of the module and require only one major array manifold and would not require a float switch, steam separator, or pump. A somewhat altered system can also be designed without a reservoir and would only require a twice yearly adjustment but this would be somewhat more costly. These newer designs would use substantial thermal storage and would be backed up in poor weather by combustible renewable or fossil fuel or off peak electricity supplied to the storage vessel.

The second type of application, combined heat and electricity production, is the subject of a current feasibility study proposal, and is already being investigated by one of Australia's largest utilities as a grid supply possibility in inland areas. At least one site in the 10-60MW array size range has been identified. Initial demonstration proposals, involving not only a 200°C array but a comparison between three locally developed heat engine technologies, would be examined at the end of 1990, for development in 1991/92. Crude, extremely simple, tracking may be justifiable on very large arrays.

It is possible the cogeneration project would increase involvement with the electrical utilities, who may subsequently be interested in downstream developments, such as the high temperature evacuated tube now under development which could allow steam production at temperatures in the range of 300°C to 500°C. The utilities finance technology using life cycle costing, which allows solar to demonstrate its true long term economy.

A large cogeneration project could attract utility support, as evacuated tube collector activity is already attracting such support in another area that is the development of a retrofit solar thermal domestic collector for home (or factory) use. Support is coming from an electrical utility because this technology would largely eliminate peaky daytime domestic grid demand, supplying cooking, refrigeration, hot water and space heating loads, using a fixed collection with seasonal output matching and off-peak backup. Such an approach also has enormous potential.

Fig. 1 Array Schematic

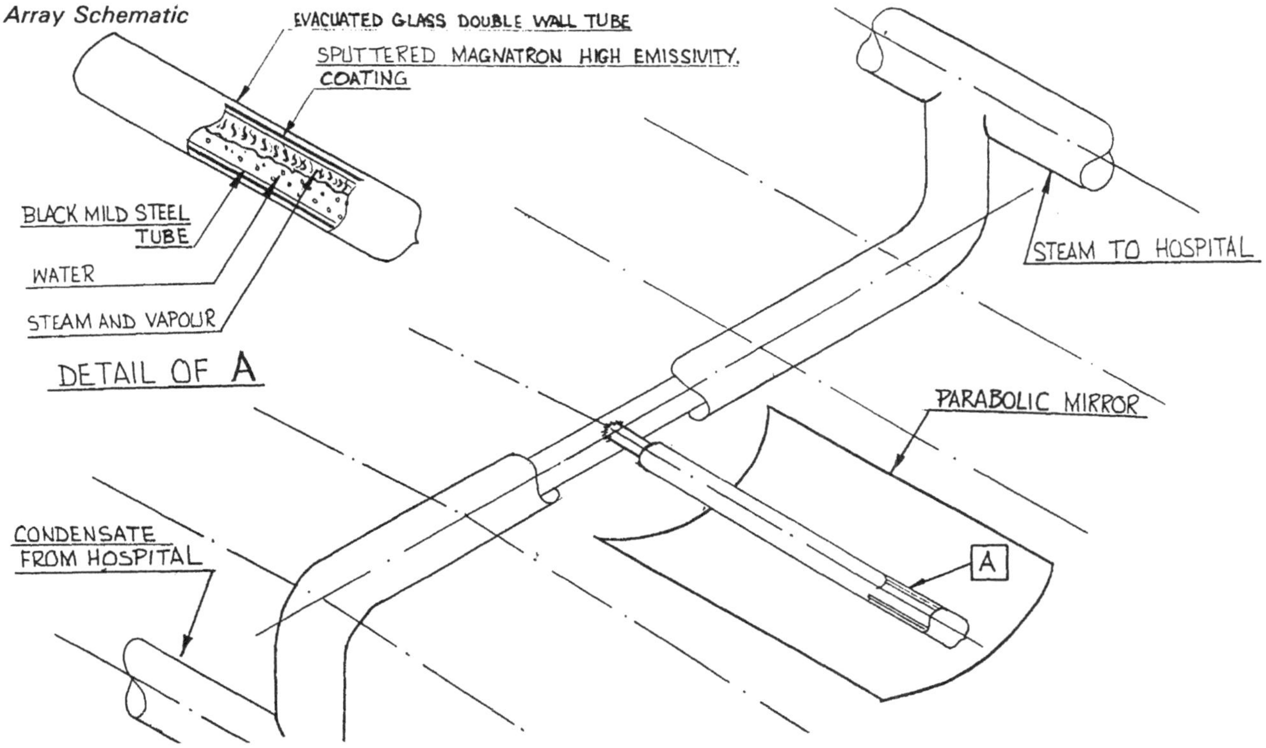

Efficient Energy Use in Hospitals Trend and Emerging Technologies

by
ing Mario de Renzio
SINERGA srl — Milano

1. Introduction

Hospitals have peculiar energy consumption characteristics when compared with other buildings. In fact they operate 24 hours a day, all year long, need high air change rates to control odours and bacteric diffusion (and therefore infection spreading), and accurately controlled microclimates to support therapies (as in operating theatres, intensive care, etc); they also need considerable amounts of energy for all the medical equipment and support activities like laundering, catering, disinfection, transports, etc.

They therefore need to have high energy demands and consumptions; also adequate reserve for emergency safety. All this means significant costs in hospital budgets. adding up to an average of from 2.5 to 5% of total expenditure, which is not far from the percentage typical of manufacturing industries.

As the main objectives of hospitals are therapies and patients care, supporting service activities are generally given less attention, with emphasis put on reliability and satefy, rather than cost and energy efficiency.

In this era of limited resources it is therefore very important to continuously stress the relevance of an efficient energy use in hospitals.

2. Energy Related Hospital Services — Forms of Energy Used

It is felt that the various energy using hospital services and some information on the kinds of energy, its vectors and their characteristics should first be summarised. More details on this subject are given in my paper presented at the 'European Hospital Conference' in Rome last year[1] and other previous papers.

These services may be listed as follows:-

* primaries:
  - lighting
  - heating
  - air conditioning
  - hot and cold water supply
* medical:
  - diagnostic equipment
  - therapeutic equipment
  - analysis equipment
  - gas supply
* auxiliaries:
  - sterilisation
  - laundering and disinfection
  - catering (kitchen, canteen, etc)
  - waste disposal and incineration
  - transports (people, goods; vertical, horizontal)
  - communications

In support of these services there are the two basic utilities: Electrical and Thermal energy supply, with their specific characteristics and equipments.

Electricity is used for:-

* lighting
* power:
  - boiler room auxiliaries
  - refrigerating equipment
  - water pumping
  - heating and air conditioning equipment
  - auxiliary services (laundry, kitchen, elevators, etc)

It is generally supplied at medium voltage; in larger hospitals it is also distributed through a main MV network to the transformer substations feeding the various buildings or departments.

For safety reasons an independent power source with an emergency generating set, plus continuity sets with inverter and batteries when needed, are also always required.

This need of an independent power source is one of the many reasons recommanding the use of cogeneration in hospitals.

The supply of Thermal power, which is both heating and cooling, is aimed at two main usages:-

- climate control (ie ambient heating and air conditioning)
- services (which account for about half of the total need)

Heating is used for:-

- ambient heating, by radiators or fan coils, or panel heating, or air heating sets;
- domestic hot water, with is used in large quantities; and
- services, as laundry, kitchen, sterilisation.

Cooling is used mostly for air conditioning, but also for refrigerating purposes.

Besides the needs below ambient temperature, there are also requirements above that level for cooling apparatuses, typically refrigerators, condensers, but also medical equipment like RX, CAT, NMR, etc.

Thermal power (both heat and cool) can be produced locally or more usually centrally, and then distributed as steam, and/or pressurised, hot or chilled water.

Two important characteristics of the thermal power supply must be emphasised:-

- temperature level at which it is actually requested, keeping in mind that above 100°C it must be steam or pressurised water. This level can vary from 40°C for panel heating, up to 140°C for sterilisation and 180°C for linen calendering; and
- duration in times: variations are both:
  daily, according to the various working hours, or
  seasonal, according to climate changes.

3. Specific Energy Consumptions: Statistical Data

To ensure the services previously listed, various levels of fuel and power demands are required, which must be well

L'EMPLOI EFFICACE DE L'ENERGIE DANS LES HOPITAUX SYSTEMES DE RECUPERATION TOTALE

Une revue initiale de l'utilisation de l'énergie dans les hôpitaux, et des differentes provenances de cette énergie est suivie de details statistiques de la consommation et des indicatifs paramètriques qui en relévent, des travaux de l'Agence Internationale de L'Energie relévant de l'emploi de l'energie dans les hôpitaux et de son Manuel d'Instruction. L'auteur termine par un discussion des techniques à employer et des développements recents relevants de la co-generation, des pompes à chaleur, des systemes à recuperation totale d'énergie l'ammagasinage de l'énergie par la glace, du controle d'operation des équipments par ordinateur (EMS).

known, both in each specific hospital and on the whole territory, to establish correct operation criteria and policy, and to identify possible efficiency improvements.

Unfortunately little knowledge was available up to a few years ago, particularly in Italy. When the International Energy Agency (an OECD body) Working Group on Energy Management in Hospitals started its activity back in 1984 little data were available on an international basis too.

Yet hospitals have high energy consumptions, with energy bills adding up, as said before, to from 2.5 to 5% of total hospital expenditures, and an annual cost in the range of from 2 to 4 million lire, hence close to a 10,000 lire a day, per bed. Also specific consumptions in various hospitals show highly scattered values. This is due to the types, sizes, locations, ages and the way the hopital and related services are managed, operated and maintained.

In order to better understand whether significant parametric indices of energy consumptions could be established and calculated, a study was made on the data collected, through different questionnaires, in two Italian Regions: Liguria (on 50 public hospitals, almost all, ranging from 30 to above 1,000 beds) and Lombardia (again 50 hospitals ranging from 50 to 2,300 beds, which account for about one third of the total).

The values collected were correlated to the number of beds and the total volume and surface; they concerned:-

- electrical energy used per year;
- maximum electric power demand;
- total thermal energy used for ambient heating; and
- thermal energy used for services.

Lacking adequate means to discriminate between the two types of heat uses, the very simple and rough criterion to assign to services the energy levels of the non heating season was chosen: the lowest monthly value was multiplied by 12, and the balance to the total assigned to ambient heating; of course the first portion would include most of the distribution losses.

This allocation was considered important because the two types of heat use follow different patterns.

Notwithstanding the very crude assumptions and the prevailing pessimism, the results of the statistical correlations were unexpectedly high. In fact the correlation factor of the assumed linear equations were found quite good, in most cases above 0.9, confirming the validity and significance of the parametric indices selected. Also the differences found between the two Regions seemed being well justified.

Without going into details, which are given in the already mentioned papers[1][2], the main results are given in the following table:-

	Lombardia	Liguria	Units
Electric Power demand	0.7	0.52	kW/bed
Electric Energy	3.3	2.2	MWh/bed.year
Total Thermal Energy	27	18	Gcal/bed.year
Thermal Energy: Services	12	10	Gcal/bed.year
Th En: Ambient Heating	58	35	Gcal/cm.year

One important finding is that the heat used for services (or better the base load which includes most of the distribution losses) accounts for roughly half of the total needs, which is more than originally expected, being, as obvious, a slightly lower percentage in the colder, and higher in the milder climates.

4. Energy Saving in Hospitals — The International Energy Agency Activity

As just mentioned, the International Energy Agency, an OECD body in Paris, among other activities including researches and demonstration projects on energy saving in buildings and communities, established six years ago an International program on 'Energy Management in Hospitals'.

The Working Group, promoted and co-ordinated by Italy's National Research Council, included USA, Canada, Germany, Belgium, Holland and Switzerland.

The aims of this activity were mainly:-

- to locate the most significant energy using areas and services, and find out characteristics and amounts of energy used;
- to define energy consumption indices and targets for comparisons;
- to determine Energy Conservation Opportunities for each area, giving indications on priorities, costs, savings, etc; and
- to produce a Manual with recommendations for energy conscious operation and maintenance and suggested modifications.

The Working Group activity was completed at the end of 1988, and the whole Manual, in six volumes written in English, was edited, tested on the field in a few selected cases, and approved a year ago. While preliminary translations in Italian and German in 'pro-manuscripto' form are available, the original English version is being printed and published by Consiglio Nazionale delle Ricerche — Progetto Finalizzato Energetica (Energy Program of the Italian National Research Council) in Rome, and available to the participating Countries.

The six volumes contents are as follows:-

(1) Generality: for both administrative and technical managers; gives instructions for the use of the manual, recommendations and details for energy accounting procedures, methods for calculating cost savings and investments pay-backs.
(2) Heat and Cold Production and Distribution.
(3) Heating, Ventilating, Air Conditionings; Domestic Hot Water.
(4) Electrical Systems.
(5) Services: Laundry, Sterilisation, Kitchen, etc.
(6) Building Envelope.

Each section gives first of all a brief description of the most common equipments and installations, emphasising the energy involvements, and points out the proper strategies to implement the energy saving measures.

Specific lists of Energy Conservation Opportunities are then given, classified in four categories:-

- operation
- maintenance
- low cost modifications
- important modifications and retrofitting

For each action indications are given on how to do it.

The manual is laid out in a practical and operative way for Technical Managers of large-medium size hospitals, to enable them to directly perform the actions suggested, or efficiently supervise and control suppliers, installers, maintenance firms or consultants implementing such actions. Even for smaller hospitals with inadequate staff it is useful as a guide for external supports.

5. Efficient Use of Energy: Trends and Emerging Technologies

Among the various saving opportunities, most of which are suggested in the IEA Manual, it is worthwhile focusing special attention on emerging technologies that are starting to be adopted in various cases and will be more and more used in the future.

5.1 Cogeneration

The combined heat and electric power production has become very popular in the recent years and is particularly well suited to the hospitals, because of their contemporary high heat and electricity demands throughout the year. Attention should be here again called to the high percentage of heat used, as a base load, for services. Also the need, for safety reasons, of an independent power source favours the installation of generating sets with heat recovery.

This recovery raises the total efficiency of a cogeneration system generally to between 80% and 90%, as opposed to the rough average of 30% for the electricity supplied by the utility at the user level (including all distribution losses). This also means that the cost of self produced cogenerated electrical energy is generally much lower then the price payed to the utility, paying back the investment costs in a relatively few years.

Without going in too much details, which can be found in other papers[3], I will just mention here the three possible alternative power plants with their characteristics, and give a few examples.

5.1.1 Internal Combustion or Piston Engines — They are the most popular power plants type, because they are normally also used as emergency sets.

They can be Diesel or gas engines ranging in power from a few 10s of kilowatts up to 1,000 kW or more. Heat is recovered from the cooling water and lube oil at temperatures between 80°C and 90°C, and from exhaust gases, generally up to 500°C; the latter can also produce steam in a recovery boiler. The total heat produced in the cogeneration process ranges around 1.5 times the electricity. Proper attention must be given to the durability and maintenance problems and costs.

5.1.2 Steam Turbines — Generally of the back pressure type, it used to be the most popular type, but now, mainly due to the low electricity to heat ratio, which ranges between 1/5 to 1/10, it is loosing momentum. Steam inlet conditions should be as high as possible, typically 50 bar and 450°C; back pressure should be kept as low as possible, compatible with the user's requirements, typically between 3 and 6 bar.

5.1.3 Gas Turbines — This is becoming the hottest item because of the high temperature heat available, small sizes and weights, lack of vibration, reasonable costs, life and maintenance charges. The large amount of exhaust gases are led to the recovery boiler to produce steam and/or hot water; careful attention has to be paid to the stack temperature, which must be kept as low as possible to obtain good total efficiency, by installing, if necessary, a large final economiser in the boiler.

The high excess of air in the gas turbine combustion, and therefore the large amount of oxygen still contained in the exhaust gases, allows burning more fuel in a post-combustor on the exhaust, thereby increasing its temperature and the content to be recovered in the boiler. The heat to electricity ratio can therefore vary from the original 2.5 up to around 5.

The number of suppliers is still limited worldwide; however, various model small gas turbine are available on the market from 500 kW upwards.

5.1.4 Examples — In the following page is a table listing a few examples of different types of cogeneration plants in Italy, with their main characteristics, designed by us; some are already in operation, some under erection and some at the contracting stage.

As a conclusion we think that every new hospital should include a cogneration system, and that retrofitting should be considered whenever possible.

5.2 Cold Production

Cold storage — Total energy systems — Heat recovery.

The extended spreading of air conditioning in modern hospitals, which is no longer confined to the special treatment areas, like operating theatres and intensive care, but extended to almost the whole volume, the trend toward the use in the building of large inner volumes requiring high ventilation rates and heat removal due to internal loads like lights, people, machines, originate increasingly higher refrigerating demands.

Ty = type: MG = Gas Engine
TG = Gas Turbine
TV = Steam Turbine

PC = Post Combustor
H.P. = Heat Pump
N = number of units

Fl. = fluid produced: S = steam
W = Hot Water

St = present situation: Op = in operation
In = under installation
Co = under contracting
D = design stage

Yet the refrigerating loads show a big difference between maximum, average and minimum values, large daily and seasonal variations, and this implies a low utilisation factor for the refrigerating machines and most of the running time at partial load, with an efficiency drop.

It is therefore very important to correctly size the machines, and pay attention to partial load efficiencies, for example by selecting variable speed drives.

Another opportunity is given by Cold Storage systems, which are also becoming popular, to level out the daily variations, consequently getting the advantages of:-

- considerably reducing installed power;
- using cheaper night electricity; and
- reserve cold storage in case of black-out.

The storage can be either by sensible heat with chilled water, or by latent heat mostly ice. Even if the major part of the known applications are based on ice (in my opinion due to the pressure put by ice systems manufacturers), I believe that, whenever space is not a problem and in new constructions, where quite often advantage can be taken of the imposed fire fighting reserve water tank, the water option is more convenient. In fact, while in chilled water storage the system still runs between the standard temperature levels of from 7° to 12°c, in ice systems the evaporator temperature of the refrigerating machine must be decreased by 10°C to 15°C, with a consequent high drop in COP or efficiency, and rise in running costs. Moreover, in spite of the much larger volume of the tank, the equipment cost is much lower, and consequently, particularly if the fire fighting reserve tank cost can be deducted, the initial investment costs are not so different.

As an example one of the very first important application in the Michigan University Hospital in Ann Arbor, USA, already in operation for a few years can be mentioned. In Italy we have designed three large water storage systems, still to be realised. In one of these the installed refrigerating machines total power was reduced from 4.5 to 3 million frigories/hour, with a 1,700 cb m tank, which substitutes the imposed 1,500 cb m fire reserve tank.

Another important opportunity is a combination of electricity, heat and cold production in Total Energy systems, which allows a good balance of the loads throughout the year and a better utilisation of the machines.

The most immediate solution is combining a refrigerating absorption machine with a cogeneration system; the temperature required by the absorption machine for acceptable performance and efficiency calls for the use of gas turbines. In such a case double effect machines with high COP values can be used, operated by 8/10 bar steam obtained from the exhaust gas recovery boiler.

One such example is given in the cogeneration list: it is

Hospital	Ty	N	Total elec. Power kW	Total Heat Recov. kW	Fl.	El eff %	Tot eff %	St.	Additional Information
Bassano del Grappa	TG	3	1.500	4.200	S/W	21	80	In	+ PC + 2 Absor. Refr.
Sesto S. Giovanni (MI)	MG	1	330	551	W	32	85	Op	
Sestri Levante	MG	2	540	900	W	32	85	Op	
Vimercate	MG	2	540	900	S/W	32	85	Co	+ 1 El. H.P. — 160 kW
S. Martino — Genova	TG	2	2.100	9.000	S/W	21	81	Co	+ PC + Absor. Refr.
Pol. Gemelli — Roma	TG	2	2.100	5.200	S/W	21	79	Co	
Ist. Ort. Pini — Milano	MG	2	900	2.470	S/W	32	85	Co	+ Tandem H.P. — 250 kW
S. Carlo — Milano	TV	1	875	7.520	S	10	87	Co	+ 1 MG driven H.P. — 500 kW
Sarzana	MG	2	500	800	S/W	32	85	In	
Catania	MG	2	2.600	4.000	S/W	32	85	D	+ 2 H.P. — 830 kW

the Bassano del Grappa Hospital, now under completion, where three 500 kW Garrett gas turbines feed a recovery boiler producing 12 bar steam, operating two 2 million frigories/hour York double effect absorption machines; two standard 1.5 million frigories/hour chillers are used for peak loads.

S. Martino Hospital in Genoa will also have absorption machines operated by steam produced by two 1,000 kW gas turbines, while S. Carlo Hospital in Milan is expected having absorption machines coupled to a back pressure steam turbine.

Combining absorption machines with gas engines is more difficult because normal engines yield only part of the heat rejected at high temperature. However a couple of manufacturers now supply gas engines with high pressure and temperature (100°C/115°C) cooling, which is well suited to the single effect absorption machine.

Another possibility is given by the direct drive of the compression refrigerating machine with a gas engine, recovering the heat for other simultaneous uses; this will be better discussed in the following paragraph on heat pumps.

One last, but not least, opportunity to be always kept in mind is the possibility of recovering low temperature heat from the condenser of the refrigerating machines, typically to preheat domestic hot water.

5.3 Heat Pumps

Heat pumps, as well known, are again refrigerating machines with an inverted function, ie heating, by pumping up with a mechanical work the heat extracted from a lower temperature source. The work required for pumping is directly proportional to the temperature difference between the heating point and the low temperature source. Therefore the efficiency or COP of the heat pumps increases when this temperature difference decreases. Hence the use of the heat pump is particularly advisable for heating domestic hot water, or for ambient heating by panels or low temperature (40/50°C) fan coils or air heating, when using external air in temperate climates or ground water, or building exhaust air or waste water. As the availability of both latter sources is high in hospitals, there are definite chances here for heat pumps. Furthermore heat pumps are especially convenient whenever there is a simultaneous need for heat and cold, because one of them, specifically the lowest one, is practically obtained free of charge, if the temperatures required meet the heat pump specifications; in addition investment costs too cover just one production, heat or cold, thereby improving the pay-back. This is again a frequent occurrence in hospitals.

In order to increase the heat gain, there is a further opportunity, as mentioned before, that is driving the heat pump compressor with a gas engine, recovering the heat from the latter as well. In this way the fuel using efficiency doubles, with PER (Primary Energy Ratio) increasing from 0.85 for the traditional boiler to 1.7-1.8 for the gas driven heat pump; more details are given in a paper mentioned in the bibliography (3).

To give a few examples:-

- the 120 kW electric heat pump for domestic hot water and panel heating, coupled with the gas engine cogeneration system now being installed in Vimercate Hospital, close to Milan;
- 500 kW gas engine driven heat pump to be installed in S. Carlo Hospital in Milan, for hot water supply, using a well water source; and
- gas engine driven 400 kW tandem unit with a 500 kVA alternator and a 250 kW compressor for heat pump on the same shaft, being installed in the Istituto Ortopedico 'G. Pini' in Milan, side by side with another 400 kW standard cogeneration set. The heat pump is used to produce both chilled and warm water, and as a supplementary low temperature source heat recovered from building exhaust air and well water is used.

5.4 Energy Management Systems

Digital control systems, using micro- or mini-computers, are now available on the market allowing with proper software to perform the following function:-

- traditional control;
- alarms managements;
- optimisation of cogeneration, refrigerating systems, heat pumps, heat or cold storage operation; and
- energy consumption and economic data processing and accounting, to compare them with design or target values.

This can ensure optimum operation of the whole installation and consequently further energy and cost savings.

These systems give also the opportunity of scheduling automatically the maintenance operations, to keep the efficiencies at their optimum levels and to provide a basis for clearer relationships with maintenance contractors.

Such systems are now being installed, for example, in the already mentioned hospitals of Bassano del Grappa, Sestri Levante, Sarzana, Vimercate, and are becoming more and more used for their usefulness.

Bibliography

(1) 'Gli aspetti energetici attuali e futuri dell'ospedale' Mario de Renzio — I Conferenza Europea sull'ospedale — Roma — 29 marzo-i aprile 1990.

(2) 'Analisi energetica di strutture ospedaliere in ambito regionale — Un caso: la Regione Liguria' Mario de Renzio — 'Tecnica Ospedaliera' — n 6/87 'HTE — Energie Alternative' — n 49 satt./ott. 1987.

(3) 'L'uso del gas per la congenerazione e l'azionamento di pomps di calore nel settore civile, terziario e ospedaliero' Mario de Renzio, Bianca Ciocca — II Convegno ATIG — Firenze — 27-29 novembre 1989.

Energy Management with Information from Building Energy Management Systems

by

Ir. H. J. Nicolaas
TNO Institute of Applied Physics (TPD), Delft
Ing LDA Van NAMEN
Sint Franciscus Hospital
Rotterdam

Introduction

In the Netherlands an organisation exists of users of Building Management Systems called 'STUGES'. A working party of this organisation is set up especially for solving user problems related to energy consumption and energy management. A very special problem from the point of view of the users is the lack of general software for energy management independent of the type of the BEM system. Only special purpose software per type of BEMS is available from the suppliers. Suppliers do not develop general software for competitive reasons.

The model for information requirements for energy management in buildings, which includes the description in the different functions of the program, will be discussed. Attention is paid to the way of presenting results independent of the BEM systems. Also overviews will be shown of the information which is needed on three distinctive levels: executive, management and technical level. Attention will be given to logical design, database choice, and connectivity problems between application software and interface software. A typical point of interest is the implementation and testing of the software in the "Sint Franciscus Gasthuis' Hospital. The introduction of general purpose software for energy management influences on a 'running organisation'.

This paper will be divided in four main parts, the Novem organisation, Energy management aspects in the hospital, the development of the software and the interfacing and the demonstration project.

Novem

As stated in the introduction the investigation was supported by the Novem, the Netherlands agency for energy and the environment. Within a framework of government energy policy Novem stimulates research and development as well as the demonstration and marketing of techniques, technologies and systems for energy conservation and fuel diversification. Novem also carries out specific assignments for the International Energy Agency (IEA). Novem further acts as an intermediary between government, industry and research. It brings government policy and market developments together and bridges the gap between theoretical knowledge and practical application. Programs of activities designed to lead to energy conservation or fuel diversification goals in such areas as manufacturing, the public utilities and the built-up environment are the basis of Novem's work. Novem drafts proposals for such programs based on the policy goals set by the government in consultation with interest groups parties in the market and outside experts, taking advantage of international developments and opportunities for international collaboration. The Ministry of Economic Affairs and any other funding bodies that may be involved then provide Novem with the financial resources required for program implementation. One of Novems programs concentrates on the built-up environments. The aim is to bring about a saving of just under 40% in non residential buildings (offices, hospitals etc). Since 1986 special attention is paid to the use of Building Management Systems.

Energy Management at the Sint Franciscus Hospital

In 1982 the director of the physical plant became responsible for the energy management program at the Sint Franciscus Hospital. An energy accounting system was set up to monitor the energy consumption and the effect of energy saving modifications. As a first step the total hospital was defined as area for energy consumption and cost reporting. Since 1982 energy consumption is being reported weekly, monthly and annually and compared with previous years.

In 1984 and 1985, the heat generation systems were modified. Production losses of the boilers were diminished by a heat recovery system and modification of the boiler control system. This resulted in a decrease of energy consumption of about 10%. A consultant investigated the possibilities for energy recovery from return air. The use of air-to-air systems appeared not to be possible due to the lay-out of the building. Airducts of supply-air and return-air could not be joined.

From 1986 on the energy conservation program focussed on the possibilities of the building management system. The TNO Institute of Applied Physics carried out a demonstration project, financially supported by Novem. In several zones, the conditioned air supply is reduced by valves in the air ducts, depending on the use of the rooms. The BEM-system controls the valves. This project was very successful, the investments paid off within two years.

In 1988 development started of software for 'real-time' measurement of energy consumption. This project will be elaborated further in this presentation. The influence on a 'running organisation', modification of plant must be planned and executed carefully. Another problem is how to convince the administration of the hospital to give (financial) support for the necessary investments. A 'critical success factor' is the attitude of the BEM-system-manager, operators and other technical personnel involved. It is one of the most critical factors in getting results.

GESTION DE L'ENERGIE PAR INFORMATION PROVENANT DES SYSTEMES DE GESTION DES BATIMENTS

Depuis le milieu de l'an 1988 l'Institut de Physique Appliqée a entamé, en coöperation avec l'organisation STUGES un project afin de développer un programme d'ordinateur général de contrôle d'énergie à utiliser pour l'interprétation des données produites par des systèmes BEM.

L'information venant des systèmes BEM sera transmisé à un ordinateur IBM (compatible). Un deuxième aspect important concerne alors la connectivité dépendante du type BEM.

Le project bénéficie d'aide financière de la part de NOVEM (Bureau Néerlandaise pour l'Energie et et l'Environnement), une organisation affiliée au Ministère des Affaires Economique.

Une demonstration des programmes généraux sera donnée dans grands bâtiments, dont un est l'hôpital 'Sint Franciscus Gasthuis' à Rotterdam.

The results of almost 10 years of energy management are shown in Figure 1.

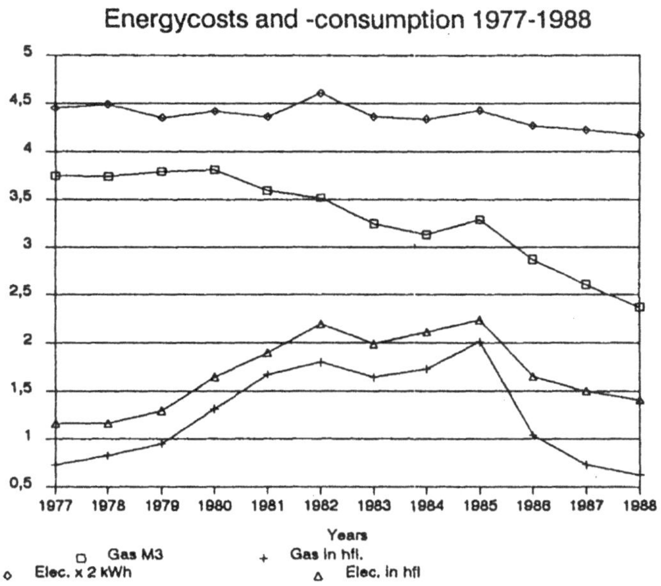

Figure 1

Developing the Software

Special software has been developed to start with energy management in buildings with Building Energy Management Systems (BEMS). This software should be used in buildings with BEM-systems of different manufacturers. For that reason the energy management information which is collected by the BEM-system is downloaded to an IBM-(compatible) PC (Figure 2). In that case one program can be developed with different interfaces to the several types of BEM-systems.

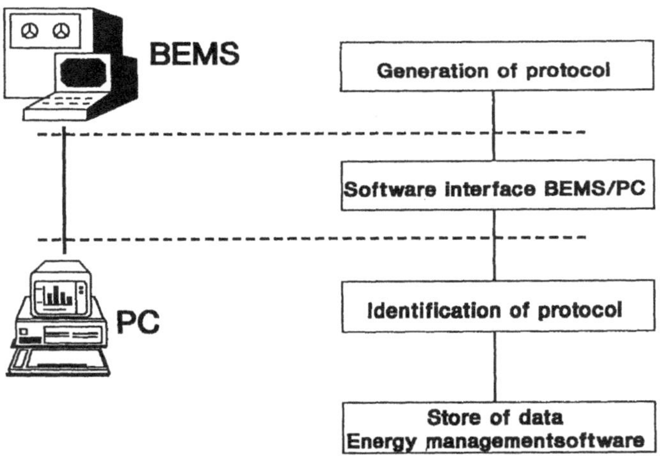

Figure 2

For the developing of the program a working party of STUGES (Dutch society of BEM-users) has accompanied the project. Representatives of the four buildings (two non residential buildings and two industries) in which the program was to be demonstrated were members of this group. The procedure was as follows (Figure 3):-

1. *List of Demands*. Wishes about the energy management features were collected from the different members of the STUGES working party. The different energy analysis methods which the members want to use, are also included in the list.
2. *Functional Design*. The list of demands was translated in functions and processes following special methods (IDEF-methods).
3. *Logical Design*. The functional design is worked out in a data structure. This represents the structure of the information needed to carry out the functions of the system.
4. *Choice of Database*. With the help of the logical design the database can be chosen.
5. *Physical Design*. The logical design can be adapted to the type of database. The result will give the physical design.
6. *Software Development*. With the physical design in hand the software specialist is able to make the computer program.
7. *Demonstration Phase*. The program is tested and demonstrated at four locations with four different types of Building Management Systems (Sauter, Honeywell, Johnson Controls, Philips).

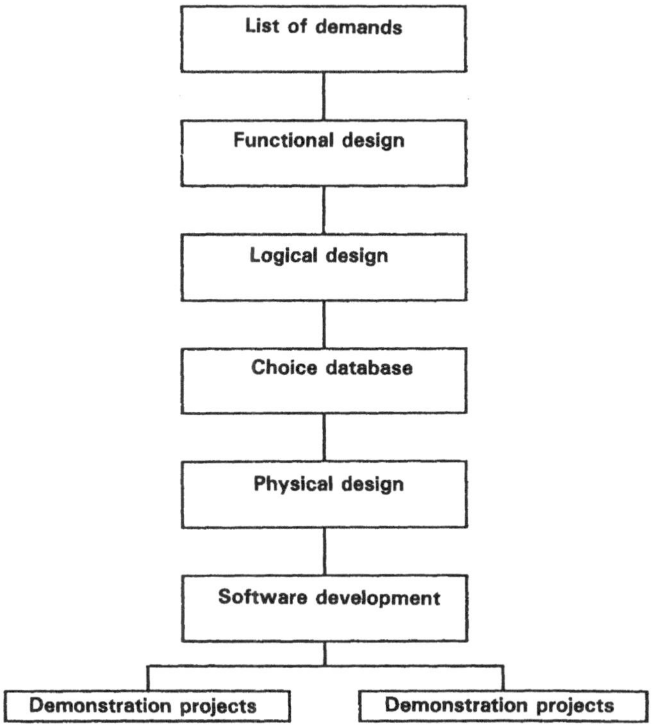

Figure 3

Targets for Energy Management

Good energy management can be reached in three steps:-

(1) Registration of energy consumption.
(2) Analysis of the energy consumption.
(3) Energy consumption reporting.

1. Registration of Energy Consumption

For the registration of energy consumption it is necessary to measure different energy flows. This means central measuring of gas oil, electricity, hot and cold water, steam and, in some cases, other gases such as oxygen, etc. Also local measurements are necessary to measure energy flows to different parts of the building complex. In case these parts have their own energy bill, other information must be available such as energy prices and special rates.

2. Analysis of the Energy Consumption

A very important point of the developed program forms the tools of the energy consumption analysis. Questions should be answered such as: 'What is normal use for the building as a whole, but also for parts of the building complex?' Can energy standards be used? With good analysing programs it is possible to make prognoses for the future, depending on the actual use of energy. The methods can be divided in:-

- prognosis based on past years;
- comparing actual energy use to energy figures from other buildings of more or less the same building type; and
- using calculation models based on mathematical relationships.

More about these analyses later on.

3. Energy Consumption Reporting

The program is designed for easy generation of reports, based on energy consumption information. These reports are produced at the following different levels:-

- executive level;
- management level; and
- technical level.

At the executive level yearly energy consumption overviews can be shown. Actual energy use compared to prognoses are also of interest at this level. Last but not least expected future energy costs can be forecast.

For the management, composition of the different energy flows in the parts of the building, during certain periods, are of interest.

For the technicians the system should be able to produce energy figures and temperatures over short periods. It should also be capable of following energy consumption of specific components in the building for monitoring and control purposes.

Energy Management Menu

The main menu of the energy management software asks for the following information:-

(1) *Definitions of:* building complex, building energy type, energy measuring point, climate measuring point, weatherstation, weekends, holidays, climate installation for each building.

(2) *Presentation of Energy Consumption Figures:* The following output is possible: tables, bars and line graphics can be given on a yearly, monthly, and daily basis. Overviews are given for energy flow type, building and building parts in more than 20 different ways with windows.

(3) *Presentation of Climate Conditions:* The climate conditions for several periods are shown in various ways. Also related values calculated from climate conditions and statistical algorithms, can be produced.

Analysing Tools

Analysing tools are of great importance for energy management. The following tools are developed:-

1. Enthalpy-Calculation: Software to calculate the energy contents (enthalpy) of the air based on climate conditions.
2. Degree-Days: Calculation of the degree days and hours over certain periods of the day or week during which the HVAC plant operates.
3. Enthalpy-Days: Calculating of enthalpy-days (cooling and or heating) for control of the HVAC-process.
4. Statistical Analysis: Software for statistical analysis with linear and non linear regression techniques.
5. Energy Signature: Calculation of energy signature following the methods described in the International Energy Agency's handbook: 'Source Book for Energy Auditors'.
6. Standards: Software based on the Dutch National Standard on energy consumption in residential and non-residential buildings.

Demonstration Project

One of the projects in which the program is demonstrated is the hospital Sint Franciscus Gasthuis in Rotterdam. The building is divided in a high rise section of 13 floors and a lower section of three floors. (Total floor area is 60,000m^2, 24 hvac units, technical staff 50 persons) every building section is supplied with one or more hvac-units. The units consists of a heating coil, cooling coil, steam moisturiser and a supply fan. The total fresh air supply to the whole building is 465,000m^3/h. Energy is delivered by three hot water gas boilers, four hot water driven steam generators and two absorption chillers.

The Building Management System

The BEM-system is a Sauter EY2400 with PLC outstations. The system contains one CPU with two displays, two printers and eight outstations. Totally 1,100 addresses are connected. This system is now coupled with a PC on which the energy management software is installed.

Energy Registration

For the registration the following meters all with pulse output have been installed (Figure 4):-

Central Meters:
Gas: Flow meter for three hotwater boilers (G1), FLow meter for the combustion furnace (G2).
Water: Central water supply meter.
Electricity: Central electricity meter (Mo).
Local Meters:
Water: Flow to different consumers of hot water (160°C and 100°C) and cold water.
Hotwater supply to the absorption chillers (H1).
Cold water delivery from the chillers (H5, H6).

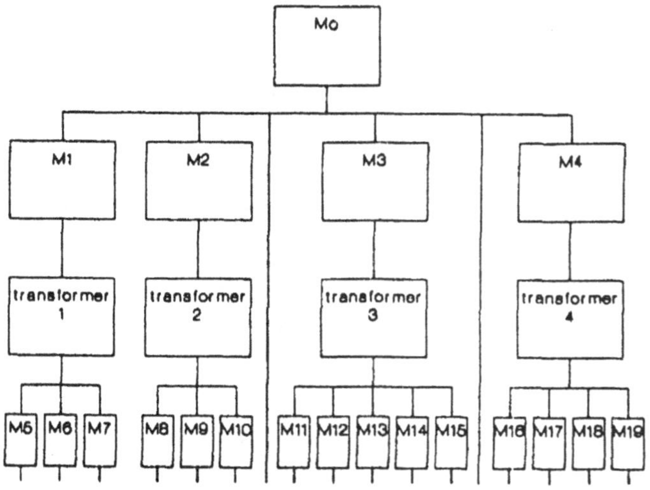

Figure 4

Warm water radiator groups (H3, H4).
Hot water for sterilisation, kitchen, hot water storage and radiators (H2).
Electricity: Each of the four high voltage transformers has its own meter (M1/M4) (Figure 5).
An inventory was made of the different consumers from each transformer. The 15 most significant electricity consumers are measured separately by its own meter (M5 to M19).
HVAC: All the supply conditions to the HVAC units have been measured.

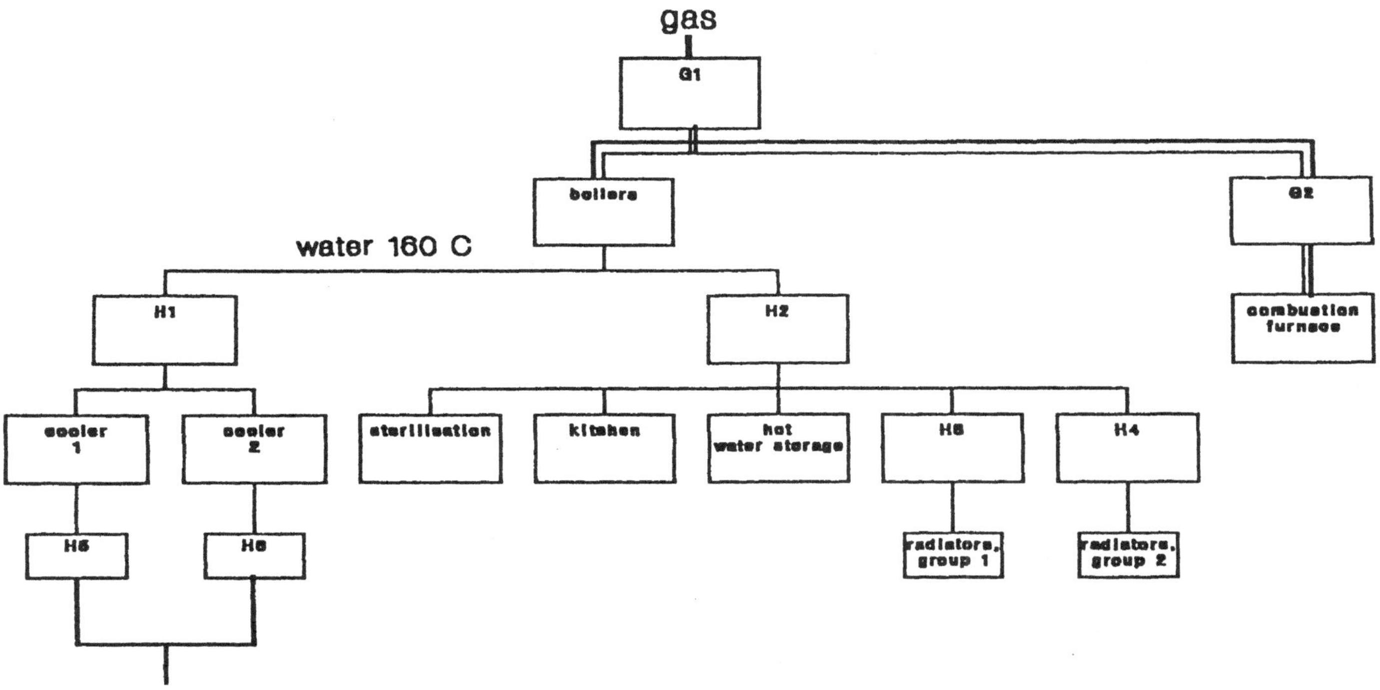

Figure 5

Status of the Project

All meters were installed at the end of 1989. The communication software and interface software was installed in January 1990. In February 1990 the energy management software was available. In June 1990 the first results are expected of the energy management software.

Acknowledgement

The project could not have succeeded without the work of many people. We will mention W. Plokker and H. C. Pietsman from the TNO Institute of Applied Physics for developing program and interface. J. Wassink from the SFG hospital for installation, and the members of the STUGES working party for their advice.

Automation with Coal Firing

by

P. Mills
Head of Industrial Sales
British Coal Corporation

Introduction

Coal plays a vital role in satisfying our energy needs. Total world coal sales exceed 3 billion tonnes per annum and a significant proportion of this is used for electricity production; 40% of the world's electricity is produced from coal. In the United Kingdom there is a substantial mining industry and coal is a recognised and accepted fuel in all market sectors, eg, power generation, industry, commerce and home heating. The majority of coal produced in the UK is used for electricity generation (75% of the UK's electricity is produced from coal-fired stations) but British Coal continues to be very actively involved in the other markets.

Automation with coal firing has been taken for granted for many, many years at power stations and large industrial sites but has only been given attention at smaller sites in recent years. This paper outlines the development and introduction of automation applied to general industrial and commercial coal fired applications.

In the early 1970's British Coal recognised the need for improved equipment in the industrial and commercial markets and began a research and development programme to improve the automation, convenience and efficiency of coal fired plant. Substantial efforts have been made to upgrade existing firing equipment such as static grates, chain and travelling grates, underfeed stokers and coking stokers. Work has also been undertaken to develop novel firing systems. It was additionally recognised that as well as developing improved combustion systems, it was also necessary to make similar improvements to all of the ancilliary equipment needed with coal firing. Much of this research and development work has been carried out in collaboration with equipment makers, and has ranged from coal delivery, reception, storage, on-site handling, boiler/furnace control and boilerhouse integrated controls to ash storage and removal. In an era when conserving and improving the environment has become paramount, much work has also been carried out on flue gas clean-up and towards ensuring that the whole plant is designed to be environmentally friendly in all its aspects.

The aim of British Coal's development programme is to provide the customer with plant which vies with oil or gas in automation, convenience, efficiency and low environmental impact.

Coal Types

In the UK two types of coal are generally supplied to the industrial and commercial markets. These are:-

(i) washed singles, a clean low-ash content coal typically 25mm-12mm in size; and
(ii) washed smalls, having an ash content in the range of 6%-10% and sized 25mm-0.

These coals are prepared for specific markets, but the detailed characteristics vary from colliery to colliery.

Coal Delivery and Reception

The majority of coal used in industry and commerce in the UK is delivered by road. The conventional tipper lorry is the type most frequently used but pneumatic delivery vehicles, which incorporate a positive displacement blower to provide the conveying air, are popular for smaller sites because the coal can be delivered directly to a storage hopper or bunker.

Containerised coal delivery, using 20 tonne capacity ISO containers is also being introduced. There would be two reception bays provided at the site, permitting the delivery vehicle to off-load a full container and then load the adjacent empty unit. After delivery, operation of hydraulic rams tip the container so that coal is discharged into the boilerhouse conveying system.

Many systems for coal reception have been used over the years and more recently additional high convenience systems have been introduced to the market, often sponsored by British Coal. Traditionally, large industrial users have stored coal in open stockpiles, but this approach is not usually appropriate for smaller industrial and commercial users. However, consumers can still obtain the benefit of low cost tipper delivery without the need for open stockpiles by utilising one of the following:-

Underground Bunkers

These have been widely used in the past, but have become less popular due to the expensive excavation and civil costs associated with their construction.

Tipping Hoppers

To overcome the construction costs associated with underground bunkers several manufacturers have developed end-tipping hoppers which provide a controlled feed from a batch of coal delivered by a tipper lorry. The tipping hopper, when in the lowered position, is a platform on to which the delivery lorry drives and tips its load. After delivery, an hydraulic jacking system lifts the hopper to an upright position and the contents are discharged by gravity into the boilerhouse conveying system. For sites with limited headroom, a side-tipping hopper has been deleloped.

Walking Floors

In this sytem the lorry is backed up to the Walking Floor and its load tipped on to the reciprocating floor of the unit. The coal is 'walked' along the length of the unit by the reciprocating action of the floor segments. There are two hospitals using this type of equipment; the first commercial demonstration unit was installed at Worcester Royal Infirmary, when an oil to coal conversion was carried out two years ago, and the other is in use at Rampton Hospital in Nottinghamshire, where a new coal-fired boiler plant was installed last year.

AUTOMATION PAR CHARBON

Le charbon joue un rôle essentiel dans la satisfaction de nos besoins en énergie. Les ventes mondiales de charbon s'élèvent à 3 milliards de tonnes par an. Une proportion importante de ce volume sert à la production d'électricité. 40% de l'électricité mondiale est produite à partir du charbon. Au Royaume-Uni, l'industrie minière est toujours importante et le charbon est reconnu et accepté comme source d'énergie dans tous les secteurs du marché (production du courant, industrie, commerce, chauffage domestique par example). La plus grande partie de la production de charbon au Royaume-Uni est destinée à la génération d'électricité (75% de l'électricité britannique provient du charbon); cependant British Coal continue à se diversifier.

L'automation par charbon est depuis longtemps considéré un fait acquis dans les centrales et les grandes industries, mais c'est depuis peu que cette possibilité fait l'objet d'un intérêt particulier pour les usine de taille plus réduite. Cet article décrit le développement et l'introduction de l'automation pour tous les utilisateurs de charbon, industriels et commerciaux.

Wide Belt Unloaders

These operate in a way similar to the Walking Floor, but use a belt about 3m wide which is carried on a chain and slat conveyor. The coal is taken to the rear of the container, where a discharge conveyor transfers it into the boilerhouse system. Little or no excavation is needed and a quantity of covered storage is available within the body of the unit. A wide belt unloader is in use at Culham Laboratory, a government research establishment near Oxford where new coal-fired boiler equipment was commissioned earlier this year.

Coal Storage

Today there is an increasing need to store coal in an environmentally unobtrusive way. Silo and bunker storage has become a popular method of answering this need, with silos ranging in capacity from 30 tonnes up to 1,000 tonnes. Economy in the use of ground space, cleanliness in stocking and convenience in retrieval from stock are obvious advantages of this form of storage.

Glass reinforced silos are available for capacities of up to about 60 tonnes, and for units up to 300 tonnes vitreous enamel-lined steel are most widely used. Silos above 300 tonnes are normally constructed of concrete.

Silos not exceeding 18m in height storing washed singles can be filled using a pneumatic delivery vehicle. Taller silos can be filled using a mechanical elevator or on-site pneumatic equipment. When smalls coal is stored, a mechanical or dense phase pneumatic system should be used. Care needs to be taken with the loading and unloading of silos to avoid the risk of eccentric loadings, which can damage the silo. Similarly, care needs to be taken with the design of the filling and emptying arrangements to minimise the degradation of the coal. The presence of fine coal particles can adversely affect the operation of the discharge and handling equipment as well as having a detrimental effect on the operation and performance of the boiler.

British Coal has produced a series of technical booklets relating to coal storage and handling systems which are freely available to users and designers of coal plant.

Coal Conveying

Conveying systems for industrial boilerhouses are either mechanical or pneumatic and the selection of one or the other type will depend on various factors including the required conveying rate, type of coal, system complexity and layout, and capital cost. Mechanical systems are generally able to convey both singles and smalls coal, although careful attention to design is needed to minimise degradation of singles and provide self-cleaning systems for small coals, whilst pneumatic conveying systems are selected according to the type of coal being moved. Lean phase systems are generally only suitable for singles but dense phase units convey both smalls and singles, although they are most suitable for smalls.

Whilst mechanical systems can generally convey coal only in straight lines, the popularity of pneumatic conveyors is no doubt due to their ability to transport coal vertically, horizontally and around bends within an enclosed pipeline. Pneumatic transfer valves are also available which give added flexibility. Although this flexibility lends itself to the aesthetic design of the boilerhouse, it must be strongly emphasised that as with all handling systems, the simplier the design the more reliable it is.

Combustion Equipment and Boilers

In recent years British Coal has been involved in the development of a range of new or improved firing equipment capable of automatic operation with part-time attendance and these have been introduced to the market place. This equipment ranges in size from small commercial units to large industrial boilers.

One such piece of equipment is a high-intensity reciprocating ram stoker marketed by James Proctor, known as the Proctor Mini-stoker. This unit is fitted to conventional three-pass horizontal shell boilers and available in the size range 1MW-2.5MW thermal. This stoker is designed to burn singles coal, has built-in combustion control and offers a good turn-down ratio. To date, some 70 Proctor Mini-stokers have been installed, many of these at public sector establishments, eg PSA buildings, hospitals, prisons, etc.

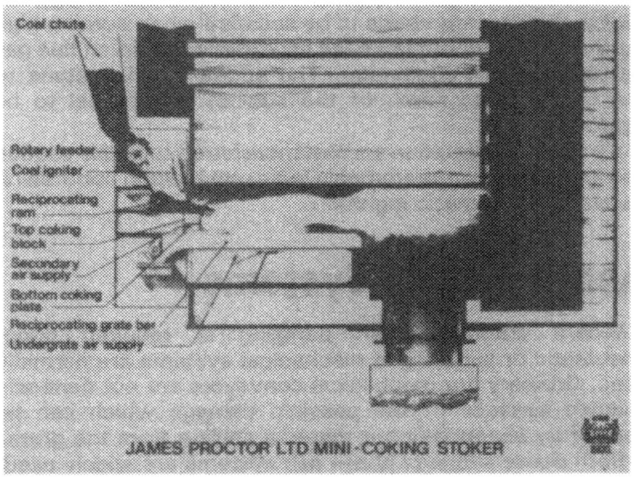

JAMES PROCTOR LTD MINI-COKING STOKER

One frequently used type of coal firing equipment used in the 2MW-6MW size range is the fixed grate stoker, with singles coal being sprinkled on to the grate via a drop tube and distributor in the crown of the boiler furnace. This equipment is available from several boilermakers and because of the many advantages of this system has proved to be very popular. Fixed grate stokers have built-in fuel feed control and full modulation but do need to be manually de-ashed once or twice a shift. In response to requests from customers, British Coal and a boilermaker jointly developed a tipping grate stoker which maintains the same combustion principles as the fixed grate unit, but enables the ash to be removed automatically by arranging for segments of the grate to tip in sequence. In excess of 30 tipping grate boilers are now in use, marketed by Senior Green.

Chain grate stokers have been used in the general industrial market for many, many years, but usually have boilermen in full-time attendance. Three years ago NEI Cochran and British Coal began the design and development of an automatic chain grate stoker for industrial applications. A prototype was built and successfully tested at NEI Cochran's works at Annan, and the first commercial Coalmaster 2001 unit, rated at 5MW, was installed at British Coal's research establishment near Cheltenham six months ago. As well as incorporating several new technical features to enable unattended operation, a completely fresh approach has been taken with the styling of the Coalmaster 2001, resulting in an aesthetically attractive boiler unit.

Another new concept in coal firing at the smaller end of the market is the Coalflow package, which is available in sizes up to 300kW, suitable for use in commercial and light industrial market sectors including small hospitals and nursing homes. These high efficiency appliances incorporate a large degree of automation so that only occasional visits are required to check the operation. Coalflow appliances have both automatic fuel feed and ash removal and can achieve very high turn-down ratios. To date in excess of 100 commercial Coalflow units have been sold by Hoval and James Scott, many to the public sector.

A new product currently under development is a 1MW appliance offering a high level of amenity and efficiency. A prototype unit is currently under test at the Coal Research Establishment and it is anticipated that the first units for commercial demonstration will be placed on the market in the next few months.

Fluidised bed combustion equipment has been available for several years and most of the 150 shallow bed units installed in the UK incorporate some British Coal technology. This combustion system is attractive to the user because of the ability to burn a wide range of coals and/or waste material, and their rapid response capability enabling variable loads to be followed and still maintain high efficiency. Most of the fluidised bed equipment installed in the UK is at medium or large industrial sites and few units have been supplied to the public sector.

With proposed legislation for the reduction of SO_2 emission from larger boiler installations, fbc technology will enable the new standards to be satisfied when burning high sulphur fuels without the need for expensive add-on flue gas desulphurisation equipment. The addition of limestone to the bed enables much of the sulphur in the fuel to be captured.

All of the combustion equipment referred to in this section can incorporate programmable logic combustion controllers, as well as automatic ingnition.

Ash Removal Systems

Where automatic ash handling is required either pneumatic or submerged mechanical systems are normally used. Ordinary dry mechanical conveyors are not generally suitable because of the possible damage which can be caused by abnormally hot material spilling from the grate.

Both dense and lean phase ash systems are widely used, but pipework and bend wear can be high unless careful attention is paid to the initial design. Conveying velocity plays the major part in setting wear rates and thus some form of air velocity control is recommended. Ash is normally conveyed from the boilerhouse to an overhead vessel prior to emptying into lorries or skips for disposal.

Mechanical systems are normally partially submerged under water. A water seal is maintained at the ash outlet from the boiler, thus isolating the combustion chamber from the outside air. Such systems are therefore inherently dust-free and any unintentional burning carbon will be immediately quenched. Both belt conveyors and en masse systems are used for submerged ash conveying.

Flue Gas Cleaning

Although electroc-static precipitators or bag filters are used for gas clean-up on larger installations and achieve very high collection efficiencies, the equipment normally used on general industrial and commercial coal-fired boilers is high efficiency cyclones or multicyclones. More stringent solid emissions standards are likely to be introduced in the UK and British Coal has undertaken an extensive programme of development work towards the production of minimum cost, reliable, low maintenance gas cleaning equipment. A number of improved systems suitable for plant up to around 10MW are under test, in anticipation of tighter legislation.

Boilerhouse Control

With the advent of microprocessor and programmable logic controls it is now possible to integrate the control of the whole plant. One control system will monitor and control the coal reception, coal transport, coal storage, boiler operation, ash removal system and effluent gas quality to achieve an operation of high efficiency and automation.

At the centre of this system is the boiler or furnace where sensors monitor the demand to be placed on the combustion equipment and initiate the changes in coal-feed and air supply required to meet that new demand. Sensors can also monitor flue gas conditions and the boil parameters trimmed to maintain optimum performance.

Similarly, in a multiple boiler complex, the control system can select the rate of firing of each boiler and the number of boilers on line to maximise efficiency. One word of warning, however, before going overboard with an all singing, all dancing control system. The greater the complexity of the system, the more difficult it is to commission and fault find. There is still a place for mechanical/electrical units integrated into such a system described above, enabling individual operations to be performed and monitored separately from the main computer control, but when proven, integrated into that system. Achieving the correct balance between simplicity and sophistication is all important for a successful boilerhouse control system.

There are many examples of automation with coal-firing at health care establishments, and it may be of interest to refer to two particular cases. One is Rampton Special Hospital where, as part of the latest redevelopment, the PSA were given a brief to install a new coal-fired boiler plant requiring minimum attendance. After examining a range of options, and inviting proposals from British Coal's technical service, the PSA selected four Hartley and Sugden boilers, each rated at 2.3MW and fired by Proctor mini-coking stokers, to be accommodated in the new boilerhouse. Coal is delivered by a tipper vehicle on to a Walking Floor reception unit and then transferred by a Redler en-masse conveyor to four storage bunkers. Secondary handling is by spiral elevators lifting the coal to the boiler hoppers. Ash is automatically removed from each boiler by a Proctor wet ash system and discharged to skips. There is a Trend building management system which co-ordinates the automatic operation of the plant, and also performs a monitoring and reporting service to the central control room. This plant was commissioned last year and we understand is providing very satisfactory service.

The second example relates to a grouping of four hospitals in the West Midlands. Towards the end of last year the Health Authority installed a new coal-fired boiler at each of four hospitals in the Dudley/Stourbridge locality. Each plant is automatic in operation with a central computer monitoring individual site performance. All four sites are supervised by a mobile operator, based at one of the hospitals, who visits the other three sites on a routine basis or on an alarm call-out. The boilers are HDS Eurotherm units fired by chain grate stokers (the sizes ranging from 1.8MW to 7.5MW) with automatic coal and ash handling. This forward-looking approach by the Health Authority clearly demonstrates not only that automation with coal-firing can be achieved but, when also linked to modern control and monitoring systems, very effective use can be made of low manning levels.

Conclusions

During the past 15 years very considerable development work has been carried out by British Coal and UK manufacturers towards the achievement of high efficiency, high reliability automatic combustion plant. The use of coal need no longer be labour-intensive and the intention of this paper has been to outline some of the coal firing plant available which lends itself to automation.

An alternative way of addressing the labour aspect is to consider contracting-out the operation and maintenance of the boilerhouse to a specialist company. There are a number of well-established and reputable heat service and contract energy management organisations able to assume full responsibility for supplying the energy needs of hospitals and other similar establishment on a long-term contractual basis.

British Coal offers a free technical advisory service to industrial and commercial energy users, including guidance on the selection and utilisation of coal-firing equipment. For those clients who would wish us to go beyond the advisory stage, British Coal is now able to offer a comprehensive contractual service through its recently formed Coal and Energy Services.

The range of expertise available through CES includes performance testing, environmental monitoring, heat service and specialist consultancy support. CES operates from British Coal's head office in London, but details of the services available can be obtained through any of British Coal's sales offices.

Acknowledgement

This paper is published by permission of British Coal Corporation, but the views expressed are those of the author and not necessarily those of the Corporation. Thanks are expressed to colleagues both within British Coal and in manufacturing industry who have contributed to the work described and the successes achieved.

Unconventional Site Energy Strategy

by

J. M. Singh CEng, MIMechE
Superintending Engineer
Department of Health
London

Background

Many hospitals in the United Kingdom exhibit the characteristic of a number of separate buildings scattered over a large site. Usually there would also be a sterilising and disinfecting unit and in a number of cases, a laundry as well. Invariably the thermal energy requirements for the site as a whole is provided from a central boiler house linked to individual buildings by a network of distribution mains. Steam was the preferred heat transfer medium as this is needed for sterilising, catering and laundry services.

In recent years rationalisation and upgrading of the estate has brought about significant changes. There is less fragmentation of individual departments and services with a consequential reduction in the number of buildings. New hospitals are much more compact and there has also been a shift away from providing, on site, support services such as laundry, sterilisation and even catering. The present trend is to centralise these services elsewhere.

These changes have in effect reduced quite significantly the requirements for thermal energy and have weakened the case for a central boiler house. Other considerations are relatively high heat losses associated with distribution mains and the low load factors these have as they remain energised throughout the year. Central steam raising boiler houses continue to be built although primarily on sites where a number of existing buildings are to be retained along with a new hospital. However there is a drift towards more localised plant sometimes sited at roof top or even within the hospital itself.

Our health care buildings rely mainly on the national grid for electrical energy and consumption has been increasing progressively over the past few years. Stand-by generators maintain essential loads in the event of mains failure, but apart form periodic testing they remain idle for most of the time. Combined heat and power (CHP) units have been installed in a number of existing hospitals but they have not as yet become a standard provision for new projects.

The trend towards smaller boiler houses in many new hospitals is likely to continue. This is being influenced by technological advances and by the on-going drive for further improvements in energy efficiency. These developments are likely to encourage the adoption of a wide range of unconventional site energy strategies for the provision of thermal and electrical energy. Indeed as CHP and heat reclaim techniques become more accepted the boiler house will give way to the energy centre. Within such a unit the supply of electrical power, thermal energy and where appropriate the destruction of hospital waste, will be undertaken not as separate processes but as a combined operation. The manner in which energy is derived at any particular time will be determined by a building management system; its primary aim being to ensure that energy is derived from the most economic source.

Energy Efficient Hospitals

In the early 1980's the Department of Health sponsored two in-depth studies into low energy hospitals. These looked at the pattern of energy consumption in a typical hospital built to standards current at the time and the variations in diurnal and seasonal loads. The studies went on to examine how energy could be reduced by conservation measures and the potential for heat recovery. An important part of this work was concerned with an assessment of the type and grade of energy used for various services, alternative methods of meeting this demand and the contribution these might make to the overall energy strategy for a hospital.

The findings indicated that by good design and with a modest increase in capital expenditure energy consumption could be reduced by in excess of 30% and fuel used by 50%; Figure 1 indicates the basic principles. These have been applied to the design and construction of two low energy demonstration projects; St Mary's a 200 bed hospital on the Isle of Wight and Wansbeck a 300 bed hospital in the north of England at Ashington in Northumbria. St Mary's will be fully operational later this year and Wansbeck is due to be completed in 1992. Although it will be sometime before the evaluation of these projects is complete the technology for the construction of energy efficient hospitals is available now and it is affordable. Therefore it is to be expected that future hospitals will use relatively less energy than the present stock.

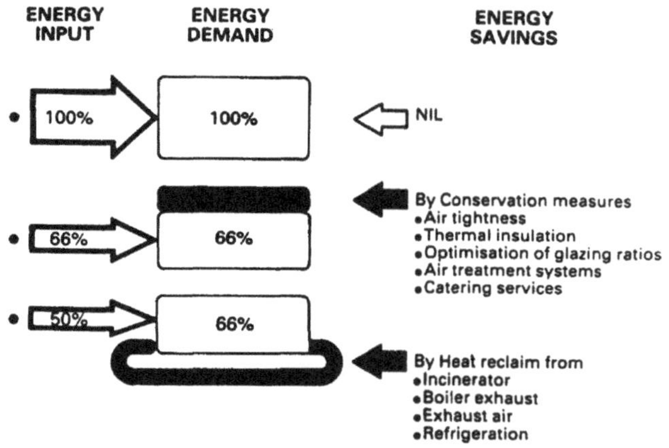

Figure 1: Reducing Fuel Consumption in an Energy Efficient Hospital.

The model on which the studies were based was a typical 300 bed Nucleus hospital, several of which have already been built and have been operational for many years. Data on energy consumption within these hospitals is being used to refine the model and to improve the degree of accuracy

STRATEGIE D'ENERGIE POUR SITE NON CONVENTIONNEL

De nombreux facteurs se sont unis pour réduire les charges thermiques dans les nouveaux hôspitaux et les méthodes de production d'énergie traditionnelles ne sont plus, dans de nombreux cas, entièrement appropriées. L'énergie thermique peut maintenant être obtenue à partir d'un grand nombre de sources grâce á des techniques de récupération de chaleur. Cette technologie alliée à la production sur place d'électricité que ce soit grâce à des générateurs auxiliaires ou à des groupes de puissance et des unités thermiques combinés offre la possibilité d'une gamme de stratégies d'énergie de substitution sur place. Des études ont confirmé la viabilité économique d'un tel projet et il a été adopté pour deux hôpitaux pilotes à basse énergie. La communication étudie ce scénario.

with which consumption and diurnal load profiles can be forecast. This level of information is essential to the development of alternative site energy strategies. Figure 2 shows the predicted pattern of energy usage in Wansbeck hospital resulting from the adoption of energy conservation measures. Energy used for incineration has been excluded.

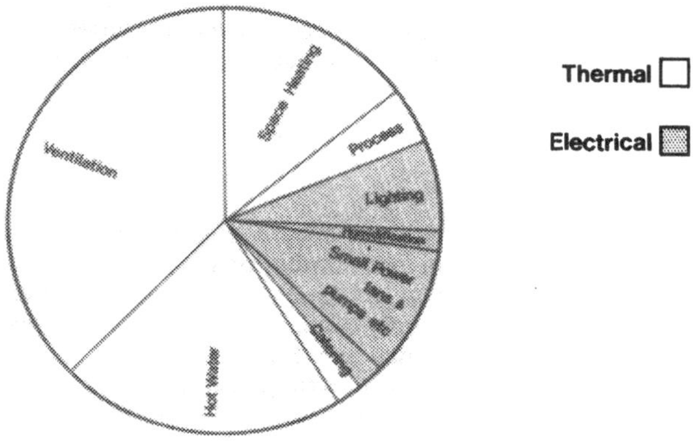

Figure 2: Annual Energy Consumption — Wansbeck Hospital.

Alternative Energy Sources

There are a number of alternative ways of generating heat and of supplying those thermal loads which traditionally have been provided from either a central or local boiler house. All involve the use of well established technologies.

Catering is a prime example of this, whether conventional or 'cook chill' food processing is adopted. The past few years have seen the introduction of improved cooking appliances such as the combi cooker and high speed steamers which are direct fired by gas and/or by electricity. Where steam is needed it is provided by a generator which forms an integral part of the appliance. This avoids mains distribution losses. For similar reasons it is preferable to utilise local steam raising plant for processes such as sterilisation and humidification. In consequence a boiler house no longer has to meet the steam load associated with these services.

A similar approach can be adopted for the generation of domestic hot water. Direct fired water heaters are now quite commonplace and overcome many of the disadvantages associated with large storage calorifiers. Several units have already been installed in a number of hospitals and so far have provided a satisfactory service.

Heat reclaim is of particular importance in the development of a viable alternative site energy strategy. Air exhausted by the hospital's mechanical ventilation systems is an ideal heat source. A significant amount of thermal energy can be recovered from this and used to preheat the incoming make-up air. Run around coils are a very cost effective method of realising this heat transfer.

Another process from which thermal energy might be harnessed is the incineration of hospital waste. This can be achieved either by an incinerator and waste heat boiler or better still by a waste burning boiler which can be operated in a conventional mode when it is necessary to do so. Over a year the waste from a 300 bed hospital can contribute in excess of 500,000kW of energy. This figure does not take into account heat which will also be recovered from fuel used in the burning of this refuse.

Small scale CHP technology is now well established and ideally suited for hospitals. Energy demand profiles are such that these units can achieve consistently high load factors through the year. Studies have also indicated that it can be cost effective to install standby generators with heat reclaim equipment. These can be operated selectively, particularly in winter, without significantly reducing the life of the plant.

Refrigeration machines which supply cooling for the air conditioning systems can also be used as heat pumps to provide thermal energy in winter. Overall cost effectiveness of this operation can be improved by using off peak electricity. Additionally, the potential for heat recovery from desuperheating of the refrigerant can be harnessed during summer and used to preheat domestic hot water. This need not compromise the integrity of the system in terms of inhibiting the growth of legionellae bacteria.

An Alternative Site Energy Strategy

The significant reduction in peak thermal loads, the availability of heat reclaim equipment and different methods of providing thermal energy have opened up the possibility of a range of unconventional site energy strategies. Table 1 summaries the maximum instantaneous demand for thermal energy for a 300 bed hospital during a peak winter day. The maximum electrical demand over this period has been assessed at 500kW. These figures are actually the resultant loads for Wansbeck hospital and take account of the contribution made by energy conservation measures.

However they are representative of any other hospital specifically designed with regard to energy efficiency. Catering, humidification and sterilising equipment are gas and/or electrically heated.

Table 1: Maximum Thermal Load-Peak Winter

	kW	Kw
Air Heating	627	
Heat recovery from exhaust air	318	
	309	309
Space Heating		278
Domestic Hot Water		339
	Total	926

The maximum demand of the hospital's essential electrical supplies is estimated to be 400kW. This can be provided by two standby diesel generators each rated at about 200kW. Each can supply approximately 300kW of thermal energy. The loads and present electricity tariffs offer the potential to operate a gas engine driven CHP unit of about 150kWe and which will have a heat output of approximately 290kW.

If hospital waste is to be burnt on site the peak thermal load in winter can be provided by a waste heat boiler, the CHP unit and both standby generators. This senario entails operation of the CHP unit for 17 hours each day between 0730 hrs and 0030 hrs and the two standby generators collectively for a total of 19 hours during the day. Waste burning must be carried out over a nine hour period from 12 midnight onwards. During this time the waste heat boiler is the main source of thermal energy as the unit cost of off-peak electricity makes on-site generation uneconomic. It will be necessary to provide some thermal storage to even out imbalances between supply and demand. Figure 3

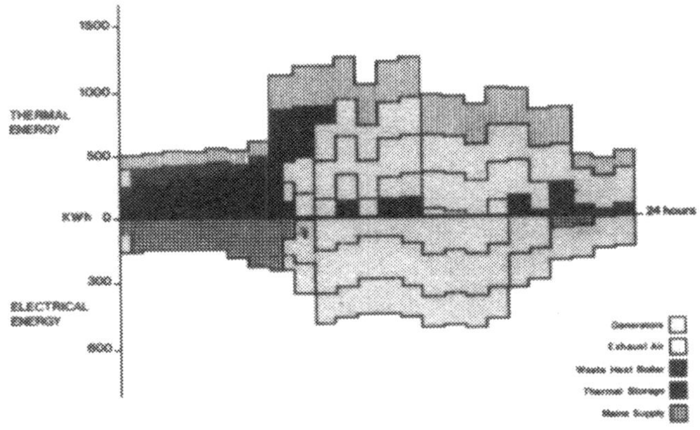

Figure 3: Diurnal Load Profile — Peak Winter Day.

indicates the diurnal load profile and the overall pattern of energy supply.

This particular site energy strategy does not rely on conventional boilers for the supply of thermal energy and as such these can be omitted altogether from the project. It is possible to do so because, by attention to design, the load in an energy efficient hospital is reduced to a level at which other sources of supply are feasible. The resulting scenario affords operational flexibility and an overall improvement in energy utilisation on the hospital site.

This basic philosophy can be adapted to suit the particular requirements of other sites. In some cases for example, it may be more cost effective to use direct fired domestic water heaters. Boiler plant will be needed where hospital refuse is to be destroyed off-site. However, boiler capacity can be significantly reduced when the plant operates in conjunction with thermal storage. Under such conditions the boiler will be able to fire for longer periods at maximum output thereby improving overall efficiency.

Standby Facilities

The adoption of an unconventional site energy strategy will necessitate careful consideration in the selection of plant and equipment particularly with regard to reliability. Energy outputs and the extent to which these can be matched to the load characteristics of the hospital are other important criteria.

Many hospitals are over-provided in terms of boilers and standby generator capacity. This is due in part to the inadequacy of design data on diurnal load profiles but other factors have also contributed to the current situation. It has for example been common practice to provide a number of boilers so that at least one is always available on standby. Additionally, not sufficient attention is being given to the practical consequences of plant failure; how this might be dealt with in operational terms and what minimum standby facilities need to be provided. The result is that, taken together, there is a significant amount of plant which is very much underused.

Better use of capital resources might be achieved if hospitals collectively contribute to a pool of mobile plant. Each can then draw from this whenever an emergency occurs or when plant has to be taken out of service for scheduled maintenance.

Conclusion

A substantial part of the energy requirements of new hospitals can be provided in a number of ways which differ from traditional methods of supplying energy. These alternative strategies not only reduce consumption but also improve the overall efficiency at which fuel is used on site. The nett effect of this is a significant contribution to improving the quality of the environment. The low energy hospital studies have confirmed the economic viability of an unconventional site energy strategy and to some extent both demonstration projects have adopted this approach to meeting the energy demands of the hospital. Both will provide valuable operational experience although the benefits from this will not be available for a few years. In the meantime health authorities should not be dissuaded from pursuing similar strategies; on the contrary. There is a need for operational experience on as many variations of the basic theme as is feasible. This will help in the drafting of guidance aimed at optimising the capital cost of energy centres and minimising revenue expenditure on fuel without compromising the functioning of the hospital.

Cogeneration in a Public Hospital

by

Denis King
CEng, MIMechE, FIMARE, SRMIHE
Chief Engineer
Dandenong and District Hospital, Victoria, Australia

Cogeneration is the simultaneous production of electrical energy and usable thermal energy, such as steam or hot water. For example, some of the best energy generated by an engine producing electricity is recovered in a waste heat boiler and used to produce steam for heating and cooling a building. Cogeneration has been in use for many years in ships all over the world and in shore establishments in a few countries, notably the USA, the UK and some European countries. It has not been economical to use it extensively in Australia for a number of reasons including the high cost of purchase and importation of capital plant and also because of the somewhat harsh conditions imposed by the local electricity authorities. An in house study carried out in 1985 did in fact confirm that a cogeneration scheme was not economical at that time, even though capital in the order of $500,000 would have to be spent on the supply, accommodation and installation of an emergency generator for the hospital and $360,000 on an extra boiler. A major factor for the scheme not being viable was the low buy-back rate offered by the SECV of 6.31c/kwh for any excess electricity exported to the grid during peak hours of 7 am to 11 pm and 09c/kwh off-peak from 11 pm to 7 am.

Background — Change of SEVC Policy

In June 1987 the State Electricity Commission of Victoria (SECV) launched a Cogeneration and Renewable Energy Incentives Package, designed to encourage the private development of new cogeneration and renewable energy projects. This incentives package forms a key part in the Victorian Government's economic development and environment protection strategies. If offers the opportunity for a limited amount of private generation of electrcity in parallel with the SECV grid, under conditions that allow the purchase of electricity from, and the sale of it to, the SECV, provided most of the obtainable waste heat generated in the process is recovered and used in performing useful work in the establishment or locality.

The Incentives

A 10 year contract with the SECV for cogeneration which includes a guaranteed buy-back rate escalated annually at a rate locked to the Consumer Price Index (CPI). The SECV sale price of electricity is also locked to CPI.

Significant improvement in the buy-back rate by the SECV from 1.04c/kwh to 9.43c/kwh for low voltage and 8.87c/kwh for high voltage buy back during peak periods (7 am to 10 pm). Off peak buy back is maintained at a much lower price of 0.9c/kwh.

SECV connection costs to be amortised over the 10 year contract period.

Financial assistance for a feasibility study on a dollar for dollar basis up to a maximum of $7,500 loan, repayable over three years if the project develops to fruition. The loan becomes a grant if the project does not proceed.

Waiving of the SECV stand by charges for the first three years. This stand by charge is based on the hospital's demand and is set at $18,720 pa for the duration of the contract period. This represents a reduction from the existing $4.43/kw/month to $2.00/kw/month.

Location

Layout

Dandenong and District Hospital is particularly well laid out for a cogeneration plant. The SECV 22 kv electricity supply is from a pole adjacent to the south east corner of the boilerhouse. A 2,900 kPa natural gas transmission line runs east west beneath the David Street footpath along the south side of the boilerhouse. The boilerhouse roof was designed for accommodating plant and has just sufficient space for a gas turbine/generator, waste heat recovery unit and the auxiliary equipment. Sufficient space exists inside the hospital boundary at the east end of the boilerhouse for the gas metering installation and the electrical transformer, switchgear and metering equipment. Figure 1 shows the general pictorial layout of the hospital and Figure 2 the boilerhouse roof arrangement. It was felt that because of the favourable layout of the hospital for a cogeneration plant, provided a suitable sized installation was possible, if it would work anywhere it would work here, because initial costs would have to be lower than most other places.

Electrical

The distance from the SECV's supply pole to the hospital's main electrical switchboard is some 400m via a 22 kv underground cable. The generator sets under consideration produce electricity at either 5.5 kv or 11 kv. By transforming to 22 kv and then metering and switching at this voltage, the existing electrical arrangements do not need alteration. Also, the SECV standby arrangements for periods when the cogeneration plant is not operating becomes a simple switching operation. Figure 3 shows the proposed electrical distribution layout.

Gas

The normal natural gas supply to the boilerhouse is via a 100mm diameter high pressure supply main (250 kPa) originating from the transmission grid some 500m to the east. The gas turbines require a gas pressure in the order of 1,500 kPa and to use the high pressure supply would

COGENERATION DANS UN ETABLISSEMENT HOSPITALIER PUBLIC

On constate qu'historiquement, la cogénération dans les hôpitaux publics de Victoria n'a guère été rentable, surtout à cause des conditions difficiles imposées par la Commission d'Electricité Nationale de Victoria (SECV). Mais le Gouvernement de Victoria a fait passert des recommendations de développement économique et de protection de l'environnement en 1987, comprenant des mesures incitatives SEVC visant à encourager les projects de cogénération. Alors que les études réalisées il y a un certain temps par l'hôpital Dandenong et District avaient démontré le manque de rentabilité de ces méthodes, un apercu des nouvelles propositions tendrait à indiquer due non seulement des économies sont possibles, mais même des bénéfices, á condition de bien planifier. L'hôpital s'est donc engagé dans une nouvelle étude approfondie afin d'établir la nature de l'installation la plus rentable. La recherche a été terminée en 1988 et démontre en effet que des bénéfices sont envisageables. L'hôpital est entré en pourparlers avec les éventuels fabricants de turbines à gaz-générateurs ainsi que des institutions financières afin de se lancer dans l'adoption de cette méthode.

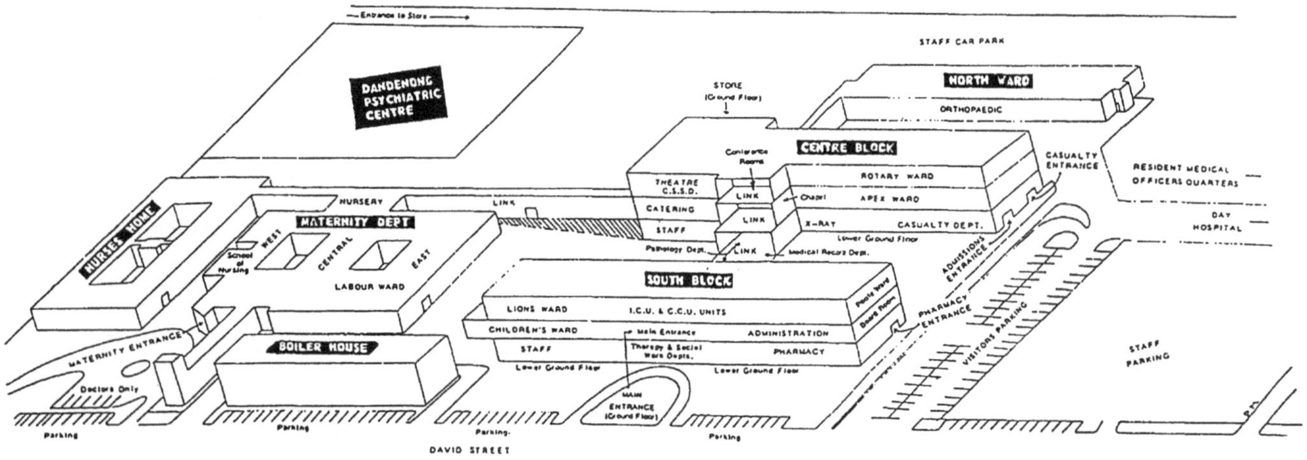

Figure 1: Dandenong and District Hospital.

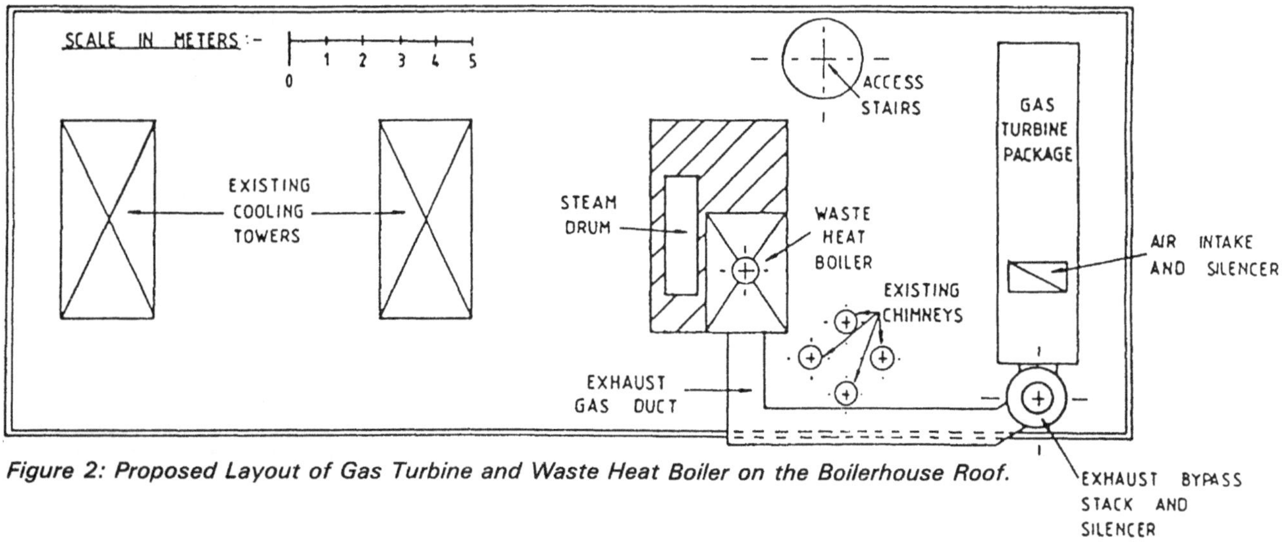

Figure 2: Proposed Layout of Gas Turbine and Waste Heat Boiler on the Boilerhouse Roof.

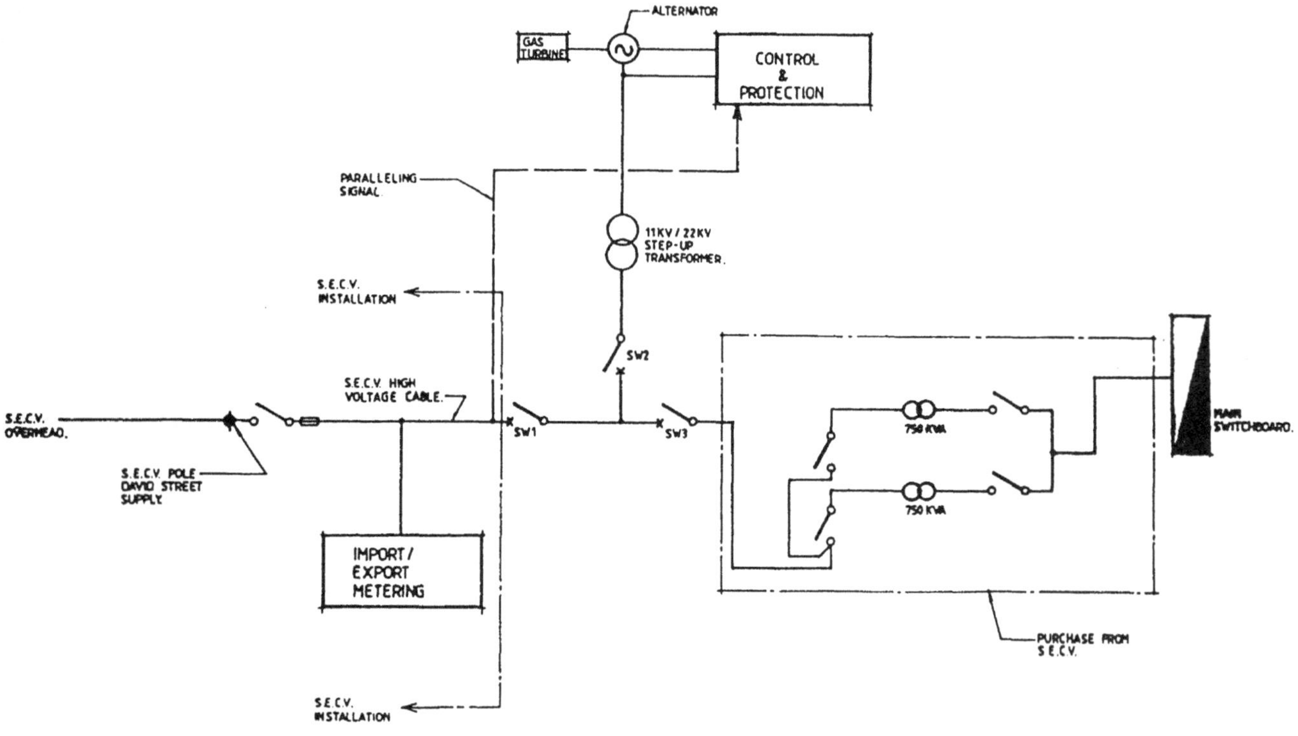

Figure 3: Dandenong and District Hospital Cogeneration Scheme – Electrical Distrubtion Diagram.

require a gas compression plant and new metering arrangements. The estimated cost of this equipment was A$245,000. It was also doubtful if the existing high pressure supply main could supply the quantity of gas required.

Following negotiations, the Gas and Fuel Corporation of Victoria agreed to permit the hospital to tap into the 2,900 kPa transmission line running past the boilerhouse. The tap in would could $21,000 and the high pressure metering equipment $118,000. The immediate advantage of this arrangement meant a capital cost saving of $106,000. The operational advantage is a more simple plant and the electrical energy required for operation of the gas compressor plant, estimated at 55kw is now available for export to the grid. Extra payback of about $18,880 pa could be expected. The removal of the need for maintenance costs for the compressor plant is an additional advantage.

Alternative Systems

Options Considered

Option A: Internal combustion engines with ebulent cooling and waste heat boilers.

Option B: A small 1.0 to 1.5MW gas turbine with waste heat boiler to supply all of the hospital's estimated electrical load and a small fraction of the heating and cooling load.

Option C: A 3.5 to 4.0MW gas turbine with waste heat boiler to supply all of the hospital's electrical load, all of the heating and cooling loads, and sale of all excess electricity to the SECV.

Steam injection to the gas turbine was a further option which would, if embarked upon, enhance the viability of the project and would probably apply to all the turbines considered under Option C.

Operating Conditions

General

A brief assessment of the steam and electricity demands shows that the selection of a gas turbine capable of generating sufficient steam in a waste heat recovery unit to satisfy all of the hospital's load ensures there is always in excess of 3,000kw of electricity available for export to the SECV grid. Given the attractive peak period buy back rate, considerable revenue is available.

On the other hand, the unattractive off-peak buy back rates indicate that the unit should be either shut down overnight or else operated at the minimum load required to satisfy the steam demand to minimise the losses.

Existing Energy Demands

The existing electrical and gas loads were obtained from the meter logs. Table 1 sets them out for the January-December period for 1987.

Table 1

Month	*Electricity Consumption (kwh)*	*Demand (kw)*	*Gas Consumption*
January	316,560	712	4,254
February	297,040	720	4,518
March	351,480	704	4,884
April	449,287	696	4,330
May	282,400	624	3,763
June	347,287	648	4,408
July	339,680	656	4,615
August	326,920	632	4,083
September	413,200	656	4,155
October	299,360	672	3,518
November	420,200	696	4,408
December	343,800	712	4,470

Projected Energy Demands

The future electrical and gas consumption figures were estimated on the basis of the existing loads and allowing for increases due to the extensions to the Accident and Emergency Department and the construction of the new North Block. These building works are due to be completed in December 1989 and July 1990 respectively. The gas consumption is estimated at 82,000 gigajoules per annum with a maximum steam demand of 8,000kg/h.

The electrical consumption is estimated at 4,600kwh with a maximum demand of 780kw and following the existing profiles. Energy costs for the hospital for 1989 are $200,000 for gas and $300,000 for electricity.

Steam Injection

Although steam injection is a well proven method of boosting power output of large gas turbines, it is relatively untried on the range of machines considered for this project. Some investigation and consideration was given to steam injection and for the Solar Contour H it is estimated that an additional revenue of A$117,000 or 15.6% is possible. In view of the lack of experience and proven track record of this technology, it was decided at this stage that down-time and extra maintenance could cancel this advantage, so it was better to be safe than sorry and not further consider this alternative in the initial instance.

It was, however, noted that development of the project should not prohibit the future consideration of this option at a later date if it develops to a more reliable status. It is also acknowledged that Ruston were persuing development of steam injection for the TB5000 model to boost its power output from 3,600kw to 4,200kw.

A second major advantage of steam injection is its effect of reducing the nitrogen oxides discharged to the atmosphere. Although this does not improve the economics, it does enhance the effect on the environment and is therefore desirable.

Environment Effects

In Victoria, the Environment Protection Authority (EPA) controls effects on the environment in accordance with the Environment Protection Act 1970.

Bearing in mind that the existing boilers are natural gas fired and will not be required with a cogeneration plant operating, and steam outputs will be the same, the exhaust emissions to atmosphere from the premises will not be significantly different whichever plant is operating. Works Approval and Licencing will, however, be necessary in any case. Should steam injection be used it would reduce NOX emissions. Noise emissions will be the critical issue, particularly during night time hours (10.00 pm to 7.00 am) when noise levels of 35 dbA at 1m distance from the perimeter of the plant is required. An acoustic screen is therefore necessary to surrond the plant, thus adding to the capital cost.

Option A

The hospital's only practical means for the utilisation of waste heat is in the production of steam. As the steam raising capability of reciprocating engines is insignificant by comparison to that of a gas turbine, it became evident early in the feasibility investigation that the use of reciprocating engines as prime movers did not warrant in depth consideration. This option was therefore disregarded as not warranting further consideration.

Options B and C

Effect of Ambient Temperature

As the only generating plant to be considered was to be gas turbines, ambient temperature would have a significant effect on the plant output.

The assumed ambient temperature at 15 degrees celcius (59 degrees Fahrenheit) which is the basis for the universally used ISO rating for gas turbines is quite close to the Bureau of Meteorology's stated average temperature for Melbourne. The assumed output from the various gas turbines used in this feasibility study are therefore close to the ISO ratings.

Economic Evaluation

Capital Costs

Capital costs estimates were carried out for one gas turbine generator under Option B and three under Option C. The Option B plant was a Ruston RH gas turbine/generator with an ISO rating of 1,590kw. The three gas turbine/generators considered under Option C were: Ruston TB5000 (ISO rating 3,670kw); Solar Centaur H (ISO rating 3,880kw) and Dresser Kongsberg DC-990 (ISO rating 4,200kw).

In each case all plant and equipment other than the gas turbine/generators is to be of local manufacture. Table 2 compares the capital costs for the four options. These figures have been loaded somewhat to prove that if a project could work with them there would be no hidden surprises in practice.

For analysis of the energy cost savings which might accrue from any proposed installation, a monthly energy use and cost model was developed based on a typical year's energy pattern. A base case of energy costs for the next 15 year period if no changes were implemented was then constructed. This base case was then used for comparison with the various cogeneration options for a number of possible varying conditions. All four cogeneration schemes have the potential to earn revenue. There is, however, a clear indication that the larger the machine the better are the returns possible.

An installation based on the Ruston RH gas turbine appears less attractive than the three larger machines. This is confirmed when the simple payback period is computed for each installation. These are:-

Ruston RH	18.5 years
Ruston TB5000	4.5 years
Solar Centaur H	5.5 years
Kongsberg DC990	5.5 years

Clearly an installation based on the Ruston RH machine did not warrant further consideration. The capital costs estimates for the options are based on budget prices and are obviously open to negotiation. This could have a significant effect on the simple pay back period of each.

An additional factor which required consideration was that one of the conditions set down by SECV was that the incentives package did not apply to government or public authorities financed schemes. In order to quality for the incentives package it would be necessary for the hospital to borrow the money needed to finance a scheme from the private enterprise money market. The gas turbine manufacturers are keen to provide the finance as their financial connection would also benefit. This situation puts the hospital in a good bargaining position as both revenue and pay back, including interest rates, could make any one of the three the most attractive.

The final part of the economic evaluation was to test the project on a 15 years discounted cash flow basis. For this exercise a capital cost loan of $A4.5M was used and interest rates of 14.8%, 16%, 17%, 18% and 20% used. As the earlier studies showed that the project would not be too sensitive to gas and electricity price variations, an electricity buy back escalator of 3% was used and an inflation factor of 6%. A capital cost of $A4.5M was used.

Although each case showed a profit over the pay back period

14.8%	A$2.89M
16.0%	A$2,25M
17.0%	A$1,71M
18.0%	A$1,16M
20.0%	A$0,40M

the return on capital investment is not worthwhile at interest rate above 17%.

Development

The hospital decided to proceed and entered negotiations with the three gas turbine manufacturers and their financial arms. Negotiations were also commenced with independent financial houses.

As anticipated, capital costs and loan interest rates were becoming very competitive and the project was shaping up better than the studies indicated.

At this stage the Health Department Victoria (HDV) decided it would carry out its own feasibility study for all Victorian Hospitals. Dandenong and District Hospital (DDH) was refused approval to proceed with the project pending the HDV's study. The HDV also decided it would bunch eight of the larger hospitals, including DDH, into one package and would carry out the negotiations and prepare contracts for the hospitals. Although DDH opposed this course, it has been forced to remain with it by HDV. The hospital is still waiting for the HDV to prepare its project.

Capital Cost Estimates and Equipment Details

Table 1

Gasturbins/Generator Manufacture and Model	*Ruston RH*	*Ruston TB5000*	*Solar Centaur H*	*Konsberg DC990*
Electrical KW Output (ISO)	1,590	3,670	3,880	4,200
Estimated Site Output	1,548	3,482	3,666	3,900
Exhaust gas kg/s at full load	7.12	20.6	17.3	20.3
Waste heat recovery unit kg/h output at full load	5,775	8,000	9,957	106,000
Gas turbine/generator ($1,000s)	1,000	1,700	1,930	2,125
Remote Monitoring and Control	200	200	200	200
Ducting, filters, silencers, bypass	25	31	31	34
Waste heat recovery unit	650	780	780	800
Feed pumps and auxiliaries	31	33	33	33
Installation	120	125	125	130
Black start	40	50	50	50
Civil works including noise suppression	40	50	50	50
Electrical Works	480	510	510	510
Gas Works (fuel)	120	120	120	120
Commissioning/ Contingency	120	120	120	120
Total Capital Costs	2,826	3,699	3,929	4,152

Cogeneration and Its Application in Hospitals

by

F. Nash, I. V. Rogerson and T. M. Buxton
McLellan and Partners Ltd

1. Introduction

Cogeneration is one of those descriptive American words written into their legislature under PURPA in the late 1970s that now has become common usage worldwide. It fundamentally covers the production of power (electricity) at high efficiency — lower limit 42.6% — in parallel with the production of heat.

Most USA schemes are industrially or commercially based and (as in the UK) its application to district heating is limited.

Cogeneration is a new name for an old practice. In 1868 the construction of a newly opened sugar beet factory was reported in the UK technical press of the time, and, whereas details of the process equipment were extensively covered, the reciprocating steam engine providing power and exhausting steam to the process attracted little comment as being normal practise. With the growth of the process industries, increased factory size and energy requirements, reciprocating steam engines were gradually replaced by steam turbines driven by steam produced in water tube boilers at higher pressures and temperatures.

By the early 1950s coal-fired boilers, generally operating at pressures around 400lb/in^2, and back-pressure steam turbines achieving overall conversion efficiencies over 75% were the norm in many companies.

In the 1960s the availability of abundant supplies of cheap oil allowed energy to be considered of little importance and cogeneration systems to become oil burning.

From 1973, with an increase in real energy costs resulting from the OPEC action, the efficient use of energy began to receive attention in all developed countries. This often resulted in tax incentives, grants and other legislation to encourage cogeneration.

These factors have however been overshadowed by the greatly increased differential between primary fuel and electricity costs caused by the world glut of oil, recognition of which finally became unavoidable in 1985. In consequence, interest in the local generation of electricity with high efficiency obtained by taking advantage of concurrent heat demands (cogeneration) has increased dramatically in the UK, as elsewhere, not only in the traditional industrial areas but also in commercial and institutional complexes such as hospitals.

2. Factors Affecting the Selection of Systems

In the 1950s system selection was easy. It was, in the main, a coal-fired boiler and back-pressure steam turbine or nothing. Today there is a wide range of equipment available and the correct equipment and system may be selected and matched to specific conditions and operational requirements to produce the most economically viable plant.

Commercial viability is always a major consideration in the selection of a system and, indeed, whether or not an actual installation results.

In general there are a number of techno-economic factors which will determine the success or otherwise of a cogeneration system. They include:-

(a) Heat and power demand of a site (normally expressed as a ratio) and the variation in these. Whilst it is possible to alleviate the worst effects of H/P ratio variations by exporting electricity, the economic returns will normally be highest with the self-use of all the power produced, so realising the full purchase avoidance cost.
(b) The type of fuel and hence the cost of fuel the cogeneration system requires.
(c) The system's fuel flexibility which allows costs to be negotiable.
(d) The efficiency with which the cogeneration system can cope with (a) above.
(e) The maintenance and operational requirements and costs of the system.
(f) The specific capital cost of the system.

System Types

Cogeneration systems fall into five fundamental categories as indicated in Figure 1.

Figure 1(a) shows the classic industrial system, still widely used today, but more and more restricted to the large

LA COGENERATION — APPLICATIONS EN ETABLISSEMENTS HOSPITALIERS

Chaleur et courant combinés, le principe de la cogénération, existent au Royaume-Uni depuis plus de cent ans dans le domaine industriel. La crise du pétrole des pays de l'OPEP de 1973 a affecté et même menacé cette pratique, d'autant qu'arrivait en parallèle l'électricité provenant d'énormes centrales nucléaires et à charbon. Il convenait toutefois de ne pas sous-estimer l'esprit inventif et la capacité d'adaptation des utilisateurs, des fabricants de matériel et des designers. C'est pourquoi 1973 a aussi marqué la début d'une période dynamique de développement de systèmes de cogénération pour tous usages. L'idée de rentabiliser l'énergie ne pouvait que recevoir l'approbation des gouvernements (PURPA en 1978 pour les Etats-Unis et l'Energy Act en 1983 pour le Royaume-Uni). Toutefois, le meilleur encouragement est arrivé en 1986, avec la chute des prix d'énergie primaire rendant la production privée d'électricité économiquement intéressante, dans le cas d'utilisation de cogénérateurs. De plus, de nombreux systèmes de la dernière génération sont d'utilisation flexible et permettent à cette méthode d'être appliquée à de grands complexes commerciaux et autres tels les hôpitaux.

Les systèmes de cogénération varient en taille depuis les grandes centrales industrielles produisant des centaines de magawatts d'électricité, jusqu'aux plus petites, se contentant de produire quelques centaines de magawatts. La majorité des hôpitaux ont des besoins en électricité se situant autour de 1MWe, bien que certains atteignent 5MWe.

Les coûts en énergie sont réduits dans la mesure où la chaleur produite lors de la génération d'électricité est utilisée au lieu d'être perdue. Plusieurs sources sont utilisables et les systèmes fonctionnent en parallèle avec des chaudières ou autres générateurs existants.

En milieu hospitalier, la sécurité du courant et du chauffage est primordiale. De plus, une grande flexibilité est indispensable, car souvent les branchements électriques et les mesures de protection sont compliqués et il faut des interbranchements et intercommunications avec les incinérateurs installés.

Cet article passe en revue les types de cogénérateurs qui sont actuellement développés, ainsi que leurs principales caractéristiques de fonctionnement. Ensuite il examine les facteurs techniques et commerciaux qu'il convient de prendre en compte lorsqu'on choisit un système. Il étudie aussi la viabilité économique des systèmes en fonction de leur taille et des circonstances d'utilisation dans les hôpitaux britanniques.

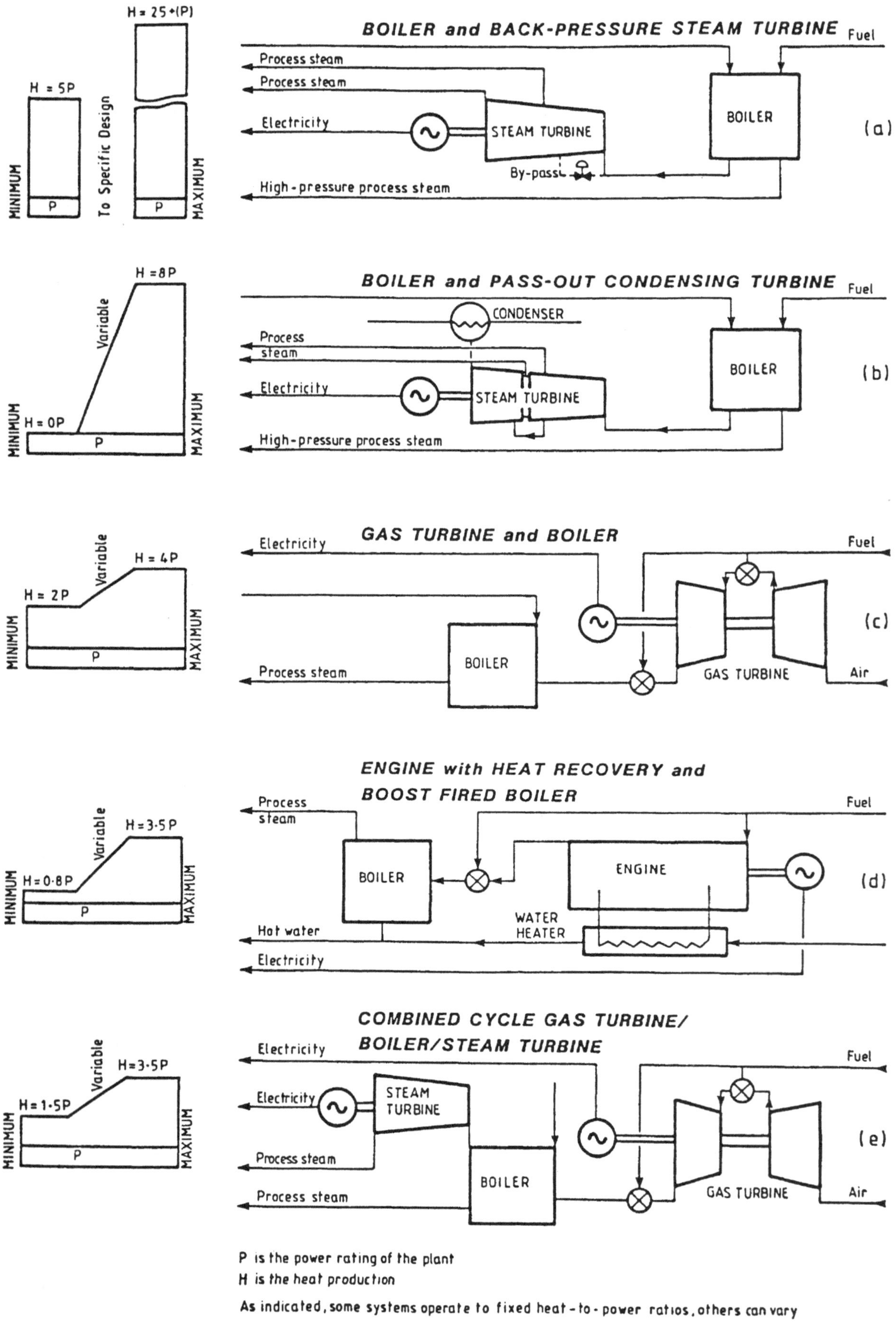

Figure 1: Types of Cogeneration Systems.

process industries. It has the advantage of being able to use any fuel but, unfortunately, the prime cost of boilers is almost always inversely proportional to the quality (and hence cost) of the fuel burnt. Furthermore, the system's design will be optimised not only against a fixed heat to power ratio but also against given demands, eg 10 MW electric and 100 MW thermal outputs, and the system loses both efficiency and value of output on turndown.

Figure 1(b) shows the standard method of providing flexibility to the fired boiler, steam turbine system by equipping the turbine with a condensing exhaust end. The heat to power ratio achievable is now variable between all the steam to the turbine being extracted (less back end cooling flow) or all steam going through to the condenser, H/P = 0. Any combination of power and thermal output is possible within the operational limitations of the turbine. Unfortunately, the conversion efficiency to useful output is normally very low for steam passing to the condenser and this detracts from economic viability.

Figure 1(c) indicates what is currently regarded as the system with most general potential, ie an alternator driven by a gas turbine with exhaust gas waste heat recovery boiler, with or without supplementary firing.

The gas turbine is very acceptable for cogeneration based on its aviation background of high power to size/low vibration levels/known acoustic treatment/high reliability/developed control and monitoring systems to minimise operation demands, and possibly most important, high availability from a quick unit exchange or major part replacement policy, operated by the manufacturers. Experience with first generation gas turbines has indicated that given premium fuel (natural gas) and uncontaminated air, maintenance costs are low.

Whilst it is almost impossible to obtain actual maintenance figures on a common basis, since even the scope of activity defined as maintenance can vary from site to site, without starting to consider different operational and accounting practices to name but three of many factors involved, experience with GTs indicates a figure of 0.15p/kWhe may be considered reasonable.

Whether this will hold true for the more sophisticated second generation gas turbines of higher efficiency but operating at increased combustion pressures and temperatures, on offer today, only some years in general use will show.

Gas turbines currently available on the world market vary in power outputs from 80kW and 203 MW with open cycle efficiencies from 11% to 37%. Steam injection can further improve these efficiencies to the order of 44% on models where this is currently available. Steam injection therefore is one form of exhaust heat recovery generating power as opposed to providing heat for process use.

In general:-

- The greater the output of the gas turbine the lower the capital cost/kW.
- For a given power output the greater the efficiency the higher the capital cost.

In the case of most installations the power output/size of a gas turbine is selected to fit the site base load power demands. This generally applies for the following reasons:-

- The efficiency falls away radically at significant outputs below MCR.
- The buy back price for electricity exported to the grid is lower than the purchase avoidance cost and hence exported units adversely affect the scheme's economics.
- Users, for instance hospital authorities, are content running hospitals and have no wish to become a utility company.

Having identified generally the output of a turbine which is suited to a specific application there is a choice of turbines available which will suit. The best can only be properly determined by considering for each machine the capital, fuel and operation costs and the heat and power demands of the site. Low efficiency turbines will give higher heat recovery potential and vice versa, but the generation of power has a greater value than the recovery of waste heat. The value factors relating to heat and power may be defined as follows:-

(1) Cost of Thermal Energy per kWh = Price of Fuel ÷ Fired Boiler Efficiency
(2) Cost of Power per kWh = Price of Bought in Electricity
Value Factor of Thermal Energy = (1)/(1) = 1
Value Factor of Power = (2)/(1) = Typically 3 to 4.5

This concept is also used in Table 3.

A gas turbine consists of three principal parts, an air compressor, combustor and turbine. The efficiency of the gas turbine is directly related to the turbine inlet temperature; the higher the turbine inlet temperature the higher the efficiency. For a given gas turbine inlet temperature there is an optimum pressure at the turbine inlet for maximum efficiency. The higher the turbine inlet temperature the higher is this pressure.

The design of turbine and compressor significantly affects the capital cost and efficiency of a unit. Table 1 shows some of the design options and their effects on capital costs and performance.

The turbine can consist of a single or several stages, each stage driving a common or separate shaft. It is quite common for the first stage to drive the air compressor and the remaining stages to be the main plant drive. Where gas turbines may be required to operate separated from the grid system the single shaft arrangement gives a more stable operation.

There is considerable free oxygen in the turbine exhaust gases and supplementary firing (boost firing) is possible, theoretically to achieve H/P ratios up to 17:1. However, physical size and cost of ducts combined with the GTs' sensitivity to increased exhaust back-pressure and type of waste heat boiler required, usually in practice limits supplementary fired systems to a 4:1 H/P ratio. As with all good general rules, exceptions are easily found; for example, where a GT is retrofitted to function as the force-draught fan supplying preheated combustion air to a boiler, furnace or dryer.

With supplementary firing the thermal output from an exhaust gas boiler can be fully varied between the recoverable waste heat and the upper limit by simply changing the amount of boost fuel input. H/P ratios below the waste heat recovery quantity can also be achieved by bypassing exhaust gas around the boiler, but this of course has a detrimental effect on system overall efficiency and the installation's economics.

Figure 1(d) indicates the same basic type of system and facilities as 1(c) above but utilises a reciprocating diesel type engine as the prime mover. This in fact changes the characteristics of the system significantly. Compared with gas turbines, engine systems have higher power generation efficiency, which is retained on turndown, and good fuel flexibility, but present more problems as regards acoustic treatment, vibration and system complication.

Large reciprocating engines currently do not have the same general acceptability as gas turbines and, although pockets of preference for engines are met from time to time, more often gas turbines are preferred on the basis (perhaps from ignorance) — 'we can start them up and forget about them'. This is certainly not true with reciprocating engines; they require regular inspection and attention, whilst maintenance involves in situ work rather than total exchange. However, given that routine actions are not neglected, it is possible that the through-life maintenance costs of larger gas engines may be comparable with those of gas turbines and those of engines using distillate and residual oils only marginally higher.

Systems using automotive type spark ignition engines are used successfully in swimming pools, hotels and other buildings; their economic viability largely de-

Table 1 — Design Options and Their Effects on Capital Costs and Performance

Item	Low Cost	High Cost	Effects on Performance
Air Compressor	Single stage centrifugal		Low pressure ratio, low power output from given turbine cross section.
			Low cycle efficiency at optimum turbine inlet temperature.
		Multistage axial	Gives high pressure ratio, high power output from given turbine cross section, high cycle efficiency with optimum turbine inlet temperature.
			Results in long air intake section and is more prone to performance loss
Power Turbine	No blade cooling and simple construction materials		Low gas inlet temperature can only be tolerated and efficiency is poor, pressure ratio is low
		Advance blade cooling and coating technology	Allows high gas inlet temperature to be used giving high efficiencies. Pressure ratios are high
	Single stage		Low efficiency
		Multistage	High efficiency

pendent on relatively low capital costs. Maintenance requirements are high, costing upwards of 0.7p/kWhe, and engine replacements' life as low as 24,000 hours.

The engine and its heat recovery equipment is modulised into a highly developed and efficient package which provides a fixed heat to power ratio somewhere between 2.0 and 2.5. Flexibility is achieved by multi-unit, switch on/switch off operation and thermal output is often only as 65°C hot water.

Small high speed diesel engines are in many ways similar to the above, although, unless significantly derated, their maintenance requirements may be even more demanding and operational life shorter. They are rarely selected as the prime mover of new cogeneration systems. Recently, however, a number of standby diesel engines have been utilised to provide a minimum cost cogeneration system. It will be interesting to see if these prove to be economic in the long term.

At the other extreme are slow speed (<350 rpm) cathedral type diesel engines which maximise reliability but are much too large and expensive for viability in a hospital environment. However, the medium speed (500 to 1,000 rpm) reciprocating engine's ability to operate on a variety of fuels at high to-power only conversion efficiencies, typically 36% to 45%, and reasonable reliability, availability and maintenance demands make it a prime candidate for such cogeneration applications. Today's base load type engines are available to operate as diesels on liquid fuels from premium diesel to the worst residual heavy oils available (up to 15 MWe output) and many gases as spark ignition (up to 2.8 MWe output) or dual fuel (up to 7 MWe output) engines.

Dual fuel engines operate using a 5 to 10% pilot injection of liquid fuel into each cylinder to induce ignition and they are currently the subject of very intensive development, possibly as a result of cogeneration requirements. Only a few years ago they were of one type only, where a methane based gas is induced into each cylinder individually, and with some notable exceptions were significantly derated to operate at a power and efficiency lower than the corresponding liquid engine. Today two more types are available, the first where the fuel gas is mixed with the combustion air prior to the turbo charger, the second where the gas is injected into the cylinder at high pressure. Both enable increased ratings and better efficiency to be achieved on an extended range of gases.

In the past engine systems have operated with waste heat recovery only where an overall H/P ratio of around 0.8:1 will normally be easily achieved but at two levels, ie 0.5:1 as steam (high quality) and 0.3:1 as 80°C hot water (low quality). It is not always easy to find a use for the latter. Variations in thermal demand above the 0.8:1 ratio level required operation in parallel of a standard fired boiler.

The development of boost firing to utilise the free oxygen in a diesel, dual fuel and some spark ignition gas engine exhaust extends the capability of systems incorporating engines (Figure 2) to H/P ratios of 4.5:1 with total flexibility,

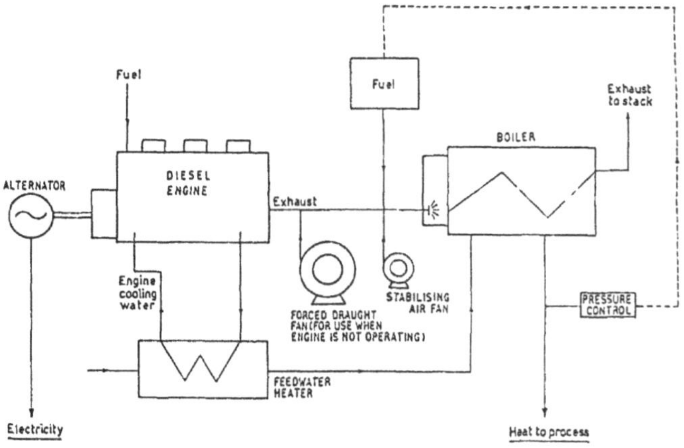

Figure 2.

and is very important to engine cogeneration systems prospects. Much will rest on the extended experience obtained from the UK Department of Energy demonstration project at Cyanamid (GB) Ltd's site, where a 3.5 MWe dual fuel (gas) engine driven alternator set is coupled to a 13,600kg/h boost fired boiler. This project has now been operating for approximately two years and in the first, 1988/89, showed a net operational cost saving over £500K against a total installation cost of £2.2 million. The boost fired technique was initially developed using a 650kW engine operating on heavy fuel oil and producing up to 3,600kg/h which is of a size more suitable to UK hospital requirements.

Last, but (certainly based on USA experience) not least, is the Combined Cycle system as indicated in Figure 1(e). In its most common form waste heat recovery, steam from the exhaust of a gas turbine is fed to a steam turbine which may be of the back-pressure or extraction condensing type. H/P ratios variable between 0:1 and 3.5:1 would be typical with a back-pressure turbine, but for ratios variable between 0.1:1 and 3:1 a steam turbine with a condensing exhaust is required. Both cases incorporate supplementary firing of the exhaust gas boilers, without which the upper limits would be around 1.5:1 fixed and 1.2:1 variable, respectively. Sometimes two gas turbines are coupled with one steam turbine but this does not affect the above.

The combined cycle extends the gas turbine capability to lower H/P ratios than if operating alone and can also provide flexibility, important if meeting thermal loads incorporating a large annual environmental element, whether this be for heating in winter or absorption chiller air conditioning, in the summer. Unfortunately, it is an expensive system and tends to be economic only at larger sizes.

Electrical Aspects of Cogeneration Plant

Cogeneration plant is normally operated in parallel with the Area Electricity Board's distribution system. This raises a number of issues which must be considered, in particular:-

- mode of operation, ie with a net import or export of power to/from hospital;
- earthing;
- increase in fault currents;
- disconnection of generating plant and board's distribution system;
- protective systems and co-ordination with existing protective systems;
- disturbance to other consumers; and
- general excitation and governor control.

Each of these areas is considered in more detail below.

Whilst the mode of operation of the cogeneration plant in terms of a net import or export of power to the local area board is determined by economic factors it does influence the generator control and protective systems.

For example, if the cogeneration plant output is always less than the electrical load the generator can be operated at its maximum continuous rating.

If there are periods when the cogeneration plant output is greater than the electrical load and it is economically desirable to avoid exporting power, the generator governor must be controlled to maintain either a small fixed or zero power import.

To avoid erroneous tripping it is essential that any protective systems installed on the connection between the cogeneration plant and the board's network must be able to distinguish between normal current and fault current.

The installation of a generator onto a distribution system will increase the currents which will flow when a fault occurs on the distribution network. The contribution to fault current by the generation plant will be equivalent to between 5 and 10 times the generator rating depending on prime mover. It is important, at an early stage in a project, to accurately assess the fault contributions from all generators operating in parallel during a fault condition to ensure that the capability of electrical equipment to withstand and interrupt fault currents is not exceeded. It is equally important to ensure that the making capacity of circuit breakers exceeds the increased assymmetrical fault levels which occur at the instant of fault.

The increase in the security of electrical supples provided by a cogeneration plant is obvious. However, to fully realise this increased security it is important to ensure that if a fault occurs on either the load or the utility's distribution system the cogeneration plant remains stable and continues to supply the essential loads during and following a fault even if operating isolated from the utility supply.

One situation which leads to isolated operation of the cogeneration plant is an interruption to the Area Board's supply. In this case the interconnecting circuit breaker between the Area Board's system and the cogeneration plant must be opened before the protective systems operate to trip the generator. If the generator output is less than the site load it is necessary to initiate a load shedding regime to maintain essential supplies.

During parallel operation the cogeneration plant would normally be earthed through the area board's distribution system. However, when the cogeneration plant operates isolated from the Area Board distribution system it is necessary to provide an alternative neutral earth.

In certain circumstances the risk of operating unearthed for short periods may be considered acceptable. This must be investigated for the individual circumstances before making a decision.

Factors Specific to Hospitals

The factors which in general control system selection as outlined in Section 2 may be distorted by special requirements associated with particular applications. For instance, in UK hospitals:-

(1) Electrical demand rarely exceeds 5 MWe and mostly is less than 1 MWe; hence cogeneration systems are small and more likely to operate on a prime fuel, ie gas or light oil.

(2) Much of the thermal load is space heating hence a very flexible system is required, ie definitely not a fired boiler and steam turbine, and a reciprocating engine system may be preferred to a gas turbine based one.

(3) There are often incinerators in the complex which might benefit in terms of emission improvements by a source of clean and preheated combustion gas still with adequate oxygen available in it for further burning, ie favours gas turbines.

(4) Security of electrical supply is of paramount importance. Whilst cogeneration reverses the norm, ie the public supply becomes the standby to the site generator instead of vice versa, it may be argued that an operating generator is more secure than one that must start and accept load in an emergency. It is also true that normally operating units must undergo regular maintenance hence multi unit installations are more secure than one single machine. With maximum generation levels of 5 MWe it is probably easier to achieve an economic multi unit installation with reciprocating engines than gas turbines.

Economics

The monetary benefit arising from energy conservation using cogeneration is enhanced because of the resultant reduction in purchased electricity of a high value factor. However, in practice, as always, there are some complications. The five major factors affecting the economics of cogeneration systems are:-

(a) The increase in overall conversion efficiency achieved by the cogeneration plant as compared with that of separate plant, see Figure 3.

Here the efficiency of the on-site separate thermal output producer will be comparable with that of the cogeneration plant but the separate system overall efficiency will be lowered by the 30% to 35% achieved by a utility power station; seen by the user as the high cost of bought-in electricity.

(b) The difference in price between the bought-in cost of electricity and the fuel used by the cogeneration system.

(c) The difference in price between the cost of the fuels used by the conventional boilers and the cogeneration system.

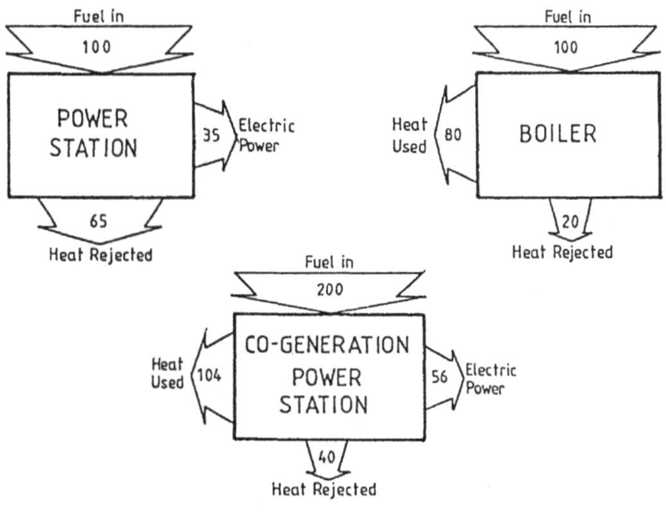

COMPARISON

	Fuel in	Electricity	Useful Heat	Conversion Efficiency
CO-GEN	200	56	104	80%
SHP	200	35	80	58%

Figure 3: Comparison Separate and Cogeneration Systems.

(d) The difference in manning and maintenance cost of the cogeneration and separate plant.
(e) The difference in capital cost of the cogeneration and the separate plant.

Table 2 indicates the average changes in typical energy costs for industrial consumers between 1981 and the end of 1989.

Using the figures recorded in Table 2 and assuming an electrical output approaching 5 MW, Table 3 computes the effects of cycle efficiency and relative energy costs for a number of systems to indicate the comparative operating cost of the cogeneration and separate plant for the years 1984 (pre slump energy cost), 1986 (post slump) and December 1989.

It must be recognised that the relative costs as calculated in Table 2 are at best only indicative since in practice:-

(a) The heat and power demands on the plant will vary.
(b) The cycle efficiency of all plants varies with changes in heat and power output.

Table 2 — UK Energy Costs

(YEAR OF PEAK CONSUMPTION)

		#1973	1981	1983	July 1984	May 1986	Dec 1989
FUEL OIL	£ per tonne (Includes Tax)	12.80	108.20	125.90	151.00	60.0	65.7
	p per therm	3.11	26.65	31.00	37.20	16.3	17.8
COAL	£ per tonne	8.90	39.90	49.60	49.80	55.0	41.0
	p per therm	3.40	15.52	19.07	19.10	22.0	16.4
ELECTRICITY	p/kWh	0.74	2.71	2.94	2.69	3.0	3.2
	p per therm	21.68	79.29	85.09	77.85	88.9	94.8
GAS	p per therm*	3.07	21.59	24.06	26.27	21.0	22.0
Ratio of Cost:							
	Elect/oil	6.97	2.97	2.74	2.09	5.5	5.3
	Elect/coal	6.38	5.11	4.45	4.10	4.1	5.8
	Elect/gas	7.06	3.67	3.53	2.96	4.2	4.3

1. All costs per therm refer to therms net CV.
2. Interruptible supply*.

(c) Interaction of electricity tariffs with load demand must be taken into account, also the extent of electrical cost that is non-avoidable.
(d) The performance of one gas turbine or reciprocating engine, etc to another as power producers are different, as is the effect they and other items of equipment have on system characteristics and these will differ again in both design and part load conditions.
(e) Operating and maintenance costs of course vary from one type of equipment and system to the next, but this is far from the whole story as they can also vary considerably from one installation to the next, sometimes for reasons not strictly within the control of the plant supplier.
(f) Last, but not least, are 'peculiar', but no less real, special factors that may apply in particular circumstances — for instance, incorporation of existing equipment into a cogeneration system, eg standby engines, incinerator, etc to minimise cost/maximise advantages.

The above makes the meaningful assessment of potential cogeneration schemes far from straightforward requiring a wide range of specialised expertise and experience, also close co-operation with the user so that his circumstances and demands are fully appreciated and considered, requirements which, if anything, are even more important through the engineering design and implementation stages of a project.

The Future

Technical Developments

One of the most significant recent developments is the steam injection gas turbine cycle. This can provide gas turbines with the flexibility to operate from a normal 4:1 heat to power ratio, to one with full steam injection of 0:1, see Figure 4, where the power can in fact be increased by 60% (ie 0:1.6 ratio) with, at the same time, an increase in

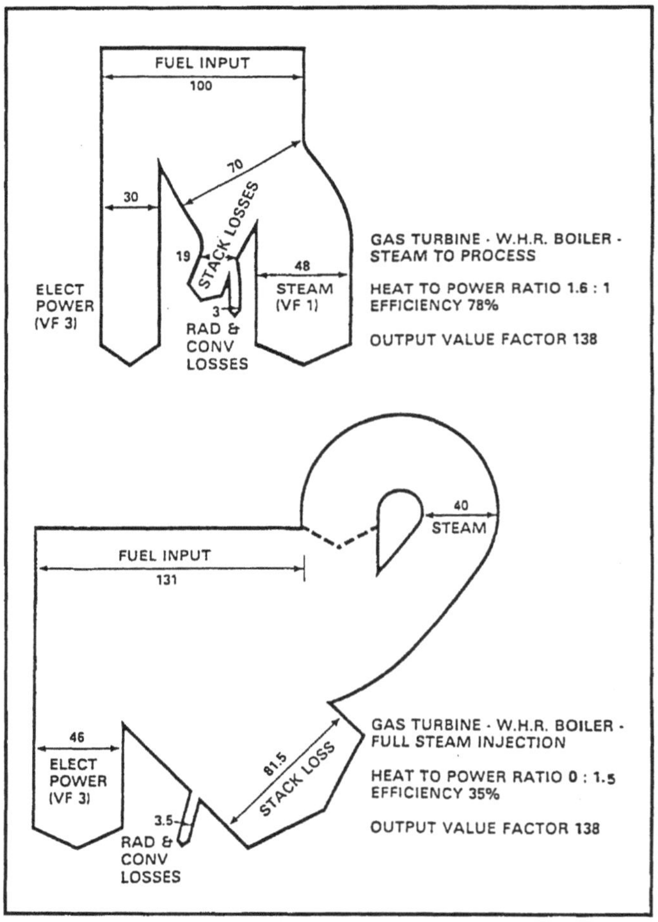

Figure 4: Steam Injection Gas Turbine — Sankey Diagram.

Table 3 — Economic Comparison of Cogenerating Systems

CHP SYSTEM	HEAT/POWER RATIO	SYSTEM ELECTRICITY	FUEL USED	DECEMBER 1984		MAY 1986		DECEMBER 1989		RELATIVE COST CHP PLANT
				FUEL COST INDEX (ELECT 4)	RELATIVE OPERATING COSTS CHP BASIC	FUEL COST INDEX (ELECT 4.1)	RELATIVE OPERATING COSTS CHP BASIC 2	FUEL COST INDEX (ELECT 5.8	RELATIVE OPERATING COSTS CHP BASIC 3	
Steam Boiler/ Turbine	8/1	84%	Coal	1	0.50	1 (HFO = 0.74 –	0.94 (0.70)	1	0.58	**2.5**
Diesel Engine/ Boost Fired Boiler	3.6/1	84%	Heavy Fuel	1.8	0.83	0.74	0.55	1.1	0.52	1
Dual Fuel Eng/ Boost Fired Boiler	3.6/1	86%	Diesel (8%) N.G.	2.4 1.3	0.61	1.25 0.95	0.70	1.5 1.3	0.65	1.3
Gas Turbine/ Fired W.H.R. Boiler	2/1	79%	Natural Gas	1.3	0.59	0.95	0.61	1.3	0.57	1
Dual Fuel Eng/ Fired W.H.R. Boiler	2/1	81%	Diesel (8%) N.G.	2.4 1.3	0.60	1.25 0.95	0.73	1.5 1.3	0.58	1.2

Basic Energy Provision - Purchased Electricity + Heat from Low Pressure Boilers

1. Basic Operating Cost December 1984 based on Electricity Cost Index 4 and HFO used in LP Boilers.
2. Basic Operating Cost May 1986 based on Electricity Cost Index 4 and HFO used in LP Boilers.
3. Basic Operating Cost December 1989 based on Electricity Cost Index 5.8 and Gas used in LP Boilers.

the efficiency of conversion to power of 18% (ie 41% rather than 35%). Theoretically an improvement in the order of 30% is possible in efficiency, hence there is still room for further improvement. These characteristics fit well hospitals and large commercial buildings with significant computer facilities and light process industries where during summer months excess steam due to higher ambient temperatures seen by the GT may be used to offset electrical generation reduction.

Boost firing the exhaust gas of reciprocating engines which provides a similar flexibility to the gas turbine system with supplementary firing and steam injection, has now been demonstrated commercially. However, there is still considerable development potential as regards detailed equipment improvement and system integration. For example, modification to the air fuel control on dual fuel engines. If bypass air is discharged into the exhaust instead of being returned to the turbo-charger inlet it would increase exhaust gas mass flow and oxygen level to allow more and easier boost firing.

However, the most pressing need for reciprocating engine systems is to match the availability of gas turbines. Achieving this will depend upon the readiness of engine manufacturers, or others, to set up on a 'national'/ 'international' scale 'maintenance contact'/'service organisations' such that on annual shutdown a team of men with the appropriate 'exchange' sub-assemblies and other items are on site ready to strip, rebuild and put the unit back into operation in the minimum time.

Conclusions

Fired boilers and steam turbines will find a niche where low cost waste or very low grade fuels are available and large scale operation is involved.

The Authors believe, however, that gas turbine plants with appropriate supplementary firing and/or steam injection will be predominant where the size of scheme and availability of reasonably priced natural gas allow, and reciprocating engine systems using gas or residual fuel oil where not.

On this basis, whilst the most spectacular cogeneration systems installed in UK hospitals will utilise gas turbine plant, the majority will incorporate reciprocating gas or oil engines.

Table 3 indicates that a good cogeneration system might in the correct circumstances reduce generating costs by around 40% and this may increase significantly in the near future if electricity costs increase and VAT is applied to energy.

Based on sound economic sense and through the more efficient use of fuels, reduced environmental damage and the conservation of invaluable fossil resources, it may be confidently anticpated that cogeneration will be a dynamic factor in working and possibly everyday life for the next 10, 20, 30, 40 . . .? years.

The Authors wish to thank the Directors and Colleagues in McLellan and Partners Limited for their help in preparing the paper.

Fred Nash CEng, FIMechE, FInstE is Director: I. V. Rogerson BSc, MInstE, CEng is Principal Mechanical Engineer, and T. M. Buxton MSc, BSc, AMIEE is Principal Electrical Engineer of the Power, Energy and Utilities Services Group at McLellan and Partners Limited, West Byfleet, Surrey.

New Integrated Gas Turbine CHP and Incinerator Plant

by

R. A. Briggs
BSc(Hons), CEng, MIMechE, MICIBSE, FIHospE
and
B. Yates
BSc(Hons), CEng, MIMechE, MICIBSE
Both Partners with Yates, Edge and Partners

Introduction

The first gas turbine based combined heat and power (CHP) project in the National Health Service is now in operation at the Queen Elizabeth Hospital in Birmingham. This plant forms part of an integrated CHP and waste disposal package that generates 3.6MW of electricity, disposes of 750kg/hour of hospital waste and produces up to 9.1MW of heat (equivalent to 14,500kg/hour of steam F&A 100°C) from the combined exhaust gases.

Background

During the early part of 1988 Yates, Edge and Partners were commissioned by Central Birmingham Health Authority to undertake two separate feasibility studies. The first study received a 50% Energy Efficiency Office grant to investigate various CHP options for the Queen Elizabeth complex. The most cost effective option was identified as a nominal 3.5MW gas turbine CHP unit with a non fired, heat recovery boiler. The second study investigated alternative incineration plant options, to dispose of the total hospital waste generated within the Health Authority. A single large incinerator with waste heat recovery boiler situated at the Queen Elizabeth site emerged as the most cost effective solution.

While investigating both studies it became apparent that, due to the space limitations around the boiler house and incineration compound, it was impractical to install both the CHP and incineration plants at this, the preferred, location. To overcome the spacial problems and to reduce the overall costs the possibility of using a single waste heat boiler to serve both plants was proposed. This development also led to the concept of recycling oxygen rich gases from the CHP plant economiser exhaust for use as pre-heated combustion air in the incinerator.

A schematic diagram of the plant arrangement is shown in Figure 1.

The Health Authority accepted the recommendation of an integrated CHP and incineration project and successfully obtained the necessary finance from two sources:-

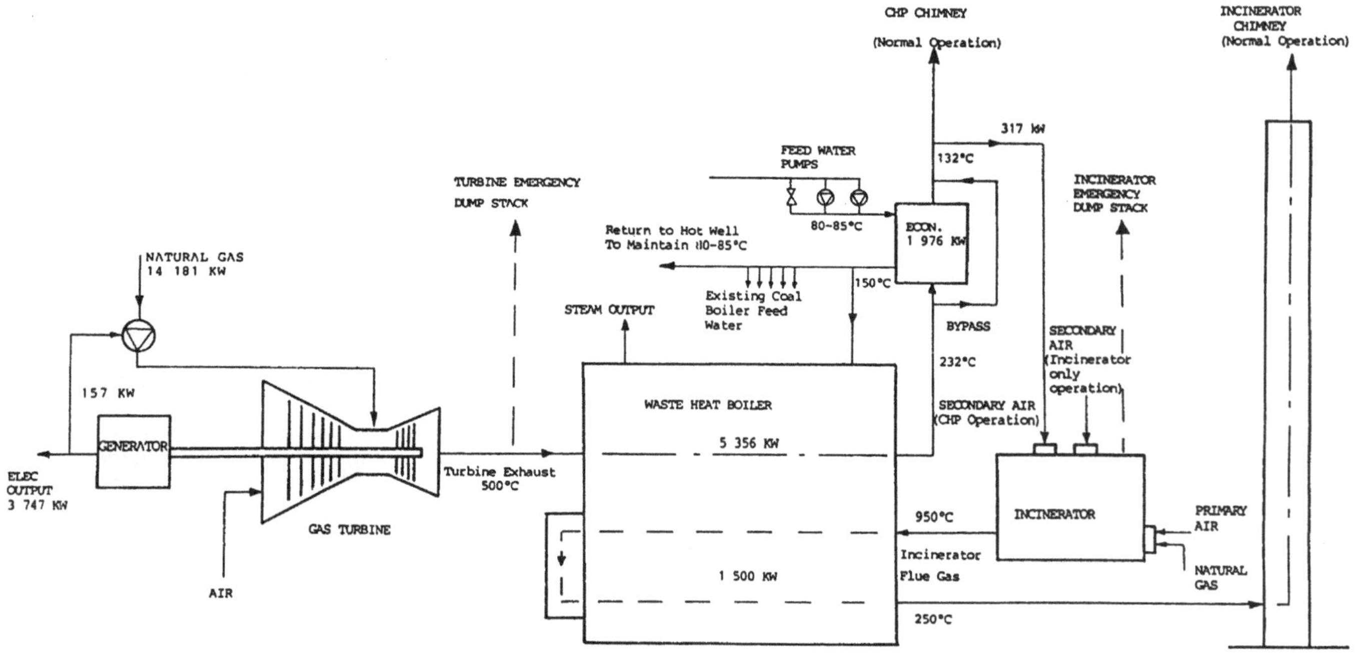

Figure 1: Schematic Diagram of Plant Arrangement.

INTEGRATION DE TURBINE A GAZ CHP ET BLOCS D'INCINERATION

L'installation mixte chaleur-courant à l'hôpital Queen Elizabeth de Birmingham constitue la première turbine à gaz CHP en milieu hospitalier en Grande-Bretagne, et elle bénéficie aussi de l'addition d'un incinérateur à déchets intégré. Ce centre générateur d'énergie produit de la vapeur à partir de charbon, de gaz naturel, de mazout ou de déchets, tout en produisant également en principe 3,5 MW d'électricité.

La turbine mixte fait fonctionner un générateur électrique de 11kV et peut opérer en parallèle avec la source d'électricité normale de l'hôpital ou seule, en fonction d'appoint. L'incinérateur de déchets utilise un container hermétiquement clos pour charger et peut traiter jusqu'à 750 kg de déchets hospitaliers à l'heure. Les gaz d'échappement de la turbine et de l'incinérateur se dirigent, individuellement ou simultanément, vers une chaudière à vapeur (chaleur résiduaire). Les besoins supplémentaires en vapeur de l'hôpital sont fournis par les chaudières à charbon conventionelles.

Cette article passe en revue les études théoriques de fonctionnement et de niveau de performance á atteindre. Il cite le concept CHP d'intégration avec l'incinérateur de déchets qui a permis l'obtention d'une bourse de la part du Département de l'Energie (Energy Technology Support Unit). Puis il évoque la planification, l'installation et la mise en opération du projet suivant et enfin parle des différentes expériences dans ce domaine.

(a) The West Midlands Regional Health Authority provided capital funding from their energy and revenue saving loan fund.

(b) Energy Efficiency Office via ETSU provided a grant under the Energy Efficiency Demonstration Scheme. The EEO grant was only available to schemes that incorporate areas of novelty or new technology. For this particular project these elements were threefold:-

- the application of gas turbine based CHP in a hospital environment;
- the combined hospital incinerator/CHP waste heat boiler; and
- the supplementary firing of CHP exhaust gases in this type of incinerator.

Having secured the necessary finance and considered both the unique character and magnitude of the project the Central Birmingham Health Authority, in late September 1988, took the decision of issuing an instruction to proceed. As the majority of the CHP revenue savings are realised from November to February each year, the instruction to proceed was given with the proviso that a fast track programme could be achieved to secure the savings available during the 1989 winter period.

Programming and Contract Organisation

The clients specified brief was that the plant should be operational by the beginning of November 1989. The design, construction and commissioning period being 14 months.

It was known that delivery times for gas turbines were at least nine months, with extended time scales for other major plant items. The problems associated with programming a £2 million engineering scheme were compounded by the building programme. The turbine hall, incinerator house, oil storage compound, gas compressor house and marshalling yard had to be constructed to accommodate the engineering proposals.

The complexity and compressed nature of the programme meant that Yates, Edge and Partners had to adopt the role of Project Management as well as Project Designers.

A critical path programming solution was undertaken incorporating all contracts and contractors requirements, deliveries, cranes etc. Furthermore, extensive and detailed schedules for installation and commissioning were developed to ensure that continuity of progress was maintained within an integrated installation in which each element relied upon another to prove its effectiveness.

Design and tender documentation of the main elements were achieved in 10 weeks. Orders for the three main plant supplies were placed on Christmas Eve 1988.

Intensive design work proceeded in early 1989 to develop the full extent of the building and engineering installation. This resulted in eight major contract elements.

The building programme did not release the site to allow the first plant to be delivered until July 1989 and the plant was handed over to the client in November 1989.

Project Content

The CHP plant consists of a gas/oil, dual fuel, gas turbine driven generator producing 3 to 4MW of electricity at 11,000 volts. The generator normally operates in parallel with the Midlands Electricity Board's mains supply and will initially provide all of the site electrical demand plus a net export of electricity. The turbine exhaust gases are directed to a single pass of a waste heat steam boiler and then to an economiser, which pre-heats the total boiler house feed water.

A new chimney was provided under this project to serve the CHP plant in both the 'dump' mode (when the turbine exhaust gases are discharged directly to the atmosphere) and the 'normal' mode (when the turbine exhaust gases are discharged to the atmosphere via the waste heat boiler/economiser).

The incinerator is sized to incinerate 750kg/h of hospital waste using a mini skip and automatic loader arrangement. The exhaust gases from the incinerator are directed to a twin pass tube bank within the common waste heat steam boiler. The incineration exhaust gases are discharged into the existing boilerhouse chimney liners. Two small liners accept the gases from the boiler while in the 'normal' mode and a single large liner accepts air attemporated gases directly from the incinerator when in the 'dump' mode.

The waste heat boiler is of a shell type construction and has been designed with the incinerator gas passes separate to the CHP gas pass such that the two gas streams do not mix. This allows each system to operate independently. The combined CHP/incinerator waste heat recovery is up to 9.1MW (equivalent to 14,500kg/h of steam F&A 100°C).

In addition a facility is provided to allow part of the oxygen rich CHP gas leaving the economiser to be diverted to the secondary combustion chamber of the incinerator where it is used as pre-heated combustion air.

Operational Philsophy

The Combined Heat and Power Unit

The CHP plant will normally operate for eight months of the year (October-May) on a continuous 24 hour day basis, both automatic and manual start up, synchronising and switching facilities are provided.

In the event of a loss of grid while the plant is operating, the statutory supply network is instantly isolated from the main hospital busbars. The site will then run in 'island' mode effectively providing primary standby generation to the site. When the grid 11kV supply is made available the CHP plant can be resynchronised with the grid without interruption of the site supplies.

Facilities are incorporated within the design to cater for selective load shedding should the site load development exceed the generator capacity in later years.

In the event of a mains failure when the CHP plant is not operating, a black start facility is provided via the existing boiler house standby generator. This allows the CHP plant to be started up on oil and to operate in island mode with the main hospital incoming switchgear isolated. When the grid supply is made available again normal operation is achieved as described above.

The CHP plant normally operates on natural gas fuel and will automatically change over to class 'D' oil, while on load, in response to a fall in gas pressure. When operating on the standby oil, an automatic sequence for on load change over back to natural gas is manually initiated.

The operation of the CHP takes priority over the waste heat boiler such that the turbine gases are automatically diverted ie 'dumped' to the atmosphere when insufficient heat sink is available.

The Incinerator

The incinerator plant is of a pyrolytic design and disposes of all hospital waste produced within the Health Authority. It operates for 8 hour/day and the resulting steam output from the heat recovery boiler matches the natural rise in steam demand during the daytime period.

During periods of initial start up, final burndown, etc the incinerator gases are air attemporated and 'dumped' to the atmosphere. Once satisfactory combustion is achieved the normal mode of operation is for the hot exhaust gases to be directed to the waste heat boiler.

The operation of the incinerator takes priority over the waste heat boiler such that the incinerator exhaust gases are automatically diverted or 'dumped' to the atmosphere when insufficient heat sink is available.

The incinerator secondary chamber air controls are arranged to automatically achieve satisfactory combustion using oxygenated gases from the economiser exit ductwork when the CHP plant is operating or ambient air during other periods of operation.

The Boiler and Economiser

When a normal boiler control limit parameter is achieved (such as high steam pressure) the CHP or incinerator plant continues to operate with the exhaust gases being 'dumped' directly to the atmosphere. Once the control parameter returns within normal operating limits the exhaust gases from both plants are automatically redirected to the waste heat boiler.

The economiser pre-heats the total boiler house feed water using recovered heat from the turbine exhaust gas after it leaves the waste heat shell boiler. A proportion of the oxygen rich gases leaving the economiser are ducted to the incinerator for supplementary firing in the secondary chamber.

Summary

Despite the complex nature of the project, the clients brief of a 14 month design and installation period was achieved within the approved budget of £2.5 million.

Early performance figures indicate that the scheme is on target to achieve the original payback of under four years.

Queen Elizabeth Hospital Installation of Integrated Combined Heat and Power Plant

Client
Central Birmingham Health Authority

Consulting Engineers/Project Managers
Yates, Edge and Partners

Architects
Temple Cox and Nicholls

Structural Engineers
Peel and Fowler

Quantity Surveyor
West Midlands Regional Health Authority

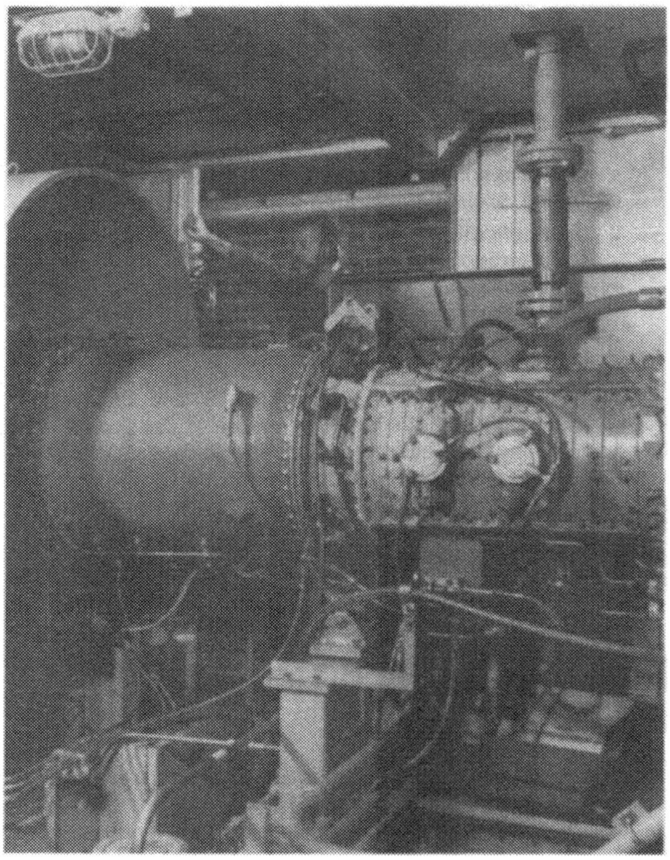

The gas turbine inside the acoustic enclosure.

Contractors
Centrax Gas Turbine Division Ltd
Beel Industrial Boilers Ltd
Robert Jenkins Systems Ltd
Midland Electricity Board
British Gas (West Midlands) plc
Mowlem Construction (Midlands) Ltd
Daly Heating Contractors Ltd (Coventry)
Atack Electrical Ltd

The Design and Construction of Hospitals in Developing Countries

by

H. Halbwachs Diplng
Deutsche Gesellschaft Für Techn.
Zusammenarbeit GTz Gmbh Eschborn, FGR

1. Introduction

The Alma Ata Conference in 1978 identified the approach of Primary Health Car (PHC) to be the key to health for all. Though curative and rehabilitative services have explicitly been included in this concept hospitals and similar health care facilities have been neglected in many countries introducing PHC. Only in recent years the important role of hospitals has been rediscovered, in particular its supporting function for PHC. This mainly includes:-

- technical support such as training and supervision, treatment of referral cases and research;
- administrative support such as supplies and organisation of referral system; and
- health education (hygiene, nutrition, child care, AIDS, Family planning etc).

The levels of care to be dealt with include the first health facility up to the second or third referral level according to the models supported by WHO:-

Higher Referral Levels
Third Referral Level (National)
Second Referral Level (Provincial)
First Referral Level (District)
First Health Facility (Subdistrict)
Community Health Activity
Family and Home

The Department of Health, Nutrition and Population Development of GTZ the official German agency for technical co-operation with developing countries for which I work, shares the opinion of many experts that hospitals exceeding 300 beds cannot be economically operated in most developing countries. For this reason and because of the apparent urgency of meeting the needs of the rural areas, this paper will only deal with health facilities below national level.

Before proceeding to the physical requirements of such health facilities, it should be remembered that circumstances with regard to technical capabilities of health staff in developing countries are far from satisfactory. When designing and equipping health facilities this fact must be taken into account.

The aforesaid is the primary reason why we have to think of hospitals in terms of a system, in which elements such as construction, energy supply, equipment and its operation and management to name only a few are intricately interrelated. Thus, planning, design and construction of health facilities cannot be regarded merely as a sequence of separate activities, but as an integrated task for a team.

2. Historical Review

In most developing countries traditional healing methods had been repressed or even demolished by external factors such as the increasing world wide contact through trade and colonisation. As a result of this process, health facilities as we understand them had been established in particular by the turn of the century.

The buildings were mainly hybrids between European standards and traditional designs and in this way captured advantages of both systems. In the years after independence, the inherited health structures were taken over without major changes and in the first instance new hospitals were established accordingly by governments and (religious) charity organisations. Between and after the world wars new demanding designs of great sophistication were introduced. Multistorey buildings with huge capacities and complicated technology were transplanted into desert, bush and jungle. Local construction techniques and ways of utilising material appropriate for the climate were abandoned and replaced by unsuitable and unsightly concrete boxes. Even development agencies of industrialised countries initially took part in this, until they realised that such facilities were doomed under the extreme conditions in most developing countries.

3. Construction and Equipment

3.1 Tasks of a Hospital in Developing Countries

In order to illustrate typical features of appropriate design and appliances, the most common hospital type, ie a 100-bed district hospital, will serve us as example. The major tasks of this type of referral facility include:-

- gynaecology, obstetrics;
- primary surgery;

LA PLANIFICATION ET LA CONSTRUCTION DES HOPITAUX DANS LES PAYS EN VOIE DE DEVELOPPEMENT

La conférence d'Alma Ata en 1978 a reconnue l'approche des Soins de Santé Primaires (SSP) comme la voie pour arriver à la santé pour tous. Bien que les services curatives et de réhabilitation ont été explicitement inclus dans ce concept, les hôpitaux et services de santé semblables ont été négligés dans beaucoup de pays qui ont introduits les SSP. Ce n'est que dans les années passées que le rôle important des hôpitaux a été redécouvert, particulierement dans sa fonction de support pour les SSP.

En accord avec les modèles préconisés par l'OMS on comprend comme les niveaux de service a prendre en charge de service de santé de base jusqu'au échelon, ainsi que le troisième échelon (de référence):-

Echelons de référence superieurs
Troisième échelon de référence (niveau national)
Deuxieme échelon de référence (niveau provincial)
Premier échelon de référence (niveau de district)
Service de santé de base
Activité de santé communautaire
Famille et ménage

Le Département Santé, Nutrition et Développement Démographique de la GTZ, l'office allemand de cooperation technique avec les pays en voie de développement, partage l'opinion de nombreux experts que des hôpitaux de plus de 300 lits ne peuvent être gérés de facon economique dans la plupart des pays en voie de développement. C'est en fonction de cela et de l'urgence apparente de satisfaire aux besoins des régions rurales, que ce texte ne vise que les services de santé en dessous du niveau national.

- emergency cases;
- equipment related diagnosis including laboratory and basic x-ray services;
- equipment related therapy;
- distribution of drugs;
- health education;
- staff training;
- maintenance of subordinate facilities;
- transport of patients and material; and
- administration and supervision of district, communication.

3.2 General Construction Features and Hospital Plants

Provided certain specific requirements and conditions are considered, the principles of hospital design in industrialised countries can also be applied in developing countries. Conditions in the majority of third world countries are characterised by extreme elimatic and topographic conditions. High temperatures and/or high humidity lead to rapid deterioration and unsuitable environmental conditions for patients and staff, unless buildings and equipment are designed accordingly. Factors to be considered are:-

- building orientation (eg east-west alignment to avoid excess of solar heat radiation);
- building shape (eg single storey buildings to avoid lifts).
- solar radiation (eg wall shading by generous roof overhang);
- ventilation (eg forced cross-ventilation);
- terrain features (eg trees for shading); and
- pests (eg protection of electrical wiring against rodents).

Remoteness accounts for difficulties in building maintenance, in energy supply, logistics etc. Utilisation of imported or scarce building material contribute heavily to maintenance and improvement problems. Also cultural and social factors determine the requirements of health facilities, for example the necessity to separate sanitary facilities according to sex or certain hygienic habits (not many people in developing countries use toilet paper!).

Some special requirements and features of hospital departments and units are described below.

Outpatient

As a rule, hospitals in developing countries have to care for a great number of outpatients. An average district hospital covers approximately 3,000m^2 of floor space. For the outpatient department between 15 and 25% of this space is required, of which the waiting, registering and circulation area should be 0.5m^2 per patient. The waiting area should be suited for health education activities. Only in smaller hospitals the emergency section may be part of the outpatient department.

Surgery

The size of theatres and its support units varies widely and depends on the specific conditions of a country. A typical size of a surgery ward for an African 100-bed hospital for example would be in the region of 300 to 500m^2. Space requirements for plaster room and theatre staff are mostly not considered. Separation of sterile and non-sterile areas is mostly not observed to the required extent. This is due to organisational and design deficiencies.

The theatre itself should be completely tiled except for the ceiling. Though sterility may not be maintained completely, a floor gully should be installed for easier cleaning. Air conditioning in hot and humid climates is mandatory. In arid areas dust poses special design problems.

Obstetrics and Gynaecology

In general, hospitals in developing countries have difficulties coping with a great number of deliveries. Efforts of health authorities to divert normal pregnancies to peripheral health facilities have not yet succeeded in facilitating this condition. This circumstance, and the tradition that pregnant women (and patients in general) are accompanied by several family members have to be accounted for when space requirements are estimated.

Laboratory

For most hospitals a laboratory space of 0.5m^2 per bed should be sufficient. Tiling up to 180cm and floor gullies are recommended. For microbiological labs various sterilising and incubating equipment may require additional ventilation of the room.

Pharmacy

For a typical district hospital which has also to back up peripheral health facilities too, 100 to 150m^2 are considered to be sufficient. In case long term storage of drugs and particularly vaccines is required, a separate cold room is recommended.

Radiology

50m^2 of space for the radiology department is considered adequate for district hospitals using the WHO-standard x-ray (Basic Radiological System, BRS). In order to meet basic safety requirements for radiation protection, solid brick or concrete walls must be provided. Wooden wall constructions and doors have to be lined with a minimum of 0.5mm lead sheeting. Separate and solid operator cabins are essential. Separate rooms for developing x-ray films are required and must be very well ventilated.

Orthopaedics and Physiotherapy

The role of workshops for production and fitting of orthopaedic appliances is often underrated. Basic rehabilitation facilities belong generally to rural hospitals as well. Most patients in this area are treated as out-patients. Again, sufficient space for these and accompanying relatives should be provided.

Wards

Wards should not have more than eight beds per room. Few smaller, separate rooms can serve as infection units. Since many patients are attended to by at least one relative even over night, appropriate space must be provided, eg extra beds which can be stored under the patient beds during day time. For easier cleaning, walls should be treated with oil or plastic paint. At least two hand basins should be installed. Forced cross ventilation provides, in most cases, sufficient ventilation. In many areas, due to religious or habitual reasons, sanitary facilities cannot be tolerated in close proximity to the ward itself or on a floor above. The single-storey pavilion type of arranging wards and hospital departments easily allows an acceptable partition of sanitary units.

It must not be forgotten that under conditions of most developing countries, a psychiatric ward is necessary too.

Mortuary, Air Conditioning and Cooling

This area is one of the technically most critical areas in third world hospitals. Poor design and management frequently leads to overload and in consequence to frequent break downs. Though split units are basically more economical to operate and more comfortable to use (noise!) single units should be preferred, since the eventual failure of one of these units does not paralyse the air conditioning of the hospital as a whole. In addition, maintenance and exchange of these units are easier and can be managed by local resources.

Cold rooms are very often established after the completion of a hospital under technically unsatisfactory conditions. Heat insulation is insufficient, problems with dampness due to condensation.

Refrigerators constitute a particular weak spot. Whether used in laboratories, blood banks, pharmacies etc or for kitchen purposes, various problems occur again and again. Two types are in use: Electrically operated compressor units and absorption units which are operated with kerosene or liquid gas. The compressor type is more reliable, provided the power supply is stable enough (< +/− 15%). Absorption units, on the other hand, can be operated under difficult energy conditions, but are rather sensitive to inadequate handling of the burner. Both refrigerator types need thorough ventilation and should therefore, but also to avoid premature corrosion, be placed on pallets.

Energy Supply

In many cases there is no external power supply or this is unreliable (unstable, power cuts, high frequency contamination). Sensitive equipment therefore need protective and stabilising devices. In-house power sources are mostly limited to (diesel) generators. Most problems with these stem from inadequate maintenance, overload and often from too sophisticated control circuits (automatic triggering etc!). Renewable energy sources are usually too expensive to buy and difficult to operate at medium- to large-scale. Small-scale applications such as solar thermic water heating, small photovoltaic units to run single equipment etc seem to be more feasible.

Water, Sanitation

External water supply is scarce and unreliable, too. Supply from the hospitals' own wells, cisterns etc tend to be insufficient or of poor quality (mineral contents, corrosive, bacteriologically unfit for consumption). Water towers should be preferred to booster pump systems. Water treatment is mostly neglected, even when a plant exists.

Fittings and sanitary installations should be available in the country to allow for easy replacement and repair. Special armatures for clinical use should be avoided. PVC tubing should not be used underground, since certain rodents take great interest in these. Waste water disposal, for ecological reasons, deserves much more attention than it is usually the case.

Sanitary installations are very problematic. A thorough analysis of local habits and designs is strongly recommended during the planning phase of a hospital.

Medical Gases

Except for countries which provide a well established technical infra-structure, central medical gas supply should not be considered. Decentralised supply with gas cylinders is much easier to maintain. Oxygen may be provided for many applications by using oxygen concentrators.

Waste Disposal

Too often the problem of disposal of hospital waste, specifically infectious waste, is neglected or not adapted to local conditions. Hospitals in third world countries do not usually possess any means to dispose of waste other than to bury or to burn refuse on the hospital grounds. Incinerators are rare and where they exist, they mostly turn out to be too complicated or expensive to run, or to be a source of heavy pollution.

Sterilisation

This area is one of the most critical in hospitals in developing countries. The failure of autoclaves, in particular if only a single central one is available, cripples hospitals frequently. Simple and sturdy design and provision of several (smaller) units in one hospital are recommended. In many cases sterilisers operated with a power source other than electricity may be preferable.

Kitchen

Many examples of hospitals which use traditional kitchen equipment such as charcoal stoves instead of the 'comfortable and efficient' machinery provided, prove that modern catering technology is prone to become unusable after a short time. It should be remembered that employing labour can be much more economic and efficient in developing countries than using fancy equipment, as for example automatic potato peelers. In some countries, kitchens are not needed, because patients are fed by relatives.

Laundry

Like kitchens, laundries are a permanent source of trouble for basically the same reasons. It is observed that old (>20 years), semi-automatic equipment does often still serve its purpose, whereas modern progammable washing robots cease to operate within a short period.

Staff Quarters

Staff quarters, though essential in most developing countries, are often not considered in the planning process, especially when foreign donors 'import' their own concepts.

Maintenance Workshop

Though mostly ignored, maintenance services are supported to play a central role within the technical management of health facilities. For the standard district hospital a minimum space of 100m^2 must be allocated, excluding an adequate open space for welding and spraying. The workshop should at least have separate working rooms for medical equipment (precision mechanics, electronics etc), hospital plants (plumbing, electrical installations etc) and carpentry. Adequate stores for tools and material and for the equipment to be serviced must be provided too. A small office should be available for the inevitable paperwork. The workshop should be equipped for two technicians and four artisans (standard staff requirement for a 100-bed hospital in developing countries).

4. Medical Equipment

This issue is too broad to give specific recommendations in this paper. The equipment situation in most developing countries is disastrous. Inoperable devices clog valuable hospital and storage space, replacement provided by donors soon give in to the unfavourable conditions. Three principal reasons are responsible:-

- operators of medical equipment are insufficiently qualified;
- after-sales-service, maintenance and repair are barely existent, equipment management not well understood; and
- equipment is insufficiently adapted to levels of care and is of inadequate quality.

Training of operators (medical doctors, nurses etc) mostly does not include technical subjects such as first line maintenance, handling and safety precautions. Equipment management is thought to be something mysterious, exclusively handled by technicians with the help of a few tools. Donors pump a tremendous variety of hospital equipment into third world countries, without much consideration for their suitability. However, it should be noted that the introduction of 'appropriate equipment' will remain a fiction even in the long run. Apart from a few exceptions, industry is not interested in investing in the development of special technology for a comparatively small market. Only standardisation and a coherent political will of the receiving governments will eventually contribute to an acceptable solution.

Selection of equipment for a specific hospital should at least be based on the following aspects:-

- country-specific data with special regard to vital statistics, epidemiological information such as prevalances and incident rates of the most important diseases, special risks of certain diseases to patients and community etc;
- staff situation, job descriptions, workload, competence, possibilities for further training etc;
- health policy related information such as catchment

areas, size of population serviced, level of health care, standards etc.

- economic situation, size of budget, budgetary control, characteristics of local currency in view of imports;
- local equipment market, maintenance provided by private sector, availability of spare parts;
- equipment management related information, role of administration maintenance and repair capacity of the institution etc; and
- data on the technical environment such as characteristics of power and water supply, availability of steam, climatic data etc.

Finally I would like to warn of overrating the impact of a 'good technology and architecture' on the quality of health services: technical solutions cannot compensate for lack of motivation and competence and for ineffective management. In other words, if health policies, administrative action and personnel resources are not tuned towards improving a health care *system*, the best and most appropriate piece of equipment will not serve its purpose.

Literature

Most information on building design has been extracted from:-

Lippsmeier, G.; Demeter, H.; Oka, K., Hospital Design in the Tropics, Edition 1988, Institut für Tropenbau, Waldschmidtstr, 6a, 8130 Starnberg, FRG.

Further information was obtained from:-

Dean, M. (Editor), The Role of Hospitals in Primary Health Care, Report of Conference held in Karachi, November 1981, Aga Khan Foundation jointly with WHO, Geneva.

Kleczkowski, B. M.; Nilsson, N. O., Health Care Facility Projects in Developing Areas: Planning, Implementation and Operation, WHO Public Health Papers No 79, 1984.

Kleczkowski, B. M. et al (Editors), Approaches to Planning and Design of Health Care Facilities in Developing Areas, Volume 1-5, WHO Offset Publications.

WHO Expert Committee, Hospitals and Health for All, Report on the Role of Hospitals at the First Referral Level, WHO Technical Report Series 744, Geneva 1987.

Frymire, T. R., MEDWORLD — A New Design Concept, Hospital Engineering December 1989, Pages 5-6.

Schmidt, H-J.; Halbwachs, H., Technical Equipment at Health Institutions in Developing Countries, To be published by GTZ end of 1990.

WHO Division of Strengthening of Health Services, Global Action Plan on Management, Maintenance and Repair of Health Care Equipment, WHO, Geneva 1987.

Halbwachs, H.; Korte, R. (Editors), Maintenance Strategies for Public Health Facilities in Developing Countries, Report on Workshop held in Nairobi, March 1989, Jointly published by GTZ and WHO in 1990.

Training Service and User Personnel in Developing Countries

by

Dr Andreas Mallouppas
Head WHO Collaborating Centre on Training and Research
Regional Training Centre
Higher Technical Institute
Nicosia, Cyprus

1. Introduction

Developing countries face major problems in the proper and effective utilisation of health care equipment due to their ineffective and inefficient management.

As a consequence of this there exists an inadequate level of health care delivery resulting in reduced standards of health care. Moreover, the mismanagement of equipment also results in wastage of limited national resources.

Factors which contribute to this waste have been identified and estimated elsewhere[1], the main ones being:-

- purchase or donation of technologically sophisticated equipment for the countries' needs and capabilities;
- shorter life time of equipment due to misuse and maltreatment by user and service staff;
- extra modifications, additions, alterations etc originally unforeseen and subsequently purchased in order to make the equipment operational;
- lack of standardisation resulting in increased spare parts and maintenance costs; and
- equipment remaining inoperative due to the inability of service staff to repair it and operating staff to use it.

The resultant wastage of resources due to the above, in some developing countries, may be up to 75% of the total equipment inventory.

As a consequence of ineffective national policy formulation and planning the proportion of money allocated to maintenance (which should include staffing of a Health Care Technical Service (HCTS), training of user and service staff, spare parts, tools, test equipment and workshop facilities and information support) is inadequate and for some items even non-existent.

The four main areas already identified[2] that need particular attention in order to improve the situation are:-

- effective policy formulation and planning development;
- existence of Health Care Technical Services;
- adequate Manpower Development and Training; and
- availability of Information Support Systems.

This paper focuses on one of the above main areas that requires attention if the situation is to improve, that of manpower development and training. Mention will also be given of basic information support systems that are a prerequisite if essential data, teaching materials and technical manuals and spare parts specifications are to be made available at country level.

However, it should be stressed, that in order to improve the situation training alone cannot solve the problem but what is required is a co-ordinated effort in all the four main areas identified previously. It is in this context that WHO's Global Action Plan[3] should be used to promote action and sensitise donors and other agencies in supporting programmes which address these issues.

2. Country Experiences

The main outcome that characterises country situation surveys is that the estimate of wastage of resources due to the above is in many cases far worse.

For many countries, in reality, an HCTS is still grossly ineffective or not even officially planned for. There are usually ad hoc, ineffective half-measures. It is true that in some countries, particularly those receiving donor support, the foundations for such a service have been laid.

However a common problem in many developing countries is the unavailability of foreign exchange. In fact the generally poor economic situation hampers all efforts to establish proper servicing or even to have an adequate purchasing policy. The availability of service workshops, particularly at district and even at provincial hospitals is very poor. At central level there is usually a badly equipped nucleus of a national central workshop, which finds itself in this state because of the lack of policy and funds allocated for its support.

3. Strategy and Approach

The field of training is an area that has received attention for some years now. In this context there have been regional approaches (such as the WHO/EMRO Regional Training Centre in Cyprus) or donor agency country projects (such as the GTZ Mombassa Polytechnic, Medical Equipment Training).

Of course training alone has been recognised as not being enough to solve the problem, that is why the training, particularly at country level, should be linked to the HCTS and to hospital practical work.

Figure 1 shows the relationship of a National Training Centre (NTC) to the Ministry of Health (policy making body) and to the HCTS (service workshops at all levels, central, provincial, district and rural).

WHO through its Global Action Plan is trying to promote various approaches which ensure that the necessary service and training infrastructure is made available or strengthened at country level.

Typical guidelines[4] to assist in estimating the number of service staff and training facilities and needs have been developed.

SERVICES DE FORMATION ET PERSONNELS D'UTILISATION — PAYS EN VOIE DE DEVELOPPEMENT

Cette présentation analyse les problèmes qu'affrontent les pays en développement dans la gestion et la maintenance d'équipements.

Une attention toute particulière est portée aux quatre points essentiels qui requièrent une panoplie d'actions cohérentes:-

Il s'agit de l'existence de:-

- *Stratégies et de planification*
- *Structures d'appuis techniques aux services de santé*
- *Formation du personnel et,*
- *Systèmes d'informations*

Des expériences concrètes ainsi que différentes startégies employées dans le domaine de la formation sont décrites.

La stratégie, dans le domaine de la formation, du Centre Régional de Formation (RTC) de Chypre, est décrite et l'accent est mis sur la nécessité d'établir des Centres de Formations Nationaux ainsi que des structures d'assistance aux systèmes de formation.

Enfin des recommendations, quant-aux actions nécessaires dans le futur, sont décrites.

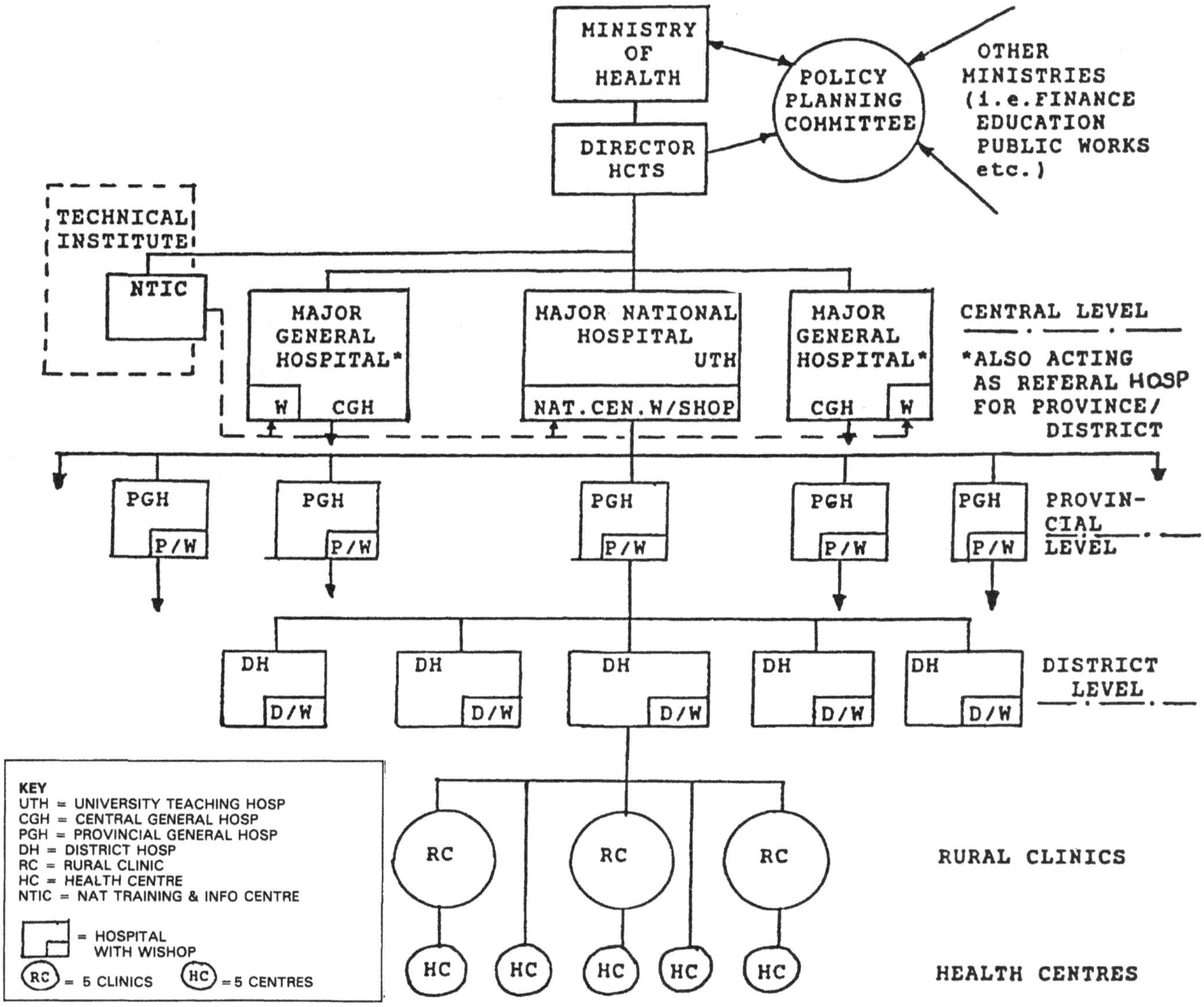

Figure 1: Typical HCTS Organisational Diagram.

4. Examples of Available Training Programmes

4.1 Regional Training Centres (RTC's)

At present there are two anglophone RTC's in Cyprus and Sierra Leone and a francophone one in Lyon.

The different RTC's cater for different levels of training of technicians. The Cyprus RTC was established first in 1978 and in 1987 was designated, in recognition for its contribution in the field of Training and Research in maintenance and repair, a WHO Collaborating Centre. It is also a Commonwealth Centre of Excellence.

A large number of different courses has been carried out and the number of students who have graduated from these since 1978 is approaching 400 from over 40 countries.

At present the Cyprus RTC has modified and updated its syllabii to run the following Advance Technician courses in:-

- Electro-Medical and Clinical Laboratory Equipment;
- Operating Theatre and Dental Equipment; and
- Diagnostic X-Ray and Nuclear Medicine Equipment.

4.2 National Training Centres (NTC)

There are NTC's in Egypt, Bahrain, Syria, Somalia, Kenya, Zimbabwe, Bangladesh, Philippines as well as in Latin America. Others are being planned for or may already be operating.

The basic starting point for NTC's is the Artisan (Craftsman) and Technician levels. The technician training is usually on the lines of the Polyvalent course initially run by the Cyprus RTC.

The majority of these training centres are linked to a nearby workshop in a large General Hospital. The aim is to carry out on-the-job training so as to expose students to the realities of the practical situation.

5. Inter-Centre Collaboration

For the first four to six years of establishing RTC's and NTC's no effective collaboration and exchange of information and or staff took place. Lately, however, this has been improved. There has been an increase in contacts made to RTC-Cyprus, for example, from interested national and regional centre counterparts, who visit the Centre and are given information and exchange experiences on formulation of courses and planning for training needs, mainly for the Polyvalent level course.

This has enabled a number NTC's to determine their requirements and programme their own training needs based on their local requirements and capabilities.

The RTC-Cyprus has also carried out consultancy services, for WHO and CFTC (Commonwealth Fund for Technical Co-operation) in the form of country surveys[5], workshops[6] and meetings[7],[2] with the aim of establishing country needs and of promoting awareness related to the issues of management of health care equipment.

6. Technical Information Support

A major area of concern is that of availability and accessibility to the vast amount of technical information that is already available in developed countries.

This issue was recognised at the Cyprus meeting[2] and recommendations were made to WHO to promote the establishment of a system for the exchange of information.

As a first step a WHO 'Health Equipment Management' Newsletter will soon be available, however a great deal more is needed. The establishment of National Information System (NIS) probably linked to National Training Centres or HCTS, at central level, are needed.

The Annex shows a very basic NIS, and as can be seen, its hardware is not very expensive and most of it should already be available in the vast majority of countries. However, a policy decision needs to be effected in order to set it up. Moreover a major consideration is the availability of software (Computer Programmes, documentation, equipment codes etc) and the setting-up of mechanisms, so that the information is disseminated to countries from developed centres. Also at country level experienced personnel should exist, being capable of assimiliating, collating, adapting and disseminating the information to the appropriate departments, within the health sector.

For all the above to materialise there is a need for international as well as national policy and action. Personnel at country level have to know how to deal with the information and on an international level the compatibility of software and hardware has to be decided upon.

7. Future Action

From present experience it appears that National Training Centres either need to be set up or strengthened, usually starting at Craftsman and/or General (Polyvalent) Technician level and should be within national capabilities and covering basic needs.

The aim of NTC's, country size and infrastructure permitting, should be to eventually upgrade the training to cover more specialised, higher level training, now available at regional level.

If National Information Systems are to be set up and become effective, then courses to train personnel on how to utilise, assess and adapt information to national requirements are needed. Such courses may commence at regional or even global level but may well be organised later on an inter-country/sub-regional level.

The need for Clinical and Hospital Engineers (and/or Technician Engineers) has been recognised and accepted[7]. Clinical Engineers should cover the Medical Equipment field but of equal importance are the hospital plants, such as boilers, kitchens, airconditioning systems, central sterilising units etc and these needs must be covered also by training Hospital Engineers.

The need for policy makers (Ministry level) and administrators of HCTS is also recognised and to cover the lack in such personnel an MSc level course in Management of Equipment is also required.

International agencies such as UNDP, World Bank, IAEA, UNIDO etc and NGO's should be sensitised by WHO to the various issues and as regards training to support such programmes as global, regional and country level which aim to fill some of the needs described above.

Inter-care collaboration should be strengthened and exchange of information and staff be supported in order to transfer information and technology.

National Professional Associations should be set-up or enhanced in order to promote the interests and standards of the profession.

In this respect Associations in developed countries, particularly International ones, should, through WHO, strongly promote such activities, as well as participate in the organisation of seminars and courses.

WHO should be encouraged to promote a standard (both software and hardware) information support system so that the vast amount of existing information be readily available to countries and adapted to their needs.

User training courses is also an important issue since a lot of breakdowns are caused due to misuse of equipment. Courses should be designed and implemented with the user in mind as well as producing self-teaching handbooks for proper use of equipment.

It should be emphasised that the above actions should not be carried out in isolation but should be part of a unified action programme which also addresses the other important issues of effective policy formulation and planning development as well as strengthening national Health Care Technical Services.

It is only through effective utilisation and servicing of equipment that the standard of health care delivery would be increased and benefit from the use of technology.

8. References

(1) Mallouppas, A., 'Background Document — WHO Programme for Support to Countries in the Field of Maintenance and Repair of Hospital and Medical Equipment' WHO, Geneva SHS/86.4.

(2) Interregional Meeting on Maintenance and Repair of Health Care Equipment, Nicosia, Cyprus, 24th-28th November 1986, WHO/SHS/NHP/87.5.

(3) GLobal Action Plan on Management, Maintenance and Repair of Health Care Equipment, WHO/SHS/NHP/87.8 (under revision).

(4) Mallouppas, A., 'Guidelines on Development and Strengthening of National Health Care Technical Services' WHO Report to be published.

(5) Mallouppas, A., 'Report of a Survey in Commonwealth South and East African Countries', CFTC Report.

(6) Report on Intercountry Workshop on Management Maintenance and Repair of Health Care Equipment, Arusha, Tanzania, July 1989 (to be published).

(7) Interregional Meeting on Manpower Development and Training for health care equipment Management, Maintenance and Repair, Campinas, Brazil, 20th-24th November 1989 (to be published).

(8) Mallouppas, A., 'Background Document on WHO International School on Clinical and Hospital Engineering' submitted at WHO Interregional Meeting, Campinas, Brazil, 20th-24th November 1989.

(9) Mallouppas, A., 'Background Document on WHO International School on Management of Health Care Equipment' submitted at WHO Interregional Meeting, Campinas, Brazil, 20th-24th November 1989.

Annex

Requirements for a National Information System

Syllabus: Subject Matter

1. Equipment Required

1.1 Computer Hardware for Data Bank
One IBM PC (AT or equivalent) with 60MB Hard Disk, 1.2M floppy.
One Laser Printer.
Fascimile (Telefax).
Heavy Duty Photocopier including Sorter, Auto-Feeder, Duplex, Editing, etc.
One MODEM to connect computer with telephone line.

1.2 Computer Software for Data Bank
Standard Data Base Package (to be adopted by WHO and other agencies.)

2. Running Costs/Year

2.1 Rentals and consumables for Fax, Telex.
2.2 Package and Postage of materials to health sector and communication with reference centres abroad.
2.3 Printer, Photocopy consumables and service.
2.4 Administrative and Secretarial Support.
2.5 Miscellaneous costs.

An Assessment of Training Requirements for Health Care Technology in the Developing World

by

Roderick T. Statham
IEng, MIHospE, MIPlantE, MBIM
Chief Engineer (Training)
Southern Regions Health Board, Tanzania
UK Overseas Development Administration

Introduction

There is an increasing amount of health care equipment of various degrees of sophistication being imported into development countries for a number of reasons; demand is created by medical staff practising their specialities in the countries' larger hospitals, the expectations of the medical staff often being raised by postgraduate experience overseas; donor agencies often give health equipment as part of an aid package, and manufacturers can identify both short and long term gains in the development world markets.

What is becoming a matter for increasing international concern is the amount of this equipment which quickly falls into disuse due to malfunction and lack of maintenance. The concern is justified when, in the context of developing countries, the equipment represents a considerable expenditure of valuable foreign exchange.

There are many issues which need to be addressed when considering the management of health care equipment. The process of equipment selection, specification, procurement, installation, commissioning, user training, and maintenance support (including spare parts), requires careful control which can only be achieved on a national scale by the existence of a Health Care Technical Service at Health Ministry level. The lack of such HCTS's, and the lack of an awareness of the issues involved, in many developing countries, is of such international concern that the World Health Organisation, in 1988, launched the Glabal Action Plan for the Management, Maintenance and repair of Health Care Equipment. Key functions of the Global Action Plan include the increasing awareness of issues involved in Health Care Equipment Management and Maintenance amongst decision makers and policy makers in Health Ministries, and support for training initiatives in developing countries.

There are many inputs into the health care equipment cycle, and many of us can identify areas where our involvement can assist in making health care equipment sustainable in the environment of developing countries. This paper looks specifically at training needs relative to health care equipment; training of technicians in maintenance, calibration and repair, training of users in the correct operation of equipment; training of managers and decision makers in controlling those aspects of the health care equipment process already mentioned.

Health care equipment needs to be maintained, operated and managed by highly skilled personnel. The ongoing process of training needs to be an integral part of any Health Care Technical Service. This paper discusses the training aspect of health care equipment management in Developing countries.

Appropriate Technology in the Developing World

There is a prevailing dismissive attitude that health care equipment in developing countries, which repidly falls into disuse due to lack of maintenance, or operator induced malfunction, is 'inappropriate'. The reaction is often that the equipment should not be there in the first place, and that less sophisticated equipment should be substituted.

However, by adapting the 'appropriate', and by implication, low, technology argument in a blanket manner across the health care sector, a paradox is being created. The issues relating to the management of more sophisticated technology, including slection and maintenance criteria, are often being avoided, and the associated learning curve which developing countries must embark upon in order to manage technology in the future, is never realised.

The greatest danger in deliberately adopting low technology in the health sector is in the continued burying of the maintenance issue; ways are being sought to avoid maintenance rather than trying to introduce the maintenance philosophy in developing countries. This is ironic in countries where even the highest technicaian's salaries represent a minute fraction of the capital cost of medical equipment.

Another problem with 'low' or 'appropriate' technology equipment is that its risk of obsolescence is inherently greater than that of more modern equipment. Equipment which is specially developed for developing countries depends on support from agencies for its development costs; there is no ready market for such equipment in developed countries and therefore ongoing support such as spare parts and technical backup, are also likely to require continued support from external agencies.

It is suggested that a more appropriate approach is to use modern equipment, with established markets in the developed world, and therefore ongoing support from the manufacturers. The approach from donor agencies and recipient developing countries should then be to build a project framework within which such equipment could be integrated into hospitals in developing countries, so that such issues as infrastructure development, manpower, training, budgets, spares support, and manufacturers agency support in the country concerned, are addressed.

Bilateral development agencies, (and NGOs), are, by definition, trying to ensure the continued development of developing nations. They will not do so by excluding

UNE ÉVALUATION DES BESOINS EN FORMATION EN TECHNOLOGIE DES SERVICES DE SANTÉ DANS LE MONDE EN VOIE DE DÉVELOPPEMENT

Cet article évalue les besoins enformation en technologie des services de santé dans le monde en voie de développement, un environnement ou des technologies plus sophistiquées deviennent monnaie courante, en particulier dans les grands hopitaux des centres urbains croissants de ces pays.

Cet article examine cout d'abord l'aspect 'Technologie appropriée', puis les phases impliquées dans la réalisation de ces technologies dans les pays en voie de développement, et enfin comment la formation, en ses différentes formes et à différents niveaux, cadre dans cet ensemble de technologies.

Cet article défie tout-un à considèrer son role eventuel au niveau formation dans les pays en voie de développement.

developing world from the technology, including the health care technology, which we enjoy in the developed world.

Training of Personnel in Hospital Maintenance

This paper is dedicated to training issues, and training is identified as a key element in the development of Health Care Equipment Management in the developing world. Training, in the context of transfer of knowledge, experience, and skills, needs to be examined in a broad context. A workshop for senior ministry officials, designed for creating an awareness of health care equipment management issues, such as the recent WHO Interregional workshop held in Arusha, Tanzania, is as important a component of the training concept as the technical training of a technician in a new place of health care technology. Management issues should be addressed as well as technical issues.

The hospitals in developing countries at the secondary and tertiary end of the health care scale are growing larger and more complex. They are required to serve the needs of growing urban populations; many are also required to fulfil the role of teaching hospitals hosting university medical schools. The management skills required to manage the technology in these establishment, including the building fabric, building services, medical and non-medical equipment, are considerable. Considering the constraints such as logistical problems in procuring spare parts, foreign exchange shortages, skills shortages, budgetary limitations, and others, it can be argued that the problems, and the management skills necessary to overcome those problems, are greater than in the developed world. Training, the sharing of skills and experience, are necessary at all levels of management, technician, and artisan, in order that the technology package can be successfully transferred to the developing world.

Skilled Manpower: Identification of Organisational Needs

It is necessary, in developing countries, to plan manpower and training needs within an organisational framework. In some countries this may involve the establishment of a Health Care Technical Service, where one does not already exist. The planning process involved in itself requires skill levels and expertise which may be in short supply in the countries concerned; the experience of running a technical service at this level is likely to be limited, and the sharing of knowledge and expertise in this field across the International spectrum can be of enormous benefit.

However, this does not necesssarily mean, nor is it meant to infer, that there is no provision for maintenance in developing countries. Building fabric and maintenance is often the responsibility of the Ministry of Works, whereas hospitals often have their own workshops and staff for equipment maintenance.

Because of the way hospitals have been built, and equipment provided, health services have often developed in a haphazard and unco-ordinated manner. Poor maintenance performance is the consequence of such a lack of co-ordination; the skills are often not available to maintain equipment and the provision of spare parts was usually not thought through at the procurement stage.

With respect to trained technical personnel in the Health Care Sector, a degree of forward planning is necessary. Health Ministries should be able to assess their current and projected asset stock, in terms of buildings, plant and equipment, and identify the technical skills, in management and practical terms, which will be required to maintain the asset sock in reasonable and usable condition.

The introduction of new asset stock, whether in terms of buildings or equipment, should be subject to the same scrutiny at the procurement stage. A donor package involving new buildings and/or equipment should include an appraisal of the sustainability of that package, and the training needs for the recipient organisation required to make the package sustainable.

There is now a shift in emphasis in the developing world; whereas buildings and equipment were provided previously with little thought for training and maintenance, the development of training and maintenance programmes are now often seen to be running in parallel with hospital rehabilitation and equipment provision projects.

The 'end result' of the identification of organisation needs, in terms of skilled manpower, will result in an organisation structure or structures, and job descriptions, which will identify the skill needs at different levels and in different sections of the organisation. This is not only for maintenance or engineering personnel; X-Ray machines require skilled radiographers and sterilisers training CSSD staff; all cadres have structured training requirements, including specific training geared to the equipment they will be using. This may appear obvious in the developed world; in developing countries it is surprising how many cadres have yet to be created in the Health sector, and training needs for those cadres identified.

Sourcing of Skilled Manpower

There are many excellent educational establishments in developing countries, with technical education often receiving special emphasis through the provision of technical schools feeding colleges. It is possible to find highly intelligent, well educated and enthusiastic technicians and engineers throughout the developing world. In the health sector, however, it is often the case that the pure theory and the practical elements of their training have not been brought together in a coherent manner. The understanding of maintenance, for instance, is often almost non-existent in graduate technicians and engineers, because they have rarely been exposed to a practical environment where maintenance is a priority.

The problem, then, is not a failure of the education system per se, but a failure of the overall training process in integrating good education with thorough practical training.

There is always a high throughput of skilled technical staff in the health care sector. Where salaries are low in comparison to the private sector, and there is an enormous demand for skills and experience in the technical field, such a high throughput is inevitable. This paradox is not exclusive to the developing world; health services in many Western countries have suffered similar problems over the years. Whereas there may be ways of slowing down such problems, such as performance incentives and structured career movement through the organisation, it is still crucial to ensure the availability of skilled personnel within the health sector by training personnel into the organisation. In the case of engineers and technicians, this involves health ministries in liaising with education ministries in establishing industrial attachments and practical experience periods within hospitals, using hospital systems and equipment during the learning process. Similarly, the continued provision of artisans is dependant upon Health Ministries offering industrial vocational training centres apprentice places within health care premises.

Many donor agencies active in the developing world have identified the sourcing of suitably trained technical personnel for the health sector as an issue with which they can provide assistance. The Government of Kenya, for instance, is working with the Austrian, German and Swedish Aid organisations in setting up training facilities for technicians and artisans throughout the country, with special emphasis on health care maintenance.

It is desirable for Health Ministries in developing countries to ensure their future availability of technical staff at all levels, by integrating their practical requirements with the education curriculum in the way discussed.

Training of Technical Personnel in Post

Where health services have suitably qualified technical staff appointed, there is still an ongoing need for training to develop the individuals in career terms. This training takes many forms, and each part should be considered a component of the process of formation, rather than an end in itself. The type of training may depend upon the cadre of person involved; there is a tendency to reserve the more expensive training such as overseas scholarships for engineers and technicians, rather than artisans.

To try and clarify a complex issue, this paper examines three main areas of training activity 'in post', that is, to qualified personnel occupying positions in a technical health care environment. Again, the criteria may equally apply to laundry managers, CSSD operational staff and radiographers as to engineering personnel. The correct operation of equipment is as crucial to its condition as good maintenance.

Area 1

'Hands-on' training, or training in the workplace. This way, or indeed should, begin with the manufacturers representative or agent providing detailed instruction in the operation and maintenance of new and commissioned equipment to both users and maintenance technicians. A properly organised equipment procurement programme will include this training component in the equipment tender.

Who will provide the 'hands on' training once the manufacturers/suppliers have left? Some of the larger teaching/consultant hospitals in developing countries may have all the services and equipment similar hospitals in the developed world utilise. This again is a matter when participation by donor agencies is beneficial. The UK Overseas Development Administration, by providing experts in an advisory role, supports local hospital engineers in a number of countries as they establish management structures, maintenance systems, budgetary control, and attempt to overcome supply and procurement and other problems. Training also includes the technicians and artisans, as, often for the first time, they carry out maintenance routines on complex hospital equipment and systems. In Mbeya, Tanzania, the UKODA have provided two hospital engineering experts in just such roles; one to develop management systems and provide management training; the other to organise maintenance and provide on-the-job training. This type of training has the benefit of forcing the trainers to work through the practical and logistical constraints of the local situation with their local colleagues, rather than merely providing western solutions which simply will not work in the developing world.

Area 2

Notwithstanding the above, there is a place for overseas scholarships and attachments, particularly for the senior cadres of staff. As part of their overall learning and development, they may require:

(1) Specialist equipment training not normally available in their own country. This may include practical attachments with manufacturers, to gain first hand experience of installing, commissioning, and maintaining the manufacturers' equipment. (2) It may include practical attachment to hospitals in the host country, to learn of the management techniques applied there and build up possible ideas for future. (3) Also it may include specialist courses at training centres, such as the NHS Training Centre at Eastwood Park Falfield. Such centres are increasingly tailoring their courses to accommodate guests from developing countries and even formulating 'packages' of courses containing a broad cross-section of topics'.

All the above 'overseas' scholarship' elements are valuable, if they are part of an overall development and training strategy. Unfortunately, all too often, the recipients of overseas scholarship awards are returned to organisations and workplaces where their overall training needs are not being thought through, and their development and career path have not been considered. In such instances, the new knowledge they have gained will soon be lost as they resign themselves to their actual environment, of which few of their lecturers and trainers of the previous months, are aware.

Area 3

The training, and guidance, of senior management in Health Ministries must not be forgotten. Whatever may happen at hospital level, it is fruitless if policies and decisions are not being formulted at the top by officials who are aware of the issues involved in the Health Care Equipment Management process. The World Health Organisation is active in the generation of such awareness amongst Senior Ministry officials, through its Global Action Plan for Health Care Equipment Management and Maintenance. Participating countries representatives are invited to appraise their own national situations in this area, during interregional workshops, and to gain information and advice from experts on policy formulation matters.

Summary

This paper has identified the components of training for hospital technology in developing countries; from senior ministry officials to artisans, from overseas scholarships to 'hands-on' training in the workplace.

There are many components of the training whole. Who should be responsible? As a profession, we should endeavour to support every aspect of Health Care Equipment Training in the developing world. The ways in which Government Development Agencies are already supporting training, in education and in hospitals have been mentioned; these should be reinforced and co-ordinated. The World Health Organisation has identified its role through the Global Action Plan. Training Institutions, such as the Higher Technical Institute in Cyprus and the NHS Training Centre, Falfield, are already accommodating engineers and technicians from developing countries.

So much has already been started. May it continue, strengthen, become more co-ordinated. In particular, let the equipment manufacturers and suppliers take their full share of responsibility for training, from the commissioning and start-up of equipment, to establishing training courses for technicians in developing countries.

Training at NHSTA, Falfield

by

Peter Lucas
BSc(Eng), MPhil, CEng, MIMechE
Estates and Engineering Development Manager
NHSTA Falfield

From Small Beginnings . . .

The origins of 'Falfield', as it is affectionately known in the NHS, can be said to have stemmed from the recommendations of the Advisory Committee on Hospital Engineering Training (ACHET) in 1967 which led to the establishment of the Hospital Engineering Training Centre at Eastwood Park near Wotton-under-Edge in Gloucesterhsire.

The acquisition of Eastwood Park by the Department of Health and Social Security in 1969 ended a long search for a suitable property or location in which to establish a national centre where training could be provided in engineering subjects which were special to health buildings and not adequately covered in the general range of engineering courses provided either by further or higher education or other training agencies.

The splendid Victorian mansion set in 216 acres of gardens, meadows and fields on the crest of a hill in the Severn Vale, to this day enjoys a location unsurpassed by almost any other training establishment. The views of the surrounding countryside are appreciated by all who visit the site and the village of Falfield is nearby. The larger towns of Thornbury and Wotton-under-Edge are within 5 miles and Bristol, Gloucester, Bath and Cheltenham are all within easy reach. It is easy to see why it was chosen all those years ago as the NHS national training centre.

The first training programme was part of the original suggestions by ACHET in 1967 but even before the 1974 Health Service reorganisation further courses were being developed in order to benefit all, what was then called, 'Works Group' staff plus courses to meet the needs of individual non-engineering disciplines. By the next round of reorganisation Falfield had become the Hospital Estate Management and Engineering Centre and was running courses for Quantity Surveyors, Regional Architects, Building Officers and Craft grades in addition to its expanding range of engineering and medical/technical courses.

Throughout this period the Director of Works Operations at the Department of Health and Social Security was responsible for the technical direction of the Centre and the Department itself was responsibile for financing it. In those days a nominal charge was made for attendance on courses but it by no means covered the true cost of the training.

1984 and All That

In April 1984 the National Health Service Training Authority assumed responsibility for all NHS training and initially requested the Department to continue its role of managing the Works training programme in collaboration with the National Staff Committee (Works) within the overall direction of the NHSTA. There followed a transition period during which Falfield was fully integrated into the NHSTA and full managerial control and funding responsibilities assumed by the Training Authority.

As is usual in these circumstances certain changes were made managerially, administratively and financially. These changes were felt to be necessary in order to bring the Centre into line with a much faster changing world than had hitherto been experienced in the NHS, to encourage the Centre to take stock of its activities and to take a more responsive stance to the emerging needs of the Service. In addition the NHSTA set self-financing targets for Falfield which meant that it had to take a much more entrepeneurial view of its activities and seriously attack issues of marketing, cost control and pricing policy that, it was felt, had received insufficient attention in the past.

It was also accepted that over the years Falfield had built up an enviable reputation for high quality and relevant training in the NHS and of course this pride in its products had to be protected and maintained. However it was also clear that the continued delivery of the traditional one week training modules would not in itself secure the future of the Centre. Thus it was necessary that the new wind of change that was blowing through the NHS should also be felt at Falfield to ensure first and foremost that the centre continued to provide training to the highest standards, to encourage the identification of new markets within the NHS for existing and new training courses, to identify new markets overseas and in the commercial world and to adopt managerial and financial policies that would ensure the development towards establishing Falfield on a self-funding basis in the future.

A Hectic Few Years!

The last three years have seen substantial developments at Eastwood Park, Falfield as it is now known. There has been put in place a new management structure.

This structure allowed for maximum responsibilities but retained clear line management principles and also allowed for the operation of separate cost centres.

Let us now take a look at what has been happening within the training area over the last year or two.

So much has happened in this area that it is difficult to know where to start. Perhaps we should start with the major part of Falfield's business — residential training courses.

Residential Training Courses

In 1981/2 Falfield offered 28 different courses for Works Staff and 12 different courses for Crafts grades. This list included five new courses for Works Staff and one new course for Crafts grades. It is interesting to note that all courses were either five or ten days long whatever the subject!

By 1985/6 Falfield was offering 42 different courses for PTB Works Staff and 18 different courses for Crafts grades. In this year the courses were divided into the following disciplines.

Electrical	17 courses
Estate Management	14 courses
Environmental	12 courses
Mechanical	8 courses

FORMATION AU CENTRE NHSTA, FALFIELD

Cet article décrit brièvement le développement de Falfield comme centre de formation pour le National Health Service, depuis le début jusqu'à la période actuelle. Les différentes formations disponibles sont classées par thèmes et il y a en outre une description des nouveaux cursus, soit à suivre sur place, soit en vue de faire l'objet de formation à l'étranger. En conclusion, l'article examine les futurs développements possibles.

Medical	7 courses
Miscellaneous	2 courses

By the way, the courses were still five or ten days in length!

By 1988/89 the number of courses listed in Falfield's training programme was 88 with 73 aimed at PTB Engineering and Managerial staff of all types and just 15 being provided specifically for Crafts grades. By the second half of that financial year, the identified themes were:-

Building Services	31 courses
Estate Management	24 courses
Medical	8 courses
Fire/Security	8 courses
Financial Management	8 courses
Sterilisation	4 courses
Energy	3 courses
Interpersonal Skills	2 courses

By this time each course had been redesigned to an optimum length and although the majority of the engineering orientated courses were still of five and ten days length, most other courses were of one, two or three days duration.

In that same year Falfield published a New Courses Brochure which listed no fewer than 28 new courses.

Hopefully, the audience will have seen our 1990/91 Residential Training Course Programme (if you haven't, please send for one!) and in there we illustrate 55 different courses for this financial year and the themes are now as follows:-

Estate Management	10 courses
Financial Management	10 courses
Health and Safety	9 courses
Sterlisation and Steam	5 courses
Medical	4 courses
Estate Maintenance	4 courses
BTEC Support Programme	4 courses
Quality Assurance	3 courses
Ventilation and Air Conditioning	2 courses
Career Development	2 courses
Lifts	1 course

Of course, all of those courses are delivered a number of times throughout the year. To give perhaps a better picture of where our current emphasis lies, the following table gives the number of course days offered in each theme this year:-

Sterilisation and Steam	245 course days
Medical	184 course days
BTEC Support Programme	100 course days
Estate Management	78 course days
Lifts	70 course days
Ventilation and Air Conditioning	60 course days
Estate Management	48 course days
Health and Safety	43 course days
Financial Management	42 course days
Quality Assurance	11 course days
Career Development	9 course days

In addition to the above, there are a number of new courses under development at present.

These include:-

The new HTM10
The new HTM22
The new HEI98
Noise Control
Electricity at Work Act
Control of Substances Hazardous to Health (COSHH)
Total Quality Management
Aneasthetic Equipment Servicing
Property Appraisal Techniques
Asset Rationalisation
Cost Analysis/Planning
Capital Charging Procedures
Estate Data Aquisition and Use
Capital vs Revenue Planning
Implications of 1992
Value for Money

These developments come out of new legislation such as the White Paper 'Working for Patients', the Health and Medicines Act 1988, new Technical Memoranda and Health and Safety Regulations and reflect current training needs in the NHS.

Clearly Eastwood Park, Falfield can no longer be considered *solely* as the place to send Craft grades for practical training. We certainly intend to maintain this service to the NHS and to ensure it is delivered with the utmost effectiveness for the foreseeable future. However the figures speak for themselves. The Centre has widened its product range beyond recognition and has thus widened its market accordingly to include all kinds of personnel in the NHS.

Locally Delivered Training

We have taken steps to make it known that some training courses can be delivered on the client's chosen own premises. This usually represents a cost saving to the client and can avoid the necessity for staff to stay away overnight.

The delivery of courses in this way has caused no great problem in cases where the required training is not based on equipment which is in regular use at the client's site. Of course portable equipment can always be transported from Eastwood Park but where it is hands-on operation of fixed equipment is necessary is it more difficult to find equipment to use. Courses which we have found are particularly suitable for local delivery are:-

Electrical Skills for Engineering Craftsmen and Plumbers (EITB scheme)
Mechancial Skills for Electrical Craftsmen (EITB scheme)
Medical Equipment Safety
Medical Gas Safety
Legionnaire's Disease
Water Management in Hospitals
Fire Safety Appraisals of Existing Hospitals
Control of Substances Hazardous to Health (COSHH)
Sterilisation
COSHH Audits

There has certainly been a definite shift towards an increasing amount of locally delivered training and while at the end of 1989/90 this aspect of our training activity amounted to a small percentage of our total volume delivery, locally delivered training activity is increasing.

Training for Overseas Healthcare Personnel

As a means of taking up spare capacity and as a way of assisting our colleagues from overseas, Falfield has increased its efforts to attract more clients from overseas countries.

The services offered to overseas clients are:-

- Attendance on programmed residential courses at Eastwood Park.
- Attendance on special residential courses at Eastwood Park which are staged specifically for small groups of overseas customers.
- Work experience and training placements in the UK.
- In-country training delivered by a team of staff from Eastwood Park.

Of course the training of overseas personnel is nothing new for Falfield. An excellent world-wide reputation has already been built up over the past 13 years in training overseas students in the fields of hospital engineering and medical equipment maintenance and this reputation has been a good base to build on.

Our major clients are the British Council, the Crown Agents, various governments all over the World, NHS Overseas Enterprises, individual hospitals in the Middle East and one or two private organisations.

The courses most in demand are Biomedical Equipment Maintenance, Steriliser Maintenance, Medical Gas and Vacuum Systems, Refrigeration and Air Conditioning.

Strategic Planning Training — Mereworth

Mereworth Strategic Planning workshops have been providing a service to the NHS since 1985.

The aims of this form of training exercise have been:-

- To encourage a multi-disciplinary approach to strategic planning for a District Health Authority;
- To provide guidance, examples and practice which leads to the successful production of a workable strategic plan together with year by year proposals for each care group;
- To test resource consequences of the planning proposals on computer programs; and
- To practice the best ways of presenting the Estate as a resource and the effects it can have on the delivery of healthcare.

The name Mereworth has over the years become part of the NHS vocabulary and by now many Districts have been through the Mereworth route and the methodology is now firmly in place in a high proportion of planning teams throughout the Service.

The Mereworth database is also undergoing radical change, change, as it must, to keep up to date with the changing world in the NHS, to ensure that strategic planning also embraces human resource development and finance, to encompass advances in information technology and not least to recognise the new legislation in the Health and Medicines Act and that proposed in the White Paper 'Working for Patients'.

Site Development at Eastwood Park

Anyone who has been visiting Eastwood Park regularly over the past couple of years cannot fail to have noticed that the accommodation and facilities have improved almost beyond recognition. Gone is the 'school dinners' approach to mealtimes together with the somewhat regimented approach to daily life.

The improvements are too numerous to mention individually but perhaps I could mention one or two. First and foremost is the undeniable and strong commitment towards a client centred orientation. These days delegates are treated as important individual customers for whom we try to provide a high quality personal service. After all we want them to come again! So we try hard to make life as comfortable and enjoyable as possible both while they are training and in their leisure time.

Thus we have a proper reception service, we address each delegate by their name, we accommodate special dietary needs and offer more flexible arrangements at mealtimes. All bedrooms now have tea and coffee making facilities and clock-radios. The decor and furnishing of all public spaces has recently undergone substantial modernisation and refurbishment.

There are still many more improvements we wish to make in order to keep pace with increased client expectations in this area and we hope that further improvements will be approved soon.

Eastwood Park can now host conferences, seminars, dinners and social events and has become a popular venue for local activities. Fees charged for these services, of course, provide a small though welcome boost to our income.

Finance and Information Systems Development

Like all parts of the NHS, the Training Authority and therefore Eastwood Park has to toe the line when it comes to systems to control finance, administration and personnel matters.

I think we can now clain to have made the transition from the previous, somewhat autonomous paper based situation to current integrated IT based systems. The site is now well equipped with Norsk-Data workstations that are linked both together and with the Training Authority's headquarters in Bristol.

Earlier in this paper I mentioned that we had taken a more marketing approach to our activities. It was clear that this had received scant attention in the past and there was strong evidence that the Centre was not getting through to as many prospective clients as it might.

During 1985/86, Falfield produced one A5 booklet about its courses plus an A5 folder listing the courses offered by each department. In 1987/88, two 6-monthly course calendars were mailed and in 1988/89, two 6-month course calendars plus two new course programmes were mailed to all Units and Districts together with full course details to all Personnel and Training Managers.

In 1990/91, the planned marketing activities are:-

- Two annual course calendars mailed twice to each Unit, District and Region.
- Two new courses brochures.
- A mailshot every month to selected target groups highlighting selected courses.
- Articles written and placed in appropriate journals.
- Advertisements placed in appropriate journals.
- Speaking at Conferences.

So — What of the Future?

This is where I have to say that Falfield's future role in the grand design of training for the NHS will become clearer as the direction of the Service itself becomes clearer.

However, in terms of training delivery at least, our course is set for the next year or two.

- Clearly we must respond to the training needs of the Service where we can assist NHS management to take maximum advantage of the opportunities presented in the Health and Medicines Act and the White Paper. Our activities over the next two or three years must reflect this.
- We must continue to support the training of hospital staff in matters that directly and indirectly affect patient safety and well being and in matters that affect the efficient operation and cost-effective use of valuable buildings and equipment.
- We will continue to provide up to the minute training on key areas of technical and medical issues in the NHS as well as new ones brought about by changes in legislation, regulations and incidents.
- We shall withdraw from delivering training that is readily available locally.
- We will be increasing the certification attached to our courses. We are already working with CGLI and BTEC and an increasing number of our courses are now being offered with optional certification at an appropriate level. Before the end of 1990 we intend to offer a 'first' — our own Certificate in Hospital Technology backed by BTEC. This is a trend we must pursue.
- We must continue to monitor the quality of our training and to ensure maximum effectiveness. We continually conduct post-course evaluation exercise on many of our courses. We want them to be as near as possible to our

clients needs and in addition want them to be good value for money.

- We will work closely with professional bodies in order to ensure that we can discuss and share a common understanding of the requirements for continuing professional development for their members.
- We will be increasing our support for local training initiatives and structures. This will mean the provision of trainer-training and ongoing support.
- We must ensure that the considerable experience and expertise of our staff is placed at the disposal of the Service not just by training delivery but also by technical consultancy and trainer support.
- We must continue to improve the facilities at Eastwood Park to reflect the increased standards now expected by our customers.

Training Authority policy over the last few months will mean that Falfield will in future be concentrating on the delivery of training that is specific to the NHS and that is sensible for a National centre to do. Other organisations will be encouraged to offer non-key training on a local basis and thus in future hospitals and Health Authorities will be purchasing their training from a range of providers.

However, the Training Authority and Falfield firmly believe in the motto 'Better Training — Better Health' and we pledge to play our part in that process.

A Systems Approach to Documenting Hospital Commissioning and Operating Policies

by

J. Kane-Berman
Medical Administration
Groote Schuur Hospital
Cape Town, South Africa
and
G. G. Jaros
Department of Biomedical Engineering
Groote Schuur Hospital
Medical Faculty
University of Cape Town, South Africa

Introduction

Groote Schuur Hospital is a 1,450 bed academic hospital situated on the slopes of Table Mountain in Cape Town. Together with the University of Cape Town Medical Faculty, it is responsible for the training of undergraduate and post graduate students in most health care disciplines and is highly regarded internationally for the research output of the medical and scientific staff who serve the Hospital and the Faculty in a joint capacity. All joint staff have patient care, teaching and research responsibilities and serve the entire Groote Schuur Hospital Region, consisting of six hospitals. The Region is managed as an integrated service by Groote Schuur Hospital's management team headed by the Chief Medical Superintendent. The patient care workload is heavy and is increasing steadily with the rapid urbanisation of the rural population. In 1988/89 96,000 patients were admitted to the inpatient facilities and 1.2 million outpatient attendances were recorded for the whole Region. Groote Schuur Hospital is fully integrated and does not tolerate discrimination on grounds of race, gender or creed.

Background to the Groote Schuur Hospital Redevelopment Project

When the original 800 bed hospital was commissioned in 1938 it was already recognised that it would be inadequate to meet the increasing needs of the citizens of Cape Town and the Cape Province.

The hospital expanded steadily in the next 40 years during which time additional land was purchased and proposals were put forward for increasing the bed capacity to 2,000. In 1979 the Groote Schuur Hospital Redevelopment Project (GSHRP) was approved by the Department of Health and Welfare and financing was authorised by the Treasury in 1982. Building commenced in January 1983 with the two main contracts, accounting for a 1,400 bed new hospital, a 750 bed multidisciplinary residence and extensive road and site works, being finally completed in December 1989, namely 71 months later. The remainder of the Project, which completes the upgrading of the old hospital buildings, has already commenced but will not be finished before 1993/94. The entire redeveloped hospital complex will ultimately contain 1,722 beds, 180,000m^2 of building (excluding the interstitial service spaces), 60 wards, 9 intensive care units containing 143 beds, 30 operating theatres, separate general emergency and trauma units, a large ambulatory care building, several large laboratories, paramedical clinical and teaching units, nursing education facilities, residential accommodation for 1,400 staff members and pre-school facilities for 240 children. Approximately half of the old main building will be used by the clinical departments in the Medical Faculty for research and teaching laboratories, offices and seminar rooms. It is a vast and inordinately complex organisation with a staff of 10,500 people and health care responsibilities which stretch beyond the borders of South Africa to our Southern African neighbours.

Architectural and Engineering Design Principles

The New Groote Schuur Hospital Consortia of architects, engineers and quantity surveyors were appointed in 1972. The consultants adopted a systems approach to the design and the construction methods for the building. Long before the clients' final brief was completed the main design concepts — insterstitial spaces between the user floors, modularity, repetitive 'H' pattern and the methods of construction — had been determined. These have been reported on previously at International Federation of Hospital Engineers Conferences and published in the Proceedings of 1980 and 1988[1, 2]. The process and system of documentation were based on Capricode developed by the Department of Health and Social Security (DHSS) in England[3].

Systems Approach to Planning

Systems theory formed the foundation of the hospital's approach to planning[4, 5]. This required a holistic approach to the hospital organisation, its environment and the interrelationships between hospital systems, subsystems and components. Understanding the hierarchical nature of systems, the relationships between inputs, processes and outputs, and the importance of feedback and control mechanisms was integral to the methodology utilised for analysing, synthesising and formulating the hospital's requirements[6]. The outcome of this process was docomented in comprehensive briefs.

MISE A L'ETUDE D'UN ESTABLISSMENT HOSPITALIER ET GESTION D'OPERATION — UNE APPROACHE PAR SYSTEMES

L'hôpital Groote Schuur est un CHU en pleines expansion et réorganisation. Il s'agit d'une organisation complex qui requiert des locaux utilisables au maximum, des systèmes d'operation, et une gestion parfaite, afin d'arriver à réaliser ses objectifs. Au cours des différentes phases d'étude, les designers et les architectes ont utilisé une approche par systèmes, qu'il s'agisse du projet global, de l'organisation ou des équipements. Cette approche se concrétise par la production d'une documentation qui décrit en détail les différentes dispositions et fonctions touchants les bâtiments, ainsi que les besoins exprimés par les utilisateurs. Une fois au stade de la mise en service, le bâtiment doit se conformer à toutes les dispositions et principles exprimés afin de garantir que l'espace, les services et les systèmes sont exploités de facon rentable. Pour fermer la boucle entre documentation et opérations, il a fallu mettre au point un système de manuels et une codification complète de ces manuels. Grâce à l'utilisation de nouveaux concepts de théorie des systèmes (Biomatrix et Teleon), il a été possible d'établir une codification basée sur les documents d'information mais qui englobe aussi tout le 'réseau vivant' de l'organisation dans sa totalité.

The Briefing Process

The hospital's briefing documentation was based on the Royal Institute of British Architects (RIBA) and the South African National Institute of Building Reserach (NBRI) guidelines[7, 8]. Many of the DHSS principles utilised in the Activity Database and Brigden's Design Briefing System were incorporated as a result of valuable contacts between members of the hospital staff and DHSS representatives[9, 10].

The Master Brief

The master brief, based on RIBA guidelines, incorporated the hospital's policies, as well as essential precepts, principles and client requirements and formed the basis for planning. This was followed by detailed descriptions of all major support systems — the result of in-depth analysis into the hospital's needs for catering, materials handling, goods distribution, communication, security and housekeeping services. After extensive research into alternatives the final decisions re these important infrastructural components of the hospital were fully documented for the planners and architects and incorporated in all departmental briefs. Many basic design principles depended on these decisions.

Departmental Briefs

The departmental briefs consisted of detailed schedules of accommodation, operational narratives and user requirement sheets.

The operational narrative was the individual user's story of how they intended their unit to function. It defined the unit's purpose, hours of operation, physical and functional relationships, departmental operating policies, goods, staff and patient movement and other information which enabled the architects to interpret the user's needs, from their input, and thence to produce a satisfactory design outcome.

The Commissioning Process

The same basic approach was used for commissioning, utilising all the preceding inputs and the processes of planning to achieve a successful outcome to the entire commissioning and activation process. British experience and literature was relied on heavily, once again, during this phase of the project[11].

The preparation of operating policy manuals was regarded as one of the most important commissioning tasks. Having based the planning and design principles on clearly defined hierarchical systems and subsystems — the operational policies for the management of the completed hospital in use had to mirror these planning and design principles — structurally, organisationally and logistically.

Policy Manual Principles

The preparation of the manuals entailed extensive, detailed revision of the policies upon which planning, design and construction had been based, to ensure that the facilities would be operationally efficient. In addition, the policies had to be documented in such a way that the resulting manuals could form the basis for all orientation, induction and in-service training courses. The manuals also had to serve as a ready reference for all staff in service and as a management tool for co-ordination and control of the building in use.

Equally important, was the need to compile these manuals so that:-

- the universal elements would be integral to all manuals, ensuring that repetitive logical order was maintained. 'Pattern Recognition' was regarded as essential for ease of transfer of personnel between units and to provide consistency and uniformity of systems and operations;
- each manual was substantive but had a logical place in the whole system — and
- each page or set of pages in a manual could stand alone as a policy statement on a system or subsystem but was an essential component of the whole manual;
- reviewing and, if necessary revising, policies and procedures could be achieved on a regular basis. Updating would be simply effected by issuing replacement pages, coded and dated, for insertion in the loose leaf policy manual binders.

Coding the Policy Manuals

It was apparent that the extensive system of policy manuals required systems based, structured codification to ensure ease of management. In the process of investigating existing coding systems and seeking the best code available, several basic principles were determined.

Policy Manual Coding Concepts

The most important requirements for the coding system were that it had to be comprehensive, systems based, matriceal, hierarchical, adaptable, expandable, divisible and multi-purpose.

Abbotts briefing documents for hospitals, developed for the NBRI were broadly based on the C1/sfb coding system[12, 13]. Abbot and Tanton adopted and expanded the C1/sfb system as the basis for their briefing guidelines, utilising a numeric, three table, three digit structure eg 400.000.000[14].

Using the structure of the NBRI briefing code as the basis for the operational policy manual coding system completed the circle from briefing to operations and theoretically linked the original user's requirements, incorporated in the operational narratives and forming part of the original brief, to the final management of the completed building and its operational systems. In practice, however, the NBRI code proved to be too restrictive despite the code's apparent flexibility.

The Biomatrix and Telsonics

In researching alternatives to the NBRI structure, recent work by Jaros and Cloete indicated an exciting development in systems theory which, applied to hospital organisation and management, opened up a new approach to the solution of the problem[15].

Jaros and Cloete emphasise the importance of processes as a starting point to any analysis of systems. In addition, they point out the hierarchical nature of things and the network (matrix) nature of the relationships between processes and things. In their terminology 'the living network of all things on earth' is called the Biomatrix and the essential, purposeful life processes are referred to as Teleons[16, 17]. An important feature of their approach is the separation of purposeful processes (teleons) into two major types:-

(1) Exoteleons, which are those purposeful processes which are directed in their purpose towards the surroundings or suprasystems external to the organism or organisation.

(2) Endoteleons, which are the teleons directed in their purpose towards the internal environment, subsystems and components of the organism or organisation.

The difference between these two types is important for a real understanding and management of an organisation such as a Health Care Region. While exoteleons exist mainly in order to ensure optimum functioning of the organisation in fulfilling its mission within society, endoteleons are or should be designed to support this role by maintaining the system with all its subsystems and components at an optimum operational level. In an organism or organisation all the endoteleons together form the endodynamics and all the exoteleons the exodynamics of the system, respectively.

Application of the Biomatrix Concepts to the Coding of the GSHRP Policy Manuals

The entire GSH Region can be regarded as a part of the Biomatrix. It is a dynamic network of proceeses and things situated largely within the geographical confines of the Western Cape but some responsibilities reach out to the far corners of the entire Province, and indeed the results of the clinical, teaching and research activities have influence internationally.

All the entities are, however, bound together by the processes of which they are part. It is only through these processes that their role becomes meaningful, thus confirming the overwhelming importance of processes within the system.

The organisation has three major dimensions that have to be taken cognisance of in the coding system, in the form of three fields.

These fields are:-

(1) Physical location of entities and processes. Such a field could, for example, indicate the Region, the hospitals, floors, wards and rooms in a large hospital or a suburb, street, building and rooms in a community clinic or even in a private home if health care activity takes place there.
(2) Entities. These could be staff, patients, equipment, consumables, funds, and other resources.
(3) Processes, which are the life force of the organisation.

The first two fields are the ones that are generally used for coding systems. They are not problematic and therefore will not be discussed further here. The process field, however, which is the main new contribution, based on the Biomatrix approach, will be discussed in detail in terms of the coding system.

The Process (Teleonic) Field

This field consists of eight Tables and has been divided into three subfields. The latter are separated from one another by a colon in order to make the handling of the code easier. The general formula for the entire field containing eight Tables, is as follows:-

n_1	$alpha_2$	$alpha_3$	$alpha_4$	$alpha_5$	$alpha_6$	$alpha_7$	$n(2)_8$
Subfield 1	:	Subfield 2		:	Subfield 3		

* alpha = alpha character.
* the subscript denotes the number of the Table, eg n_1 is the numeric character for Table I, $alpha_2$ is the alpha character for Table II.

•() indicates the number of characters in the table.

The contents of the various tables are as follows:-

Table I (n_1): Main Grouping — This table forms the top of the teleonic hierarchy. Apart from the two main groups, viz, exodynamics and endodynamics, it also contains the code for the overall governance which is essential for the organisation to function as a whole.

Example 1: Table I for Main Grouping.

Table I — Main Grouping

2 = Exodynamics
3 = Endodynamics
4 = Overall governance

Table II ($alpha_2$): Functional Subgroups — For each of the main groupings there are different subgroupings. Two examples are given:-

Example 2: Table II for exodynamics (ie 2⌴) contains the main exodynamic functions ($alpha_2$).

Table II: 2⌴ — Exodynamics

A = Patient care
B = Education
C = Research
D = Community Service
E = Public Relations
F = Medico-Legal
.
.
.
W = Exodynamic Governance

Example 2a: Table II for endodynamics (ie 3⌴) contains the main endodynamic functions ($alpha_2$).

Table II: 3⌴ — Endodynamics

A = People
B = Buildings
C = Technology
D = Information
E = Materials
F = Services
G = Security
.
.
W = Endodynamic Governance

Tables III-V ($alpha_3$, $alpha_4$, $alpha_5$: Finer Teleonic Groupings — These tables define the Divisions, departments and units which form the clinical service structure of the GSH Region.

Example 3: Table III for exodynamics (2): patient care (A) (ie) 2A:⌴) contains the clinical Divisions ($alpha_3$).

Table III: 2A ⌴— Exodynamics: Patient Care

C = Paediatrics and Child Health
M = Medicine
P = Psychiatry
S = Surgery
N = Nursing
W = Obstetrics and Gynaecology
.
.
Z = . . .

Example 4: Table IV for exodynamics (2): patient care (A): Division of Medicine (M) (ie 2A: M⌴) lists Departments ($alpha_4$).

Table IV: 2A:M⌴ — Exodynamics: Patient Care: Division of Medicine

C = Community Health
D = Dermatology
G = Geriatrics
L = Medicine (Units)
M = Medicine (Clinics)
N = Neurology
.
.
.
Z = . . .

Example 5: Table V for exodynamics (2): patient care (A): Division of Medicine (M): Department of Medicine (M)(ie 2A:MM⌴) lists Units or Sections in Departments ($alpha_5$).

Table V: 2A:MM⌴ — Exodynamics: Patient Care: Division of Medicine; Department of Medicine (Clinics)

A = Cardiac Clinic
B = Respiratory Clinic
C = GIT Clinic
.
.
.
Z = . . .

Tables VI and VII and VIII (alpha$_6$, alpha$_7$, n(2)$_8$: Description of Teleonic Activities.

Example 6: Table VI for all exodynamics (2): patient care (A) all Divisions; departments and units (XXX) (ie 2A: XXX) contains the facilities within which the major patient care activities take place (alpha$_6$).

Table VI: (2A:XXX:$\underset{\wedge}{\sqcup}$) — Exodynamics: Patient Care: All Divisions; Departments; Units

A	=	Wards
B	=	Clinics
C	=	Emergency Units
D	=	Theatres
E	=	X-Ray Suites
F	=	Radiation Therapy Suites
G	=	Laboratories
H	=	Therapy Suites
J	=	ICU's
K	=	Day Wards
L	=	Special Wards
M	=	Dialysis Units
.		
.		
.		
Z	=	. . .

Table VII consists of generic activities that take place in all facilities.

Example 7: Table VII for exodynamic (2): patient care (A): All Divisions; departments and units (XXX) and facilities (X) (ie 2A: XXX:X$\underset{\wedge}{\sqcup}$) is the description of the activities (alpha$_7$).

Table VII: (2A:XXX:X$\underset{\wedge}{\sqcup}$) — Exodynamics: Patient Care: All Divisions; Departments; Units; Facilities

A	=	Unit Management
B	=	Patient Management
C	=	Public Management
D	=	Diagnostic Services
E	=	Therapeutic Services
F	=	Medical Services
G	=	Paramedical Services
H	=	Pharmacy
I	=	Social Support
.		
.		
.		
Z	=	. . .

Table VIII defines the activities listed in Table VII in greater detail (n(2)$_8$).

Example 8: Details of exodynamic (2): patient care (A): all Divisions; Departments and Units (XXX): facilities (X); patient management (B) (ie 2A:XXX:XB$\underset{\wedge}{\sqcup}\underset{\wedge}{\sqcup}$).

Table VIII: (2A:XXX:XB$\underset{\wedge}{\sqcup}\underset{\wedge}{\sqcup}$) — Exodynamics: Patient Care: All Divisions; Departments; Units; Facilities; Patient Management

10	=	Special Patients
20	=	Referrals
30	=	Admissions
40	=	Transfers
50	=	Deaths
60	=	Discharges
70	=	Patient Emergencies
80	=	Notifications
.		
.		
.		
90	=	

Comment

Because of its size only a small portion of the system has been illustrated. The system is still being developed as details are incorporated into the existing framework. This expandability is one of the major advantages of the system.

A further advantage of the coding system is that each subfield can be used on its own or in combination with another or both remaining subfields, to provide a concise, general reference system for all hospital files, correspondence and documentation. This is possible because of the unique character of each subfield ie Subfield I = n × 1, Alpha × 1; Subfield II = alpha × 3; Subfield III = alpha × 2, n × 2.

Conclusions

The structure of the documented policy system not only reflects the briefing systems concepts, utilising the basic structure of the NBRI briefing code, but also incorporates the Biomatrix systems concepts. Objectives, structure, process, people and things are woven together into a framework which can accommodate and co-ordinate the complex network of the Biomatrix. The total system provides the governance which is essential for the management of complex organisations.

As the policy manual system is gradually constructed in the process of commissioning, the degree to which the coding system meets the stated objectives becomes steadily more apparent. The method of codification which has been developed is proving to be fully comprehensive, systems based, utilises both matrix and branching tree structures hierarchically, is very flexible being both expandable and divisible and serves many purposes.

References

(1) Shapiro B., du Toit G. A., Hospitals: Modular Design and Structure — An Integrated Approach; Proceedings of the 6th International Congress of Hospital Engineering, American Society for Hospital Engineering, Washington, 1980.

(2) Shapiro B., du Toit G., Design and Construction of the New Main Building at Groote Schuur Hospital in Cape Town. Paper presented at IFHE 10th World Congress. 17-22 July 1988. Edmonton, Alberta, Canada, 1988.

(3) DHSS. Capricode, Capital Projects Code: Hospital Building Procedure Notes 1-5. HMSO, London, 1969.

(4) Von Bertallanfy L., General Systems Theory. George Braziller, New York, 1968.

(5) Kast F. E., Rosenzweig J. E., Organisation and Management A Systems Approach. Second Edition, McGraw-Hill Kogakusha Ltd, Tokyo, 1974.

(6) Kane-Berman J., Ward Design for the New Groote Schuur Hospital: How to satisfy the users: Process and Outcome. Paper presented at the International Hospital Federation Congress, Lausanne, 1983.

(7) RIBA. Architect's Job Book. London: RIBA Publications Ltd, London, 1973.

(8) Woolley J. C., The Architectural Brief and Planning Information (Hospital Design 9). National Building Research Institute Bulletin 59, CSIR Research Report 277, Pretoria, 1970.

(9) Brigden R., Personal Communication, 1983.

(10) DHSS. Guide to A and B Activity Data Sheets and their use in Health Building Schemes, HMSO, London, 1982.

(11) Millard G., Commissioning Hospital Buildings. Third Edition. King Edwards Hospital Fund, London, 1981.

(12) Abbott G. R., Briefing and Design Guide. General Ward. Health Care Building Series Report Number 2. Council for Scientific and Industrial Research, Pretoria, 1983.

(13) Tanton J., Personal Communication, 1985.

(14) RIBA. C1/sfb. Construction Indexing Manual, 1976 Revision. RIBA Publications Ltd, London, 1976.

(15) Jaros G. G., Cloete A., Biomatrix: The Web of Life. World Futures, 1987; 24: 215-236.

(16) Jaros G. G., Teleonics: The Study of Process-based Systems in Proceedings of the XI IFAC World Congress, Talliun, USSR, 13-17 August 1990 (in print).

(17) Cloete A., Jaros G. G., The Biomatrix: Optimisation and Efficiency of Teleons in Lasker, GE. ed. Advances in Systems Research and Cybernetics, International Institute for Advanced Studies, Windsor, Ontario, Canada, 1989.

The Westminster and Chelsea Hospital Project

The Experience of Commercial Design and Development Techniques on a Large NHS Project

by

R. Wheeler
CS Project Consultants (Project Managers)
S. Webster
Sheppard Robson (Architects)
and
R. Evans
Donald Smith Seymour and Rooley
(Services Engineers)

Introduction

The North West Thames Regional Health Authority together with the Riverside Health Authority evolved a concept that at the time was visionary but has since proved to be the pathfinder in the brave new world that the Government has decreed for the British National Health Service.

During recent years pressures have been increasing on Health Authorities to trim their budgets as inflation has risen, labour and equipment costs increased, patient numbers grown and medical and communication technology advanced.

In response to these pressures the NWTRHA, as part of their Regional Strategic Plan, identified the need for the redistribution of resources from the Riverside District to the Shire Health Authorities. The Riverside Health Authority responded by proposing the rationalisation of their acute services and in 1987 together with the NWTRHA carried out an option appraisal that would lead to the closure of five hospitals and the building of a new General District Teaching Hospital.

The Westminster and Chelsea Hospital from its conception has established itself as an innovative project, breaking new ground in many ways. Perhaps the most significant being the adoption of methods used in the commercial development world to finance and procure a project quickly.

The progress of this new hospital is being watched closely and the level of its success will and has already, without a doubt, led to the development of other NHS schemes being progressed along similar paths. The impetus perhaps being generated by the publication last year of the Government's White Paper 'Working for Patients'.

The project, at present, is two and a half years into its four and a half year programme and some 14 months into its 37 month construction period. This then is an interim report.

The Concept

The preferred option that emerged from the appraisals and feasibility studies was to retain the Charing Cross and develop the site of the existing St Stephen's Hospital.

This rationalisation of acute beds would realise significant savings of many millions of pounds per year which then could be redistributed within the Region. What also became apparent was that if this re-organisation could be achieved in the sort of time frame undertaken by commercial developers then the revenue savings would be made much earlier and the Regional Strategic targets be reached much sooner than could have normally been expected.

The target therefore was to plan, design and construct the new hospital in four and a half years. A timescale, that to my knowledge, has never been achieved for a major NHS hospital. (See Fig 1).

It is interesting to note that this proposed programme offered not only the early release of resources but the opportunity for the traumatic period of decanting and decommissioning to be kept to a minimum limiting, hopefully, the inevitable loss of morale and uncertainty that is the usual consequence of a major re-organisation.

It must be emphasised that from a very early stage this radical programme was agreed in principle by both the Regional and District Health Authorities and the Department of Health. This was vital for the project as the DOH was to play a very important role in accepting a flexible approach to procedures and processing the AIP in a relatively short period.

Having set target dates, financing the project was considered. A new large complex hospital requires high capital expenditure over, what in this case, would be a very short period. Included in the early studies was the consideration of what was termed 'unconventional' funding — that is the 'up-front' sale of existing properties within the Region with a phased handover to a developer as they became vacant thereby generating income. A joint venture with a commercial developer (including land swap) was also seriously considered but at that time the DOH and the Treasury raised concerns at such methods.

The concept was now in place . . . how then was it to be implemented?

Procedures — A Flexible Approach

Conventionally health building projects in the United Kingdom have had to be fully designed and signed off by the design team before the works could be tendered as a lump sum contract. This has resulted in periods of 10 to 12 years for the completion of a new hospital.

It was necessary therefore to look to the commercial world and the use of fast track planning, design and construction techniques and to consider running the 'Capricode' stages concurrently.

During the feasibility studies the Department of Health procedures were investigated and analysed. Capricode is a check list itemised into various stages that monitor and

L'APPLICATION DES TECHNIQUES COMMERCIALS AU PLANNING ET A LA CONSTRUCTION DU GRAND HOPITAL DES SERVICES DE SANTE PUBLIQUE ANGLAISES

A la suite de la Directive du Governement Brittanique les services de santé publique ont dû revoir leur méthode d'operation, leur organisation, leurs revenues, et leur gérances des equipment et de leurs biens mobiliers.

La necessité d'avoir à exercer leurs fonctions dans des batisses agée et maintenant inaptes, pose un lourd fardeau sur leur budget.

Récemment certains de ces Autorités ont eu recours aux sources commercials pour des moyen alternatifs de financer et de construire de nouveaux hôpitaux.

Nous avons, dans le cas de l'Hôpital de 'Westminster and Chelsea', une méthode radicalement nouvelle de planning et de construction d'un grand hôpital sur un site restreint à Londres (GB) avec l'emploi des techniques commerciales rapides.

cross reference the briefing, design, cost control, tendering, construction, commissioning and evaluation activities in a logical sequence. It is this logic that gives the code its strength and enables it to be used in a flexible way.

Programming

In determining that the project should be carried out under a fast time table, that the Capricode stages should run together and that the design and construction periods should overlap it was necessary to 'map-out' the sequences in a logical manner to establish critical areas and activities. The Management Control Plan was prepared. With the preferred option established the briefing and initial design work (stage 2) took place at the same time as the preparation of the API (stage 1). Full planning consultation was carried out during this period.

It is important to understand that as stages 1 and 2 were being carried out concurrently, cost checks against the developing AIP were essential. Following the completion of the planning consultation and the AIP, detailed design (stage 3) was started before Budget Cost. During this period the tender documents for early works packages were prepared and work started on site following the completion of the Budget Cost.

The MCP formed the bases for other more detailed programmes such as the design, construction and procurement programmes. This method of very detailed planning enables the Design and Construction teams to work in a very disciplined but flexible manner.

As the design period was short it was necessary to further separate and overlap this process. The form of the proposed building and its structure was conceived at an early stage. The development of the shell and the internal departmental planning (medical planning) was carried out at the same time by separate but co-ordinated teams.

The Management Contractor had been appointed during the stage 1/2 period to enable buildability, market costs and material availability exercises to be carried out during the early design development stages.

This then was the strategy . . . what of the philosophy and operation?

The Problem

The problem facing the design team was how to accommodate 88,000m^2 of scheduled usable area plus the associated circulation, communication and plant space on to a site of 2.84h in a central London site in four and a half years.

The Architectural Intentions

The architects wished to break down the barrier between a hospital as an institution and the everyday environment in which it was located. Not by means of scale but by function, by incorporating shops along the frontage of the Fulham Road. At the same time they wished to make the best use of the usable space on the site rather than waste it on left over lightwells and courtyards which over time would be built over, and in the meantime would not give any benefits to occupants. The third objective was to have a legible building.

These objectives were reached through the transfer of the concept of an atrium from other building types to a hospital.

Mechanical ventilation had been developed for the atrium. However, it was not possible to reach agreement with the DOH regarding the fire principles of this area and so the design was amended to an earlier concept of a natural ventilated covered courtyard.

As yet unpublished studies based on research in Canada indicate therapeutic benefits are derived from an atrium hospital. The architect suggests that this may be because it allows for the popular sport of people watching which would relieve the enforced tedium of being confined in in-patient accommodation or waiting in large waiting areas so common in many of our larger buildings, not just hospitals! Opportunities have been sought therefore to create spaces on the bridges linking departments across the atrium to provide places to step aside and watch the activities of the rest of the hospital. The privacy in the rooms around the perimeter of the atrium has been taken care of in the design and specification of the windows themselves which permit views out while strictly controlling the view in cue. Another subliminal therapeutic benefit is given by the colouring that is given to the space. There is a perception that light, bright colours indicate cleanliness and health and these have been deliberately selected in the development of the interior, which is generally in high-key colours and filled with daylight coming from the large roof above.

At this point, it may be as well to give some statistics about the building and the atrium. The main building itself is 156m long by 84m wide by 31.5m high. The atrium is enormous, 116m long by 52.8m wide by 36m high. It is longer than a football pitch and has the area of 17 tennis courts. The volume of air in the atrium is equivalent to 1,000 houses.

Constraints

In achieving these architectural objectives a number of constraints have had to be met. As a teaching hospital the Westminster and Chelsea hospital does not come under the control of the local planning authority but has a special procedure set out in the DoE Circular 18/84 which requires the usual consultations, the same documentation, but takes away from the local authority the ability to sanction the scheme. This is substituted by a right to object or not object. In the circumstances, the Royal Borough of Kensington and Chelsea insisted that the development conform to their usual site plot ratio of 2.521. Policies on parking, waste disposal, incineration, traffic and pedestrian movements all had to be agreed with the local authority and, as the Fulham Road is a designated road, also with the Department of Transport. The unstated constraint was that a large hospital of irreducable size had to be inserted into a residential neighbourhood. It was therefore a problem of reconciling the client's brief with community interests so much so that a major redesign was undertaken in July 1988 which effectively took out six months from the time frame. The proposed completion date stayed the same.

The major constraint fashioning the design of the atrium has been the health services 'Fire Code Policies and Principles' and 'HTM 81'. These documents give guidance to hospital designers to provide a suitable escape strategy. It was decided to transfer the concept of escape commonly found in contemporary city office buildings to the hospital as this offered the advantages of the smaller compartments, shorter escape distances to a point of safety and quicker evacuation. This pattern of a series of external escape towers and a race track plan of interlinked compartments on every floor to allow progressive horizontal escape has also been adopted in hospitals in other countries. The designers excpected to be able to build on this experience.

Because there is a large volume of air enclosed under the roof surrounded by a large building constantly losing heat to the environment, the atrium tends to operate as a natural engine. The internal ambient temperature is controlled by natural convection from air intakes below the lower ground floor but fire separated from the basement by two fire resisting constructions and there is a range of louvres that occupy the entire perimeter of the building above the uppermost occupied floor.

Operational Policies and the Activity DataBase

Because it was intended to build the hospital in four and a half years and carry out the entire planning and building in

54 months the usual consultation followed in this country had to be modified. The project speed dictated that the brief used for the various departments in the hospital should be based on standard existing policies in the NWT Region and upon the activity database sheets prepared by the DOH. This proved a less than perfect approach because there were difficulties in briefing the designers about the new technologies required in the building. For example, the idea of the digital imaging in the radiography department which is being proposed, DINS/PACS, and with the Cook/Chill kitchen proposed rather than a more conventional 'cook-on-the-premises' kitchen. There were also difficulties in using the activities data for the academic departments.

The Building Process

Another technique transferred from other building types was the idea of using fast track construction principles.

The concept was to build the envelope of the building as quickly as possible using steel frame, light weight steel sheeting and concrete floors, standard service cores etc, enabling the fast erection of the external cladding and roof so as to allow the fit-out of the hospital to proceed in dry conditions. For the services the idea of 'Shell and core' was introduced from office buildings.

Services Design

The services design solutions for the Westminster and Chelsea Hospital are a radical departure from the established United Kingdom public sector health care norms. The fast track construction requirements and the building design with its large atria has dictated some changes while the location of the building on a congested inner city site have necessitated other changes to control the environmental impact. The emergence of new technology and the drive to control energy usage have also resulted in the evolvement of new design solutions.

Fast Track Requirements

As expected in order to design and construct a 655 bed teaching hospital in four and a half years early programming indicated the necessity to complete the design and commence installation of some of the services distribution while in some areas planning and design was still continuing. In order to enable this process to happen in addition to letting the services contracts in a number of packages it was decided to adopt a commercial shell and core plus fit out approach and alter the philosophy for a hospital services street.

Instead of the primary services distribution being at high level above the main hospital communication routes a system of distributing all of the primary services vertically through a number of services risers was adopted. These services together with all of the principal plant rooms were incorporated in a shell and core package and has enabled the main services distribution to be prefabricated and installation has commenced following erection of the steel work and the pouring of slabs on a zone by zone basis significantly reducing construction time.

Energy Conservation

A thermal analysis and detailed studies of electrical load profiles were prepared and a running cost and capital cost analysis of all of the alternative systems compared. (See Fig 2 and 3). On a cost effective basis the final design solution was a combined heat and power system with electrical energy being generated from two 1.5Mw gas turbines providing high grade heat for process steam, absorption refrigeration machines, heating and hot water service requirements. (See Figs 4 and 5).

The system is driven by heating requirements and in times of low electrical demand surplus electrical energy is sold to the grid. The turbines are dual fuel fired and capable of running in parallel with the National Grid thereby providing a high level of supply security and avoiding the need for local standby generation and dual electrical feeds reducing capital costs and maintenance requirements.

Further energy saving measures include a controlled naturally ventilated atria, air to air heat recovery utilising plate heat exchangers and the use of low energy motors, transformers and light fittings.

In order to maximise the operational efficiency of the engineering systems control is effected by a database management system allowing the operators total flexibility in system and plant selection.

Fire Engineering

An integrated building design and fire engineering philsophy has been adopted after detailed analysis of fire loads within all areas of the building and the study of fire reporting evacuation and control procedures.

The entire building is monitored by an addressable smoke detector system providing various levels of information from the fire control point to nurses stations and operating smoke control regimes within the atria and ventilation plant.

The majority of the building, with the exception of certain clinical areas such as operating theatres, is covered by a sprinkler system integrated with other fire control regimes this has allowed a reappraisal of normal hospital fire fighting policies and obviated the need to provide a hose reel system.

Environmental Design

Careful consideration has been given to the design of the internal environment and the impact of the building on the external environment.

Internally the large naturally ventilated atria with the provision to control the air flow rates in winter and summer has provided a cost effective and energy efficient solution to a large part of the internal environment and has obviated the need for air conditioning to the atria and many of the surrounding areas of accommodation.

The CHP system utilises base energy at high efficiencies leading to the lowering of the overall CO_2 emissions. Dry air coolers are used to dissipate the heat of rejection from the absorption refrigeration plant. These coolers are acoustically treated to limit the impact on the external environment and avoid the need for evaporative cooling and associated problems of legionella pneumophila.

The adoption of absorption cooling avoids the need for refrigeration plant operating with CFC's. Building construction elements and insulation materials have also been selected that do not contain or require CFC's in their manufacturing process.

New Technology

As well as the use of the latest technology for the control and optimisation of the building services systems much of the plant being used in the building contains the latest technological developments. The gas turbines in particular are of a new design providing significantly higher efficiencies than was hitherto attainable with machines of their size.

It is proposed that diagnostic medicine will be assisted by the use of a digital X-Ray system and digital Nurse Call and music systems are also incorporated in the design.

Conclusion

This short progress report has hopefully given an insight into the Westminster and Chelsea Hospital project and the commercial approach to health care building.

WESTMINSTER AND CHELSEA HOSPITAL

TIMETABLE FOR THE FAST-TRACK HOSPITAL

Feasibility study complete	November 1987
Appointment of Project Consultant Team	December 1987
Concept in Place	December 1987
→ Commencement of detailed briefing and planning layout	January 1988
Planning Application Submitted	April 1988
Appointment of Management Contractor for pre-construction phase	June 1988
Approval in Principle ; submission to DOH	July 1988
Revision to Design(due to planning requirements)	July 1988
Planning Approval received	December 1988
DOH Approval in principle	December 1988
St Stephens Hospital decanting commences	January 1989
Decanting complete	March 1989
Budget Cost	March 1989
→ Demolition & Construction works commence	May 1989
Handover of department for early fit-out (Radiology Department/A&E Rooms, Computer suite)	October 1991
→ Practical Completion	June 1992
Main commissioning and fit-out of Hospital Services commences	June 1992
Hospital open to first Patient	October 1992

54 Months; 4.5 Years; 37 Months

Figure 1: Time table for the fast track hospital.

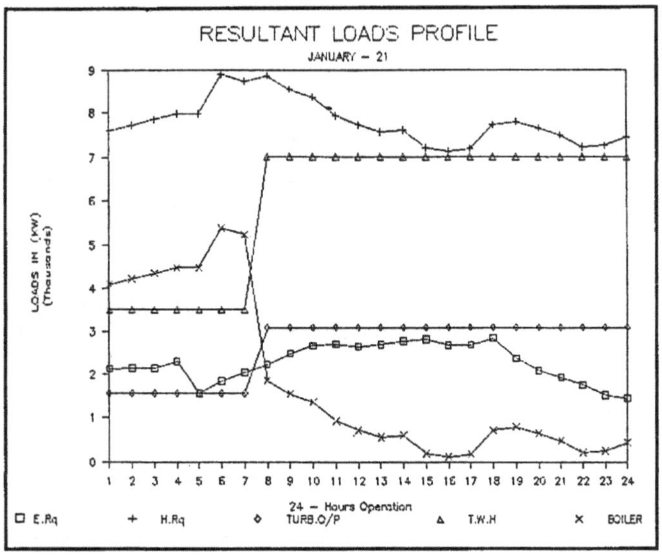

Figure 2: Resultant loads profile (January).

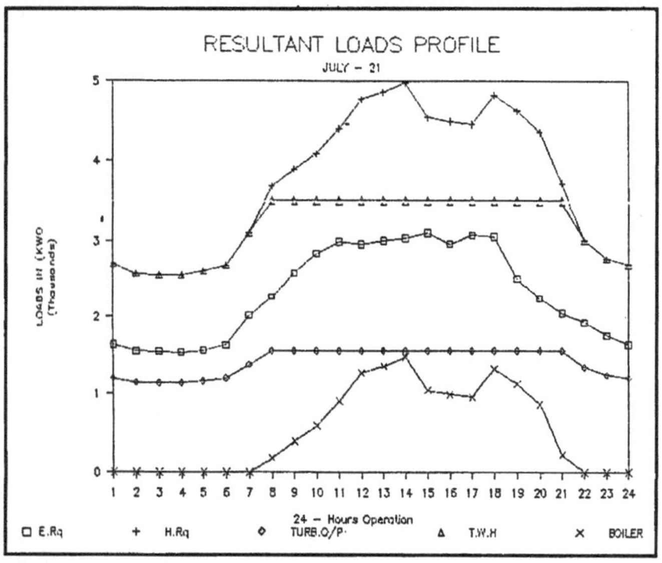

Figure 3: Resultant loads profile (July).

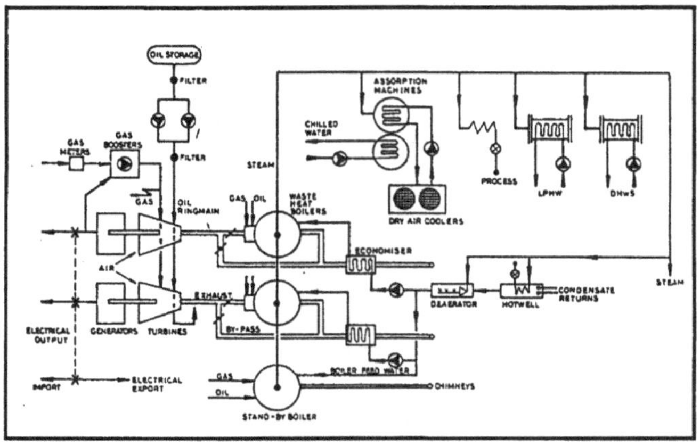

Figure 4: Thermal Schematic CHP System.

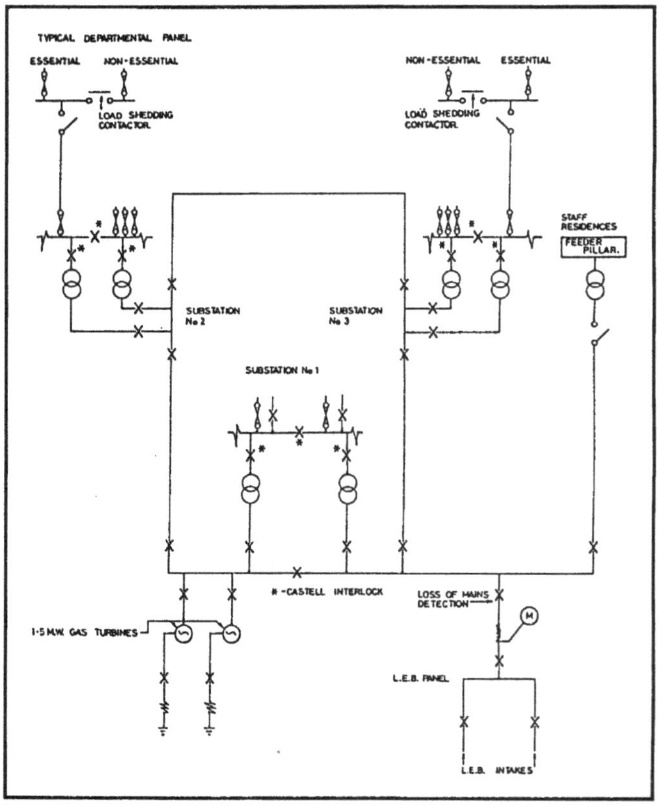

Figure 5: Electrical Schematic Combined Heating and Power System.

Integrated Resource Based Planning and Design for Primary Health Care Buildings

by

G. R. Abbott and M. D. Steyn
Division of Building Technology, CSIR,
PO Box 395, Pretoria 0001, South Africa

Introduction to the Health Care Problem in South Africa

In common with many developing countries South Africa is faced today with a troubled economy, a burgeoning population and a low rate of growth. With the high rate of urbanisation it is said that greater Durban has become, after Mexico City, the fastest growing city in the world. Other centres throughout South Africa are not far behind. Those responsible for health services are facing their greatest crisis yet. The clamoring demand for health services is fast outstripping our ability to provide services from the relatively diminishing resources at our disposal[1].

South Africa at present spends approximately 5.4% of its GNP on health[2]. This is over the target for the year 2000 of the WHO of 5% GNP per annum and high compared to many other countries with a similar GNP per capita. As a proportion of GNP per capita this has grown marginally over the last decade. However this could change as, in common with other countries with a high population and low eceonomic growth rates, the population growth rate is outstripping the economic growth rate leaving, in effect, less money for more people.

We have inherited and built on a fragmented delivery system with different authorities having responsibility for different sectors of health care. It is an extremely complex environment with overlapping spheres of responsibility where integrated planning is difficult to achieve. Within authorities, planning is often based solely on capital level expenditure as in many cases there is no mechanism for planning co-ordination between capital and operating expenditure.

There is currently also an imbalance in health services favouring higher, curative level care — only 4% of health expenditure is at PHC level. However the new national health strategy[3] places the highest emphasis on the need to ensure the provision of primary health services within reach of all in South Africa.

Finally, as in the provision of health services, there are many different authorities involved in the provision of health buildings. Standards of provision and design vary considerably from those that are underplanned to the over-designed.

While highlighting many of the problems inherent in the health delivery system in South Africa it would not be right to conclude this section without paying tribute to the dedicated health professionals and workers who are providing a high level of care and without noting the improvements that have been achieved in the health status of the population in general. Most WHO target health indicators for the year 2000 have been achieved for all sectors of the community, many are indeed comparable to those in the developed world[2]. That there is, however, still room for improvement is acknowledged and perhaps the key factors in achieving an improvement in health status are:-

- more effective management aimed at an equitable distribution of resources (financial and manpower);
- the development of a uniform approach to the provision of services through which both national goals and the specific needs of the community served can be considered; and
- the development and use of uniform standards of provision and design.

Framework for a Solution

In looking for a way to approach the provision of health buildings it is tempting to start from too narrow a point of departure and focus on a symptom rather than the problem as a whole. Control over what is built has been approached through fixed need, area and cost norms (eg provide one nurse examination room per 2,500 population at a maximum area and cost of 60m^2 and R27 300 respectively). Such national need norms do not, however, make provision for real regional differences in epidomiology, service expectations, available resources or, unless regularly updated, for change in service level necessary over time. Fixed area and cost norms have, in addition, been found to be counterproductive resulting in more expensive buildings[1]. The point of departure, we believe, should rather be from a more general problem definition, ie the provision of a health service that is effective, equitable and affordable.

The degree to which a health service can claim to be effective could be related to the level of improvement over time in the health indicators of those served. An equitable service could be defined as one displaying a balance in the level of service provided to different regions and communities. However while it would be a laudable and desirable goal to provide a fully comprehensive and equitable health service to all members of the community, what can be provided is limited, in practical terms, by the resources — including both capital and operating funds as well as health staff — at the disposal of the providers. The service must also be affordable.

As building professionals our focus must be on the building process. The most important resource implication decisions are taken during the planning stage before the design team normally becomes involved. Fig 1 illustrates the involvement of the planning and design teams and the relative cost consequences of decisions at various stages.

The decision to build has service, staffing, capital and operating cost consequences. The proper determination of 'need' for a facility is therefore of paramount importance. This can best be done by developing and implementing effective resource planning that will place the incentive with

PLANIFICATION ET DESSIN A RESSOURCES INTEGREES — BATIMENTS POUR SOINS DE SANTE DE BASE

Des conditions économiques, démographiques et d'autres liées à une attente toujours plus exigente en ce qui concerne les soins de santé entrainent de plus en plus de pressions sur les responsables de planification et de dessin qui travaillent sur les équipments de soins de santé. Il faut absolument une structure de gestion ainsi que des outils de planification efficaces pour permettre aux professionnels de réconcilier de facon aussi satisfaisante que possible les besoins et les ressources disponibles, en évitant une distribution inéquitable dans des conditions où les moyens sont trop souvent limités. Le designer d'équipement de santé a lui aussi besoin de pouvoir disposer des services d'expertise disponibles. Les recommandations de planification et dessin à ressources intégrées, élaborées par la Division of Building Technology visent à offrir cet outil indispensable de travail.

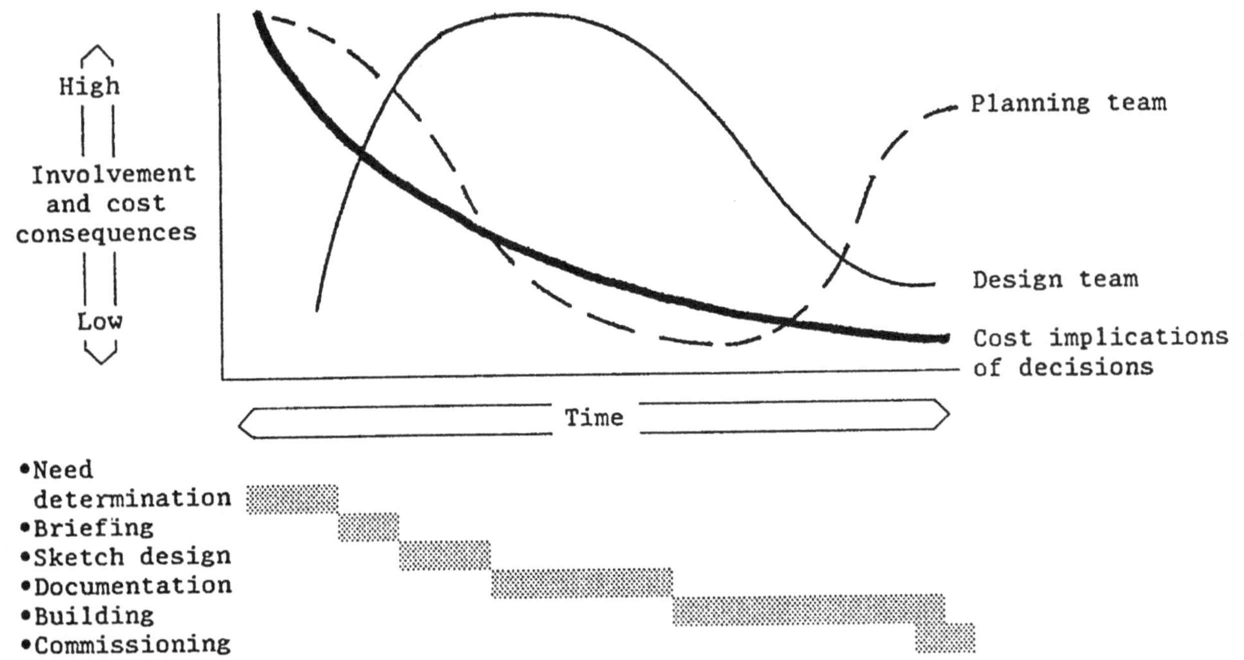

Figure 1: Involvement of planning and design team and cost consequences of decisions during building procurement process.

the user organisation to develop innovative strategies for the best use of scarce resources, especially of finance and staff. Buildings, equipment, staff, running costs and other variables must be considered holistically and it must be possible to evaluate alternative health delivery strategies simply and quickly.

While there is an urgent need for the adoption of a co-ordinated national health strategy we believe that, at the same time, a 'bottom up' approach should also be adopted where, through a managed approach to project planning, the climate can be created for a more rational approach to the allocation of resources on a regional and national basis.

DBT has proposed, on previous occasions[(5),(6)], an integrated management system that would assist those responsible to view the problem holistically. Further work has been undertaken in the development of this system, particularly for local or project level planning.

Development and Validation of a Holistic Approach to Planning and Design

After preliminary work had been done on the development of a planning and design strategy for primary health care, DBT was fortunate to be commissioned to undertake the planning and prepare sketch plans for a large community health centre in Meadowlands West in Soweto, a vast dormitory town on the outskirts of Johannesburg. This provided the opportunity to further develop and to test and refine our proposals.

Throughout the planning and design process we worked closely with a planning team made up of respresentatives both from the client department head office and from the end user groups.

Meadowlands West Planning

The following process was followed during facility planning for Meadowlands West CHC:-

- problem definition (catchment area, population, existing health buildings and service);
- setting of project goals;
- strategy development;
- strategy evaluation and selection;
- needs approval; and
- briefing.

Catchment Area: Before planning per se can take place the environment within which the health service must operate must be clearly defined. The first step is to identify the catchment area for the community that is to be served by the proposed facility or group of facilities. Both hard boundaries such as geographic features (eg railway lines) and soft boundaries such as an imaginary line between facilities, were used to define the catchment area.

Population: Reports of an influx of people into backyard shacks gave rise to unofficial population estimates up to twice the official figures. Clearly without reliable population data it is not possible to make sound planning decisions. In communities where rapid urbanisation is a fact of life official census statistics taken at long intervals are unreliable as the population changes too rapidly. A useful technique, used in this case, is photo-interpretation based on aerial photographs that can be completely up to date. House types were categorised and counted and from sample ground surveys average household sizes established for the various house or shack development categories. Population projections were based on an analysis of undeveloped land, its potential for development and potential increased density[(7)].

Existing Health Buildings and Service: The existing health buildings in the community were identified and analysed in terms of the number of usable spaces (such as examination rooms), maximum desirable use and state of repair. Statistics were also gathered on the level of service currently provided to the community in terms of number of contacts. Using the population figures these were translated to a service rate of number of contacts for each service type (general consulting, physiotheraphy, dentistry etc) per person per year. The number of births was also established both at PHC and hospital level from which ante- and post-natal statistics could be developed.

Project Goals and Service Projections: Once the current operational environment was defined, the next step was to set new service goals in consultation with the planning team. These had to relate to the type of community, to the level of service in neighbouring communities and to national goals. Using this data and the population projections, new service levels (ie anticipated number of contacts) were computed. Using a set of activity levels for different services (eg average number of contacts per nurse per day) the number of primary service rooms (eg examination rooms) or planning units (PUs) required for the community as a whole could be calculated.

Strategy Development and Selection: Once the projected service need for the community as a whole had been established a suitable site was identified and an exercise undertaken to establish what part of the service could remain in the existing clinic and what would be included in the new CHC. From earlier calculations, which had established an estimated capital cost per PU, the projected capital cost could then be calculated. Projected operating costs were established from comparative overall service costs for neighbouring health centres.

Where more than one site is available alternative strategies for the subdivision of the service could be considered and evaluated in terms of capital and operating costs and of staffing requirements.

Planning Brief: Once the service plan had been approved by the user department and the co-ordinating authority, the next step was to establish a schedule of accommodation required to support that service level. A series of meetings were held where standard schedules of accommodation were used as a check list and the resulting net area controlled against a net area guide established earlier from the number of planning units required.

Meadowlands West Design

Existing design standards required by public sector user departments were, we believed, unnecessarily high. Accordingly one of our objectives was to critically look at current area standards. Some key rooms were identified and the activities analysed and layouts generated using a computer aided design (CAD) programme with minimum space for the performance of each activity. These tests showed a consulting/examination room could easily be fitted into a 12.5m^2 space as compared to the 16m^2 originally required by the user department (Fig 2).

Full Scale Room Mock-Up: In discussion with the planning team it was clear that there was unhappiness about a smaller consulting/examination room. Accordingly both in order to test the proposed consulting/examination room layout fully and to demonstrate it to the user department, a full scale mock-up was built on the CSIR site. Walls and doors could easily be moved and all furniture and curtain room dividers were provided.

Representatives from the user department were invited to view and 'test' the room. Changes were made and as a result of a new requirement that two large cupboards be added to the room for dispensing of drugs, the room was increased to 13.5m^2 (Fig 2). Although no other rooms were tested using the mock-up facility, different designs were analysed and layouts generated using CAD.

Design Game: An important feature of our approach to the design was to develop the design interactively with the planning team representing the end user. The correct number of the various spaces required by the schedule of acommodation were plotted, cut out and stuck onto stiff cardboard, forming a set of 'jig saw pieces'. After developing a first design ourselves based on zoning diagrams prepared in collaboration with the planning team, we took the design and room blocks to a meeting with the client and set out the design on the conference table. The planning team were then able to comment on and suggest improvements to the design by moving room blocks around. In this way information about the desired relationships between rooms and work flow patterns was obtained while we were able to see that building design requirements were not compromised. This process led to the development of a new design which was 'owned' by both the planning and design teams. Fig 3 illustrates the main site and building layout developed for the sloping site while Fig 4 shows the layout developed for the midwife obstetric unit.

The validity of this approach became apparent later when, on submission for formal approval, only two minor changes were required to the design (the moving of one door and the addition of a cupboard) in contrast to major redesigns required on other occasions.

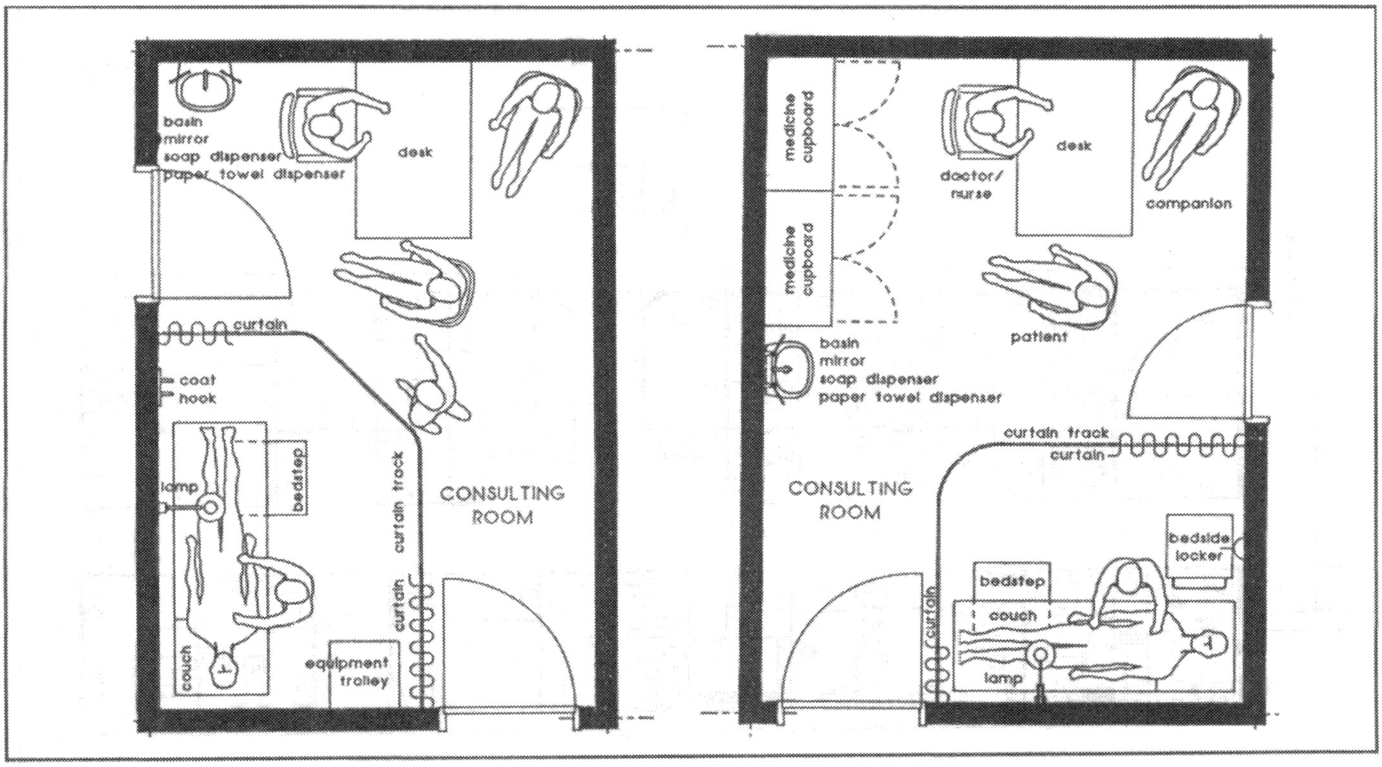

Figure 2: General consulting and examination room — 12.5m^2 and Meadowlands West CHC general consulting and examination room (including space for dispensing cupboards) — 13.5m^2.

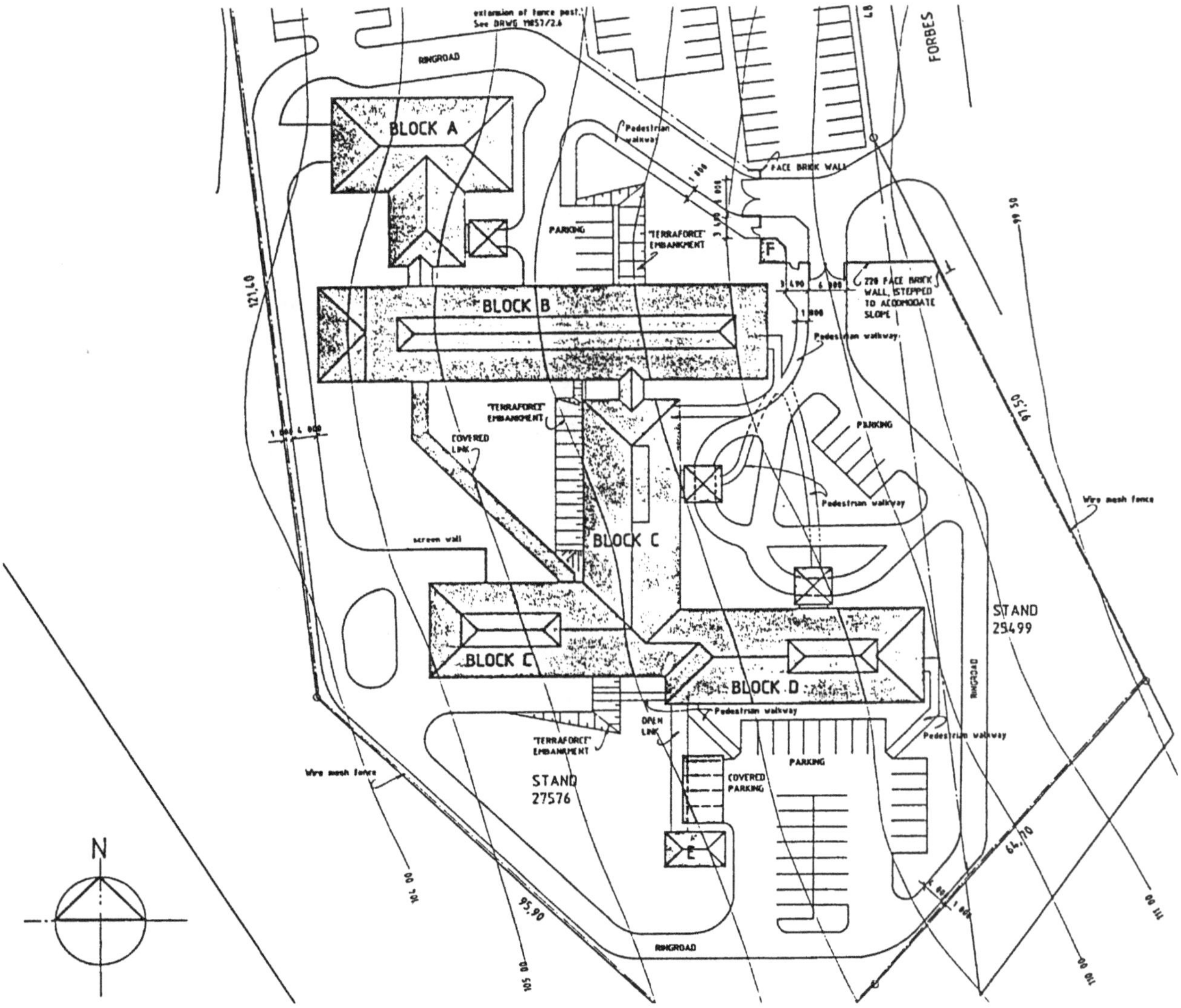

Figure 3: Meadowlands West CHC site and building block plan.

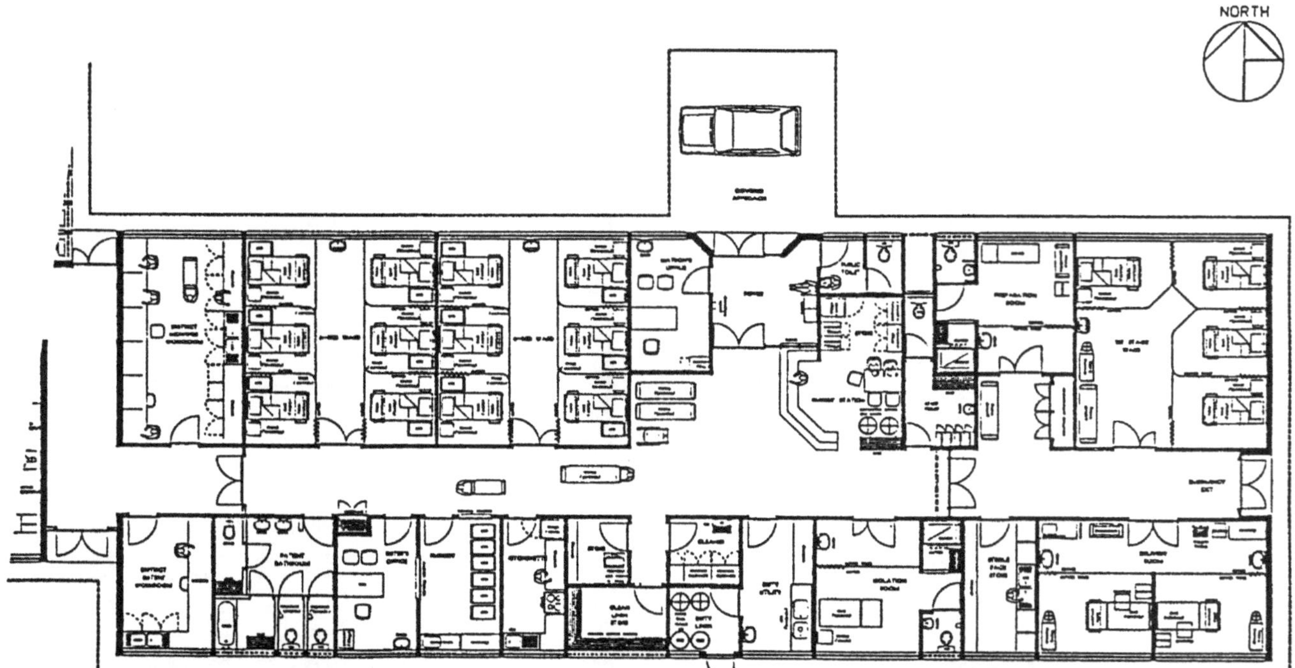

Figure 4: Meadowlands West CHC — Midwife Obstetric Unit.

Planning and Design Guides and Computer Aids

At present there is no standard system in South Africa for the development of a health strategy in response to a voiced need. One of the major problems currently facing planners and designers is the varied approach to planning and design of the many health authorities. This has led to different standards being accepted by authorities serving neighbouring communities or even to different levels of service offered in the same community.

There is a need for a uniform, standardised approach to planning and design. DBT has gathered the information developed on the Meadowlands test bed into separate but co-ordinated planning and design guides for primary health facilities.

Primary Health Care Planning Guide

Two versions of the PHC planning guide are being produced. The first is in the form of a booklet with a series of questions and tables which can be filled in during the planning process while the second is in the form of an expert system programme which can be run on a standard PC. In both a major consideration is simplicity and ease of use. Both versions of the guide are supported by explanation or 'help' sections where the rationale behind the strategy can be checked or additional information gathered. The planning process used is illustrated diagrammatically in Fig 5. A measure of iteration is allowed for as, during resource reconciliation, it may appear that a goal or strategy needs to be refined or redefined.

During the planning stages of Meadowlands West CHC a set of computer based spreadsheets were found to be particularly useful, especially during goal setting and the development of a service strategy. As new service levels were fed into a set of spreadsheets at a team meeting, it was possible to assess the resource consequences immediately and to tune the mix of individual service goals to obtain a balanced service within projected available resources. This interactive planning is a useful feature and cannot be replicated in a workbook of questions and static tables. But it is aknowledged that occasions will arise when a computer based model is inappropriate.

In most cases as changes in population served and services required are not entirely predictable extreme accuracy is not necessary. What is important, however, is that decisions are based on a realistic assessment of the consequences of a particular policy.

Two levels of output come from the planning guide. The first includes sufficient summary data from the various levels of investigation to provide the co-ordinating health authority with a minimum of comparable data to evaluate the development proposal, while the second is a schedule of accommodation based on approved planning units and matched to the area and cost guides developed earlier in the process. In developing the schedule of accommodation, reference can be made to layouts and operational policies included in the standard design guide (Fig 5).

Primary Health Design Guide

The second part of the integrated planning and design system relates to the physical design of primary health buildings. As indicated earlier there are many authorities responsible for building health facilities. Not only do differences in standards occur between departments but also within departments due to personal preference of advisors. The standard design guide seek therefore:-

- to introduce minimum acceptable ergonomic standards;
- to simplify the design process through making sufficient background and detail information available to the designer;
- to make alternate design options available to meet differing service needs; and
- to provide a data bank of economic design solutions.

The guide comprises five sections:-

- understanding the organisation;
- generic design data;
- common activity spaces;
- linking activity spaces; and
- evaluation of alternate design solutions.

Understanding the Organisation: This section includes information on the principles of CHC design, operational procedures and policies and their impact on design and an analysis of the services which can be provided at PHC level. The various activities which are required in these services are identified and activity sequence patterns and relationship diagrams included (Fig 6).

Generic Design Data and Common Activity Spaces: Using the activities and their interrelationships identified above activity spaces were developed and linked into common activity spaces. A number of different layouts were developed based on different operational policies and preferences.

Linking Activity Spaces and Evaluation of Alternate Design Solutions: This section includes suites of rooms developed from the activity sequence patterns and common activity spaces. A number of alternate design solutions, where groups of spaces are joined into suites are offered and evaluated. Fig 7 illustrates a suite of duty station, urine test, sub-waiting and consulting/examination rooms developed from the library of standard activity spaces and rooms.

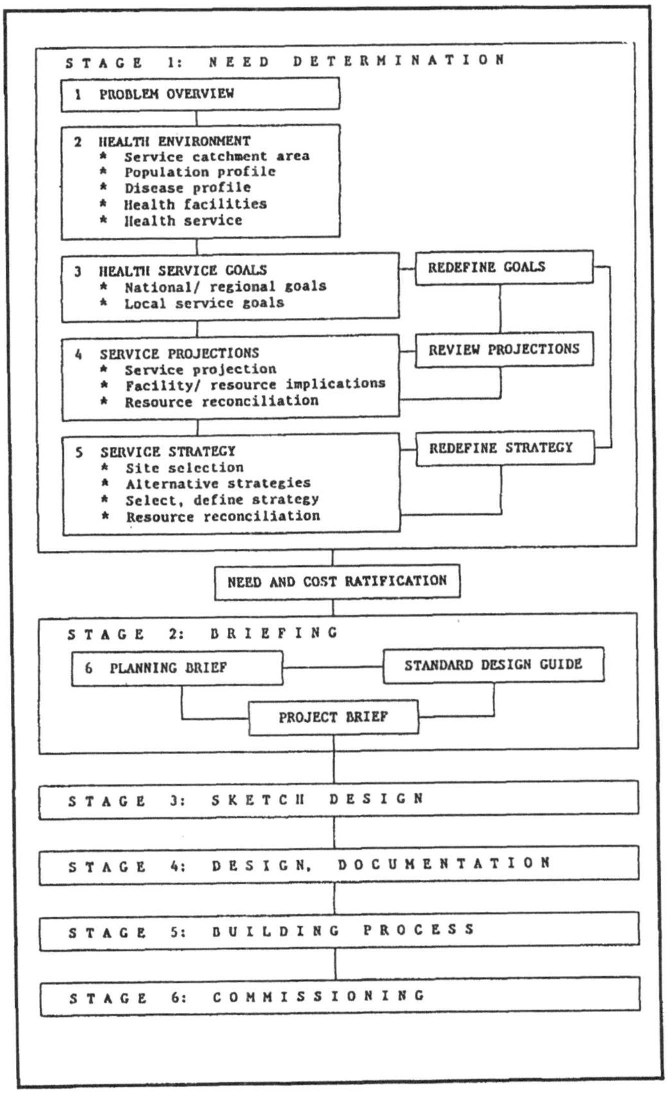

Figure 5: Standard primary health care facility planning guide: Need determination and briefing process.

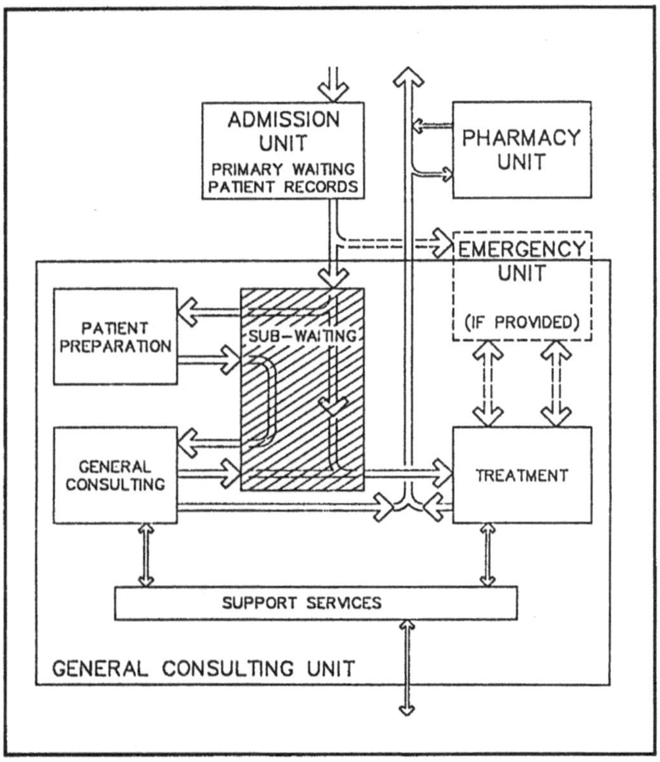

Figure 6: Standard primary health care facility design guide: Activity sequence patterns.

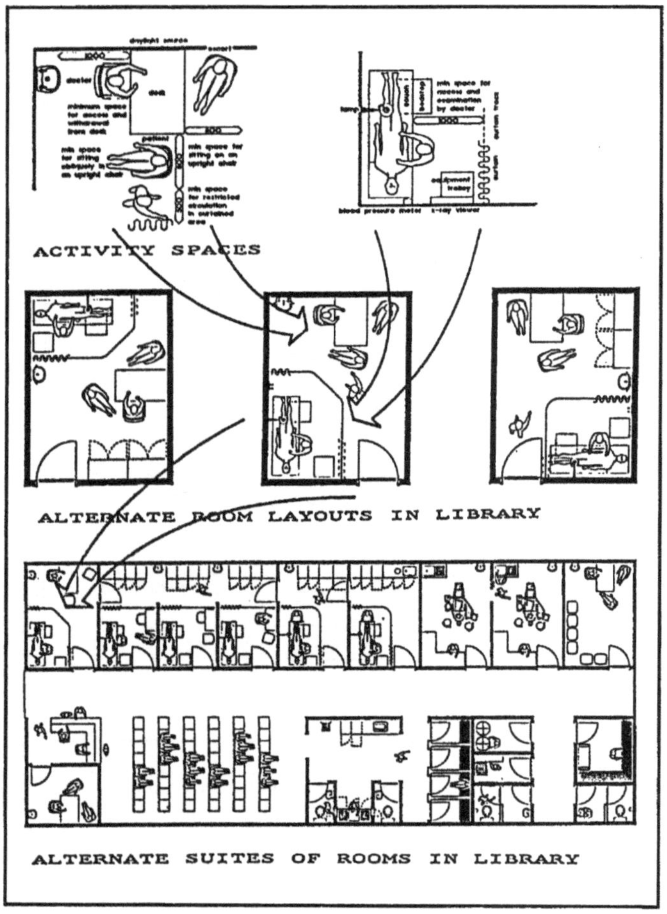

Figure 7: Standard primary health care facility design guide: Development of suites of rooms from library of activity spaces and alternate room layouts.

CAD Files of Activities and Activity Spaces: As for the planning guide two versions of the design guide are available: as a manual and as a floppy disk version compatible with the most widely used CAD systems in South Africa. The advantage of having the library on computer is that the user need merely copy and manipulate the parts as desired speeding up the design process considerably.

Conclusions

If the overall objective of health service planners and designers is to provide a health service that is effective, equitable and affordable, it is essential that the environment be created in which it is possible both to measure the current service as well as to plan for a future service in terms of these objectives. From the response of those involved in the planning and design team for Meadowlands West CHC it is believed that the system developed by DBT provides just such a structured approach in which the service needs of the community can be matched both to the goals of as well as to the resources available to the health authority. Further, by using such a system, it is possible to collect data for a variety of regions on a uniform basis which will improve the quality of later planning decisions.

In developing the most effective and equitable health strategy within economic and manpower constraints it is essential that the correct decisions are made at the right time in the procurement process. In order for this to occur the planner must have ready access not only to a structured process but also to sufficient planning and design data. As many different, and often inexperienced, planners are involved in the provision of health services to closely related communities it is important that the planning system used can provide answers simply and consistently. It is suggested that an expert system can provide just such a framework for effective, efficient and affordable planning.

Similarly it is important that planners are aware of the design and building implications of the options available before final decisions are taken. The standard design guide is designed to provide this link between planning and design phases of the building procurement process. In addition, the design team is provided with uniform information which can be used directly or, if a better approach can be motivated, could be superceded.

References

(1) Abbott, G., Cowan, D. Norms system and application — an alternative approach. Paper presented to the Congress of the SA Federation of Hospital Engineering, Durban, September 1989.

(2) Department of National Health and Population Development. Health trends in South Africa. Pretoria, 1989.

(3) Department of National Health and Population Development. A National Health Policy and National Health Objectives ('n Nasionale Gesondheids-beleid en Nasionale Gesondheidsdoelstellings). Pretoria, 1990.

(4) National Plan for Health Service Facilities. Issued by the Department of Health and Welfare on behalf of all health authorities in the RSA. Pretoria, 1981.

(5) Cowan, D., Raddall, J., Abbott, GR. Basic considerations in planning for developing areas — a challenge to management. Paper presented to 23rd International Hospital Federation Congress, Helsinki, June 1987.

(6) Raddall, J. Jig-saw puzzles management and computers. Paper presented to the International Congress on Progress in Architecture, Construction and Engineering, Johannesburg, July 1987.

(7) Division of Building Technology, CSIR (Housing Policy and Strategy Programme). A survey of population in Meadowlands West with the aid of photogrammetry. Project report for the Chief Director: Works, Transvaal Provincial Administration. April 1988.

Planning a Regional Burns Centre — The Trials and Tribulations

by

Michael F. Green
MB BS, LRCP, FRCS(Edin), FRCS(Eng)
Consultant Plastic Surgeon
Welsh Centre for Burns, Plastic
and Reconstructive Surgery
St Lawrence Hospital, Chepstow, Gwent, Wales

The Regional Burns and Plastic surgery provision for South Wales, with a population of two and a quarter million, is currently provided at St Lawrence Hospital, Chepstow (Figure 1).

Originally an EMS Hospital, it was built in 1942, to take the transferred wartime Gloucester Plastic Surgery Unit after the war. I am not an engineer but a consultant plastic surgeon, and have been involved in the planning of the relocation of the Unit from its current site at the eastern end of South Wales to a more central position and this paper is presented from that view.

Welsh Regional Burns and Plastic Surgery Centre: Workload

	Current	Proposed
Plastic Surgery		
Beds	130	90
Discharges 1988	3,862	
Burns		
Beds	35 (9 + 26)	32 (10 + 22)
Discharges	551	
Outpatients 1989		
New	3,475	Day cases 1,235
Total	22,916	

Figure 1

The Plan

The original plan was to relocate the Unit at the Welsh School of Medicine at Cardiff. This having failed, an option appraisal, carried out by the Welsh Office, altered the site to the Nucleus Hospital development at Morriston Hospital, Swansea some 70 miles from the present Unit (Figure 2).

A planning group was set up of Medical, Nursing, Planning personnel, Architects and, in no way last, Engineers as an important part of this development was to involve engineering. The meetings of this group have highlighted details in design that are specific to the Burns environment and very different to the standard concepts of hospital design. The members of the group overcame their initial natural reluctance and found seeing actual clinical cases helpful in understanding the clinical problems presented.

Relocation Plans

Year	*City*	*Date*	*Specialities at SLH Plastic Surgery +*
1958	Cardiff	Sometime	Gen Surgery, Medicine, and Orthopedic Geriat. Paeds
1974	Cardiff	1978-9	Ortho. Geriat.
1979	Cardiff	1984-5	Geriatric.
1983	Swansea	1991-2	Only Plastic Surgery
1988	Swansea	1994-5	? Community Hospital

Figure 2

The Burn

Burns are an emotive subject. Each one of us will at some point in our lives burn ourselves, or a relative, to a greater or lesser degree. It may be against a fire, or with hot coffee, and it may be catastrophic. Because of the nature and the length of treatment required to heal burns, a working environment is required that not only physically enables the necessary treatment to be carried out but also supports the psychological state and morale of both patients and staff.

The clinical treatment of burns may be simplified into three phases:-

(1) The initial resuscitation;
(2) The maintenance of life and morale;
(3) The healing or replacement of the skin loss.

Each requires a different design solution of structure and engineering provision compared to that expected in the standard hospital.

The resuscitation period after arrival at hospital needs the provision of adequate space to allow the medical teams to maintain the body's vital systems. The temperature control of this room needs to be able to maintain an equable state and able to cope with the wide and intermittent use extending from empty, to full, ie with a stripped patient and six-seven working medical attendants. Burning flesh produces fear in all animals, including man. The smell of the burn is not only a reminder to the patient, but is extremely unpleasant to the staff, even accepting their professional ability to ignore it. It is necessary therefore that the ventilation system within this resuscitation room is able to quickly remove the air and with it any smell, whilst not altering the air flow patterns throughout the rest of the Unit.

The next phase in the treatment of the burn may extend from days to months. The human body remains at risk whenever its surface skin is lost. The loss of energy, body fluid, and protein may be compared to the heat loss from a house with no windows or doors. The design for the Unit has to allow for maintenance of ambient temperature and humidity, to help limit this loss in situations as varied as the patient being either exposed or completely dressed in enveloping wool dressings on a bed producing heat.

The burn is effectively sterilised at the time of injury and the risk of infection in a Burns Unit is different to that which the lay-person might expect. All burns become colonised with bacteria and the most likely sources of these are the

PROJETS POUR UN CENTRE RÉGIONAL DE GRAND BRÛLÉS, LES DIFFICULTÉS

Une équipe multi disciplinaire, chargée de l'étude de ce projet a examiné la possibilité de déplacer le Service des grands brûlés régional de l'extrême est du Pays de Galles à la ville de Swansea, situèe plus au centre du pays.

Les blessures provoquèes par les brûlures sont frèquentes et variables en taille et profondeur, elles peuvent être mortelles et nécessitent les soins d'une équipe de médecins et infirmiers spécialisés. Les conditions envıronnantes peuvent soit améliorer, soit compliquer la rapidité de la guérison et donc les propositions en ce qui concerne plans et installations doivent en tenir compte même si le plan peut paraitre contraire aux plans hospitaliers tranditionnels.

Malheureusement le plan proposé a été du être changé par, le contrôle administratif due projet, ayant retardeé celui ci Nêanmoins, un plan a été mis au jour.

patient's own commensal organisms from their mouth and bowels. Hopefully they are reasonable immune to these, and so it is the risk of other bacteria to which they have not had previous contact that is the concern. Hospital-type antibiotic-resistant bacteria provide a further complication. The burn is an excellent culture medium and a breeding ground for many bacteria, thus the patient becomes a risk to other patients to whom the bacteria may be transferred. Ideally therefore burns are nursed in an area specifically designed for their needs.

The presence of various toxic gases following burns, for example the sponge in upholstery, or wood in house construction may produce a far more significant metabolic respiratory problem for the patient than the apparent burn. The risk of cross-infection and the difficulties in decontamination requires the size of each room, in which this stage of the burn care is carried out, to be large enough to cope with the range of facilities required for life support systems and monitoring equipment that may be needed.

Infection in burns due to air-borne spread is unusual. It is more common for the spread to be passed by the physical activity of staff dealing with the patient in one form or another. The building design should therefore limit the likelihood of this form of transference. Major burns of the type envisaged for this care are probably not going to be mobile enough, certainly in the first 48 hours or so, to consider using a normal toilet. Provision therefore has to be made for the removal of liquid and solid excreta, plus clinical wastes, without producing contamination of the staff or the Unit itself.

Once the life threatening period is over, the second phase of treatment, the preparation of the wounds for skin grafting, requires rooms of less sophistication, yet maintaining the cross infection control. These rooms are also usable in the final recuperation phase.

The third phase in the treatment of burns, the replacement of the skin, cannot occur until the burn, either naturally, or by surgical procedures is prepared for skin grafting, our attempts to reglaze the house. Repeated dressings associated with operations for the removal of dead tissue and/or for the replacement with skin grafting need to be carried out. Therefore specialist facilities are required to enable this. These may require specified engineering provision, for example the large Arjo bath which enables complete immersion of the patient, and requires specific water pressures and room humidity control.

The Opposites

The Burns Theatre/Dressing Room complex provides a major design problem. The overall size of the operating theatre needs to be larger than normal as more than one side of the burnt patient is operated upon at the same time. Additional operating theatre lights, and space for the extra staff and equipment are required.

The normal operating theatre is designed in such a way that it is perhaps the cleanest place in the hospital world. The air is normally at a positive pressure in the theatre relative to the surrounding area and may pass from the theatre into adjacent rooms. However, in burns, the moment the dressings are taken down to enable any procedure to occur, the room is flooded with bacteria and the Theatre/Dressing Room becomes the dirtiest place in the Unit and thereby a major cross-infection risk. Barclay and Dexter in the Wakefield Burns Unit[1] showed that the one requirement for dressing rooms and theatres was that the air should not leave the theatre towards any other clinical areas but should be exhausted from the theatre immediately. This has been the pattern that was used in the current St Lawrence Hospital dressing rooms and theatres, since it opened, without a single incident of cross-infection being linked to either the theatre or the dressing room suite.

Ideally, the Unit should divide in such a way that it can be used in a reduced form whilst work is carried out to disinfect or repair any shut down area. Without this facility, a contingency plan is needed that enables two Burns Units to be functioning, in an overlap, if the problems of resistant infection are not merely to be transferred from one Unit to the other.

The requirements for the Burn Unit may be summarised as the maintenance of temperature, humidity, and air flow patterns whilst a wider than normal variation of working patterns takes place and the air flows may be different to normal hospital practice.

The Concepts

The concept of the planning group was to take the design features of the present Unit that had worked satisfactorily and to correct those areas of concern (Figure 3). The present Unit at Chepstow has a simple system of rooms with negative air pressure relative to the corridor.

Technical Details Engineering Present Burns Unit

Full air conditioning capable of providing ward conditions of between 16 C to 26 C at 30% to 65% RH at any normal seasonal outside condition.

Air conditioning provided by a main air plant capable of heating, cooling, removing moisture and cleaning incoming air.

A single duct distribution system to smaller additional air plants (each supplying two wards) providing humidification and additional heating.

Figure 3

The initial plan for our new Unit was to have a simple concept of a clean corridor, a dirty room and a dirtier corridor and an airflow pattern that would have maintained the clean corridor clean, and accepted a degree of air passage into the outer corridor (Diagram 1). This would

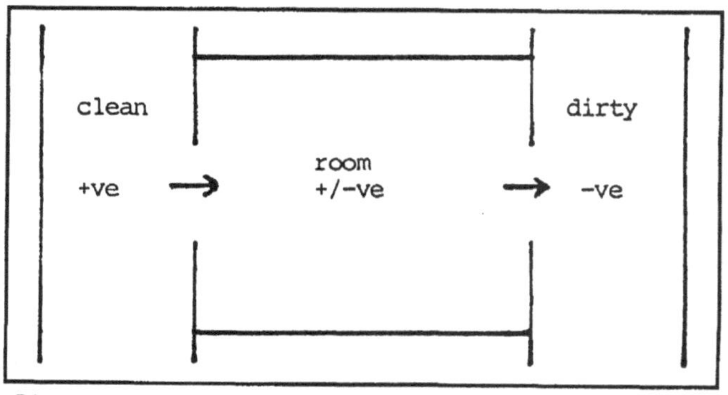

Diagram 1: Users Room Design and Air Pressures

have enabled clean dressings, etc into the rooms, and dirty dressings and excrement to leave via the far corridor. Unfortunately the problems of the design control plan of the Welsh Office which was based on the option appraisal, in which the users had great misgivings, now began to occur. A suitable initial plan was considered by the Welsh Office to have too large a floor area to comply with the option appraisal, so the Dirty corridor was removed (Diagram 2).

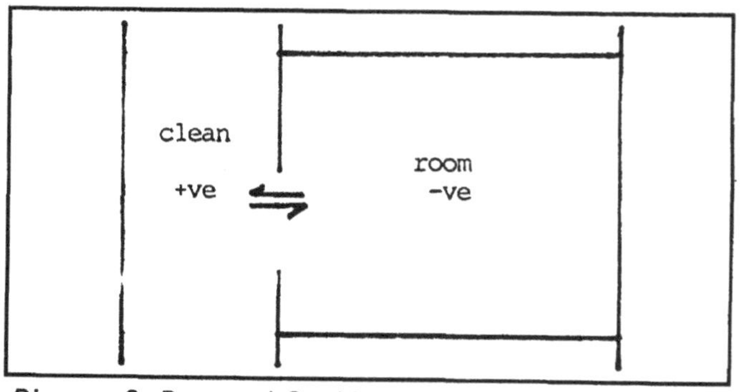

Diagram 2: Removed Corridor (= present unit)

This left however the risk of air in the room being able to pass back into the clean corridor. To prevent this, small 'lobbies' were developed at the beginning of each room to enable staff entry, and a satisfactory design completed (Diagram 3).

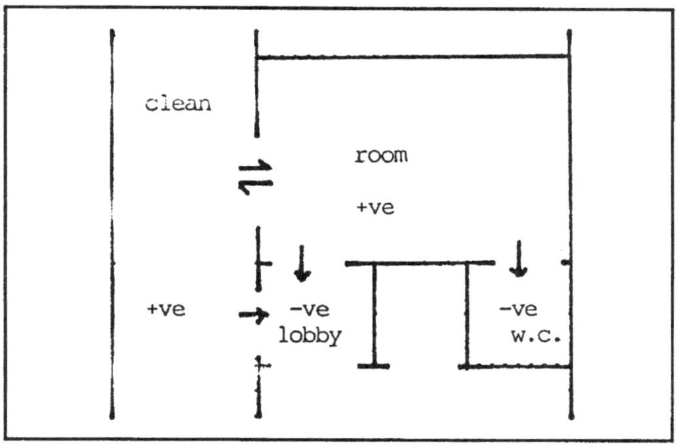

Diagram 3: Agreed Plan = Small Lobbies

The Outsiders

The plans were sent only at this stage by the Welsh Office to an external assessor for advice. The person concerned had little or no experience of the design planning that was used and was not associated with the current management of burns patients. However, on the basis that the air flow in normal operating theatres was not the same, was unhappy to accept the design as it stood. It became necessary therefore to provide a negative pressure lobby to act as a sink, thus enabling the rooms and the corridor to be at positive pressure, so producing isolation of the patient (Diagram 4). This requirement applied equally to the theatre, dressing room complex and the acute rooms (Figure 4 and 5).

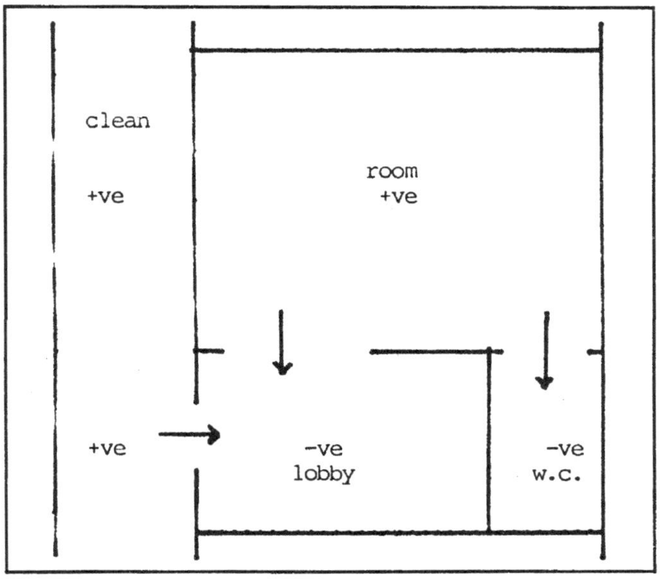

Diagram 4: Large Lobbies

Air Flow Patterns

	Corridor	*Room*	*Lobby*	*Corridor*
Present	Pos	Neg	XXX	XXX
Users	Pos	Neg/Pos	—	Neg
Agreed	Pos	Pos	Neg	XXX
Lobbies	Pos	Pos	Neg	XXX

Figure 4

Burn Intensive Care Complex (Approximate sizes)

	Room Lgth × Brdth	*Lobby* Lgth × Brdth	*Toilet/Sluice* Lgth × Brdth
Users	4.700 × 4.500	XXXXXX	XXXXXXXXX
Agreed	4.700 × 3.200	2.100 × 1.500	2.100 × 1.400
Lobbies	5.500 × 3.800	3.600 × 2.200	2.100 × 1.400
Future	6.000 × 4.300 & 5.800 × 3.800	3.600 × 2.200	2.100 × 2.00

Figure 5

This may be right for the bacteriological control but it will lead to additional psychological problems because of the isolation for the patient and the need for additional nursing staff.

This complicated system of lobbies has now increased the area of the Unit beyond that which was discarded in the initial plans as being too large (Figure 6).

Escalation in Floor Area of Intensive Burns Unit

Present Unit	715 sq m^2
Users Initial Plan	905 sq m^2
Lobbies Plan	1,495 sq m^2
Users Plan	1,470 sq m^2
Future Plan	?1,510 sq m^2

Figure 6

The Tribulations

How has a situation arisen that after many years, numerous meetings, multiple redesigns, and a massive escalation in cost, we have ended up so far from our initial concepts? (Figure 7).

Escalation of Costs

1981	Option Appraisal	£5-6 million
1985	Initial Planning	£13 million
1988	Budget Submission	£21 million
1990	Inflation Cost of Delay	£N/A

Figure 7

It has not been problems within the group actually planning the Unit particularly the unstinting support of the design engineers through all the changes, but in the planning system used by the Civil Service on the administrative side. It has been a 'ladder' system and everything decided by the users has had to be passed via a third person to above and decisions made by the Welsh Office were returned via the same route. No representation of the clinical 'users' occurred at the top. However, unfortunately there was effectively a tripartite planning process but with a linear control. Consequently the final decisions on the design of the Burns Unit were made by a committee on which nobody, to my knowledge, had any current burns management experience.

An example of this effect — the users at the initial meetings considered that there was little need for toilets in the acute phase rooms as the patients are unable to use them, yet at the insistence of a nurse manager, not associated with current burn management, they were reinserted into the final plans without further discussion with the users. The insertion of the lobbies and the toilets, without an increase in the overall size of the Unit, led to the situation where the individual intensive care rooms were reduced in size. One of these rooms, when viewed in mockup (to prove to the users that they were large enough) was shown to be not only too small for the functions that are necessary within it, but worse, it was in fact smaller by 500 millimetres than the recommended minimum size for an ordinary single room in a National Health Service hospital.

The value given to the medical advice may be interpreted

from the attitude of the Welsh Office towards the costs incurred by the various participants within the planning group (Figure 8). No financial allocation was made either to the consultants personally or to recompense their Units for

Financial Cost to Date

Planning	£)	Based on the Budget cost submission
Architects	£)	(Fee element £3.08 million)
Engineers	£)	A notional sum of £750,000 of would
Other costs	£)	have been expended to take the
Consultancy	£)	scheme to budget cost stage.
		NB: Medical Advice = £00.00

Figure 8

their absences on the necessary planning committees. The clinical commitments of the consultant medical advice have still to be covered by staff at a junior level or if these are not available, by cancellation of patients. Perhaps if the authorities had been committed to pay the rate the consultants would have received in private practice, then their opinions might have been more valued. Over 100 meetings which have taken place would have cost at least £100,000.

I originally submitted this paper in mid 1988 when I thought the plans were complete and before the 'outside' expert opinion was obtained. This was too optimistic and in the second week of December 1989, after many alterations with the administrative side, the medical users presented a redesign of the Unit that solved some of our functional clinical concerns. Meetings were held over Christmas and in the first weeks of January 1990 and an acceptable plan able to comply with the third party's advice yet fulfilling the users requirements was completed.

The final design incorporates larger acute rooms protected by individual lobbies, with integral toilets and bed pan sanitary units, necessitating a further increase in floor area.

This may be all to no avail for a meeting between the British Burn Association representatives and the Society of Hospital Infection (including the Welsh Office adviser) has stated that the rooms and theatres should be negative relative to the rest of the units, that is to say, back to how the users and the engineers had originally planned. This failure of planning control has left the engineers, like the rope in a tug of war game, being pulled in both directions at the same time yet liable to be blamed if the system does not work.

The design of a Burns Unit is difficult in the first place because the complexity and variability of the burn patient necessitates a wider range of ventilation and engineering solutions for the environmental conditions that will be required (Figure 9).

The best efforts of a users group to produce a centre for the 21st Century able to treat patients in the best clinical and psychological way with the aid of a dedicated design team have been delayed and effectively thwarted by a management process. There has been a heavy cost in financial, personal and patient care terms with loss of morale leading to resignations from the Health Service.

Technical Details Engineering Proposed Burns Unit

Five air conditioning plants dedicated to various areas of the Burns Unit template.

All air plants capable of providing heated, cooled, cleaned and humidified air to the various room requirements, via a dual duct (hot and cold) mixing box distribution system.

The single bed acute wards will have provision at the mixing boxes for additonal heating, cooling and variation of humidity. This will provide room conditions of between 16 C to 28 C at 30% to 65% room humidity at any normal seasonal condition. Each ward will be independently controlled of all other rooms.

Figure 9

The Message

It is not the failure to design a Regional Burn Centre, for I am certain that this Unit, when finally built will be world class. But to emphasise the need in specialist medical fields for the design team to include whatever technical or clinical experience may be needed at the beginning and to ensure that theirs is the defined line of command and with a definitive end date for completion.

The brief for the architects and engineers must be to provide the necessary physical conditions to enable the burnt patient to be treated and to limit by the design process any potential risks. The clinician's only requirement must be to be able to take a severely burnt patient and return them to the highest possible level of functional, cosmetic and psychological health.

The understanding of each others problems, aided by involving the design engineers in seeing actual patients improves the final result for the design, and more importantly, for the client who matters, the patient.

Reference

Infection and cross-infection in a new burns centre. T. L. Barclay and F. Dexter. Brit J. Surg 1968 55:3, pps197-202.

My thanks to all the members of the 'users' planning team, representing: Anaesthetic Medical Staff, St Lawrence Hospital; Bacteriology Medical Staff, Morriston Hospital; Nursing Officers, St Lawrence Hospital; Nursing Officers West Glamorgan HA; Welsh Health Common Services Authority and West Glamorgan Health Authority Planning.

Hospitals Should be Beautiful As Well As Functional

by
Mr M. F. R. Miles and Dr J. H. Baron
British Health Care Arts Centre

A New Policy and its Basis

Health Building Note 1 represents a new policy. Before seeing how it may be implemented, we may establish some of the reasons for the policy, and how it makes economic as well as aesthetic sense, and may make clinical sense.

The Benefits of a Well Designed Environment for Healing

An example of the cost-effectiveness of an attractive environment has been found with patients recovering from surgery. A study (by R. S. Ulrich) was based on patients recovering from gall bladder surgery, some of whose beds overlooked trees, others only a brick wall: those looking at the trees 'had shorter post-operative hospital stays' as well as needing less medication. This seems common sense — a positive state of mind can assist recovery, and a brick wall is not a happy metaphor in such circumstances, but we have many hospitals without such therapeutic views, and landscaping is often cut from a project budget on grounds of cost. Yet a shorter period of hospitalisation represents considerable saving. Landscaping, and presumably attractive interiors including plants, are conducive to healing. It is less likely that the ubiquitous bare gloss walls, linoleum with cigarette burns, discarded lockers and trolleys, or plastic chairs in mismatched hues, will help patients feel well. In the long term, attractive buildings and landscaping may be highly cost effective as well as pleasant.

The area of a hospital experienced by most people at some time is the Outpatient Department. Frequently such areas are filled with broken chairs, redundant posters, and a sense of despair which concentrates the mind on human frailty. Everyone arriving for an appointment will be frightened — of disease, pain and death — it is entirely natural. They will also need to remember to tell the consultant the exact symptoms of what is wrong. Having arrived early (in order not to be late), found their way through a labyrinth of corridors, negotiated some humanity from a reception desk, they will wait, perhaps for an hour or longer, in dismal surroundings. As their stress rises, it has physical effects, and the patient's memory may become increasingly confused so that they are less likely to recall their detailed symptoms. How in such circumstances can there be accurate diagnosis? Yet inaccurate diagnosis can hardly be cost-effective, and there are alternatives, such as the excellent new outpatient clinics at Hammersmith, designed by John Weeks. In 1989, the Department of Health established five 'Demonstration Projects' in Outpatient areas (at Leeds, Nottingham, Gateshead, Liverpool and London), and invited the British Health Care Arts Centre to be consultants on the visual aspect of each site.

Beautiful hospitals are not a luxury. They help patients regain health, and staff work more efficiently. Industry has given considerable thought and money to the design of factories and offices, not for any altruistic reason, but to gain the most from the workforce. Local government has found that carefully designed public buildings and places are rarely vandalised, whilst neglected spaces often are (which causes expense). Everyone likes to work or linger in a place which they can feel is 'theirs', by differentiation from other spaces, and art is an effective way to do this, not always involving purchase. There are several picture loan schemes, such as Paintings in Hospitals, or others operated by the Arts Council and its regions, from which hopsital staff might select works they like. Staff who feel at ease in their workspace generally are more productive.

We have sketched some arguments for art in hospitals on economic and other pragmatic grounds. Perhaps we should not overlook that there is another argument based in the 'aesthetic dimension'. Art is a way of giving form to feeling. Patients may find the hopsital routine, and the clinical efficiency required, leave little room for feeling. It may be that art, and growing things — plants and wildlife gardens — become essential vehicles for feeling which enable the patient (and perhaps the staff also) to attain a balanced and humane state of mind. We do not live in laboratories, yet a hospital may seem like one and increase the natural fear a patient carries with them. Whilst the routine may be necessary (and has emotional as well as clinical reasons), it leaves a gap in terms of 'normal life'. Art and craft, because they are unique things made by peoples' hands, can restore some of the quality in life. Let us not overlook that the Beautiful commuicates more directly than verbal description, that small and private moments of reverie occasioned by works of art may be the most valued moments in a day. Such things cannot be measured. It is necessary, in the end, simply to assert that we believe in a quality of life, and the role of art and things of beauty within that. If our world were to be composed only of balance sheets, and the ground of the spirit be completely built over by the metaphorical equivalent of the multi-storey car park, we should surely be impoverished.

Implementation of the Policy

It is important that, to achieve a well designed interior, all aspects of the visual environment are co-ordinated, and this is best done in the design stage of a building. Cosmetic solutions only distract from underlying problems. Prints in the corridor are fine, but if all the other visual messages declare institutionalism, the environment will remain depressing.

There are three particular areas in which the policy may be interpreted: the quality of the environment, the sense of locality, and the place for the personal. All these may be reflected in methods of commissioning a building and its interior.

A Concept of Quality

The 'quality' of something is perceived in the sum of its

L'HOPITAL DOIT ETRE PLAISANT A VOIR AUTANT QUE BIEN FONCTIONNER

L'auteur revoit les raisons financiers et pratique pour la création d'un environnement plaisant, et fait le compte des départements de l'hôpital ou les bénéfices sont les plus marqués, il considère les avantages d'une aesthétique bien appliquée pour les soignants et les malades.

Il continue par une revue des moyens nécéssaires à cette création, ce qui requiert un sens des impératives de la qualité, de l'environnement, et des besoins humains, il cite un nombre d'exemples ou ces objectifs ont été atteints, il termine en appuyant sur l'importance de la participation du personnel au planning de l'hôpital.

parts, and may be, figuratively, more than merely the sum. It is the combination of elements in a whole. The notion of the 'whole' is not without interest in the context of 'health', since the two words share an origin. Perhaps we should look to hospitals which express health. This implies the sharing of a common vision by all those who contribute to their design: the architect, engineer, landscaper, interior designer and artist. As we have said, they need to collaborate in the design stage of the building. This should be reflected in the building's budget, with safeguards for landscape and art if the project goes over budget. A percentage of construction costs set aside for Art may be a useful mechanism, ensuring that art and landscape have funding on the same basis as drains and electrical work. Just as no hospital would be commissioned without drains or electric sockets, so it should not be devoid of art or landscape, as, indeed, hospitals rarely were until recent times — look at the beautiful tile murals in several Victorian hospitals such as the Royal Infirmary at Newcastle or St Thomas' in London. Unfortunately these elements are often marginalised today and are reliant on external funds, either from the hospital's endowments or from sponsors. Even in such a prestigious and widely publicised project as Richard Burton's low energy hospital for St Mary's, Isle of Wight, the proposed landscaped lake and wildlife enclosure was cut from the budget and restored only by the intervention of a sponsor. It would be unfortunate if the Poor Law ethos remained in effect by default because such essential elements are not safeguarded in budgets, and if we have a concept of a whole hospital, how can they be regarded as marginal extras? Besides, for a very small outlay, art and landscape may confer the identity of the site and prove an excellent investment, focusing the building as an entity of quality.

If the budget includes art and landscape, then this will reflect the desire that all the visual messages given by a hospital shall relate to a quality of life. The further implication is that such elements be designed into the building at the beginning as they were in Edward Cullinan's recent West Dorset hospital, in Dorchester, featured by the Prince of Wales in A Vision Of Britian, and have been in the new hospital in Bournemouth, where blacksmith Richard Quinnell MBE made a Tree of Life.

Cullinan designed West Dorset hospital around a series of courtyards; one contains a sculpture of Queen Victoria loaned by the Arts Council; another is being made into a beautiful garden; a third contains a waterfall-sculpture made by Hamish Horsley from 20 tons of Portland stone. It took a year to make, and each of the receding pools is carved at its edges, in some cases reminiscent of ammonites — a local reference since the Dorset coast is well known by fossil collectors. Its cost was around £20,000 including all materials and the artist's fee, which, compared with the overall building cost for any project, is not a great sum, yet one which has produced the hospital's most prominent landmark and an image, both beautiful and therapeutic, which the patient, visitor or member of staff will remember. The use of brick rather than concrete, and the wide, carpeted and well-lit corridors also help give a feeling of ease, something we more often associate with a hotel than a hospital. It is not meaningful to consider separately the elements of materials used in construction, provision of courtyards, growing and flowing things, light and colour, and the collection of contemporary art and archive photography on the walls, since these all contribute in their way to the ambience of a building of quality. Pervading the whole is a sense of human scale, and the feeling that those who made the building were concerned for the well-being of those who use it.

A Sense of Locality

There is no formula for quality in a building, and much may depend on relating to landscape, vernacular styles and materials, and the history of the locality. A visual link between a hospital and the geography and geology of the area in which it is situated helps make the building less frightening, less remote. Sometimes a link with a local museum may provide visual material, such as old photographs or artefacts, which can be displayed and engender reminiscence in patients and visitors. Museums often have a policy to reach a wide audience, and the whole community uses its local hospital, so the link may serve the interests of both parties. In any case, culture is a useful way to make a bridge between a hospital and where it is.

West Dorset shows the use of traditional shapes and materials, in a building which is at the same time innovative, renewing rather than copying tradition. In contrast, many hospitals built in the 1960s or 1970s use materials, and a scale, quite out of keeping with their locality — Southampton General, Belfast City, or St George's, Tooting being examples of hulks 'beached' amongst streets of small houses. They appear quite separate, as places apart which require the patient to leave the familar and the normal behind at the entrance. On the other hand, the scale of Homerton hospital in East London relates well to its catchment area, and is reassuring.

Homerton is a good example of an art project based in a sense of locality. The building itself, with its courtyards and gardens, and well designed interior, assists the art to be effective, but the local nature of much of that art also helps link the hospital to the daily lives of its patients. The nearby Whitechapel art gallery provides professional advice to the hospital's art committee, and changing exhibitions of work by local artists. The art covers a wide range of styles and subjects, and because exhibitions are temporary some risks can be taken, but there remains a natural reflection of the locality in the work of artists who live there.

The art committee has commissioned several major works for specific places. For example, Jane Gifford painted a local scene for the accident and emergency waiting area, and Linda Schwab another for the ante-natal clinic. Andrew Darke made a 'Branch Library' by binding cut logs like books, for the teaching wing. Care is taken that commissioned works, both painting and sculpture, are well placed and well lit, and that detritus such as notices and advertising do not interfere with the visual statement of the building and its interior. The result is a place which has a clear identity, a strong sense of where it is (and familiarity for local people), and an exciting range of art by local artists which engages the attention of those sitting waiting, or walking the corridors (which of course are wide and well lit), and takes their minds away from illness and fear, towards health and ease.

Locality may provide ideas for visual themes picked out in decorative details, or for the materials from which a building is constructed, or for the overall shape of a building. The ideas promoted by Leon Krier for urban planning and architecture may be equally relevant to hospitals, and tend to centre on such notions of local appropriateness, in feeling as well as material elements.

A Sense of the Personal

A large district hospital may admit 75,000 people a year and they may receive 300,000 visitors, which is a major cross-section of the local population. There may be 4,000 staff, who will wish to influence their environment. The lesson of art in local authority commissioning is that greater consultation usually leads to work being better protected against vandalism, and that people can be articulate in expressing their taste. In the case of a hospital it seems vital that staff in all sectors have a say in the appearance of the building, and that feedback is taken from patients and visitors so that an art project may develop along constructive lines.

Staff may bring into their place of work visual items which they value — a favourite picture, of whatever sort — and these should not be excluded for the purity of the designer's view. All sorts of small things become valued by personal association, a quality utilised by Hannah Collins in a series of colour transparencies for Colindale hospital. These borrowed one item from each of a group of elderly patients, which had a symbolic value, standing perhaps for an important memory, and arranged them on shelves to be photographed. Hence a visual trace of that temporary community of patients became a kind of minor monument, to the feelings of ordinary people. This kind of art brings the domestic into the institution as well as being a vehicle for deeply personal feelings.

At St George's, Tooting, another aspect of the personal was achieved by the sculptor Peter Randall Page, who made three landmark structures in Welsh slate to draw attention to the main entrance. The works are obviously hand-made, as opposed to the mechanical blandness of the buildings, and give an intermediate scale, between the building and the spectator. The sculptures were constructed on site, so people walking past could see the artist at work. Sometimes the value of art is as much in its process, or in the unique perception of each spectator, as it were completing the work through their interpretation, as in its finished objects.

Any art or craft work has a personal dimension, deals with feeling and expression, which may be legislated out of the clinical routine. As such art and craft, made by hand and with emotion, unlock creative and emotive responses in the recipient. This experience may be important in keeping a balance of mind, and a sense that the patient is an individual not a statistic of illness.

Methods of Support

To support an environmental project a nucleus of staff from within the hospital is necessary, and should represent all sectors — administration, medical and nursing, works, and voluntary groups, and be formed into a committee. They will be able to draw up a policy and form a confident overview of the visual needs of the hospital, from which they can contribute to any brief given an architect, engineer, designer or artist involved in major refurbishment or a new phase of building; they will, as a committee, be in a stronger position to appeal for funds from external agencies or the hospital's own trusts and endowments. Where they need professional advice on visual matters, they may seek it from local galleries or museums, the Arts Council (and its regions), or from the public art commissions agencies (such as Public Art Development Trust) who are knowledgeable in such matters as selection processes and contracts. In the case of a new building (or extension), it is advisable to invite the responsible engineer to join the art or environment committee, not least to ensure that where art works are to be installed they will not be in visual competition with fire hoses or electric sockets, or be banished by radiators, and that if water sculptures or fountains are planned there will be a source of water. It is often what seem small, functional matters that enable an arts project to succeed.

The British Health Care Arts Centre is the national organisation (established by the Health Service and charities such as the Kings Fund) which can assist hospitals in forming a policy, initiate liaison with local cultural provision, advise on the selection of artists, and monitor and evaluate a project as it develops.

The first step is the most difficult, and hospital staff who wish to take an initiative, or engineers concerned for a better environment, may feel isolated. Yet the move towards hospitals which are attractive as well as functional is gaining pace, nationally. Successful precedents exist in other countries, in Scandinavia especially. The concept of a beautiful hospital may be a vision, but it is not a dream or an illusion. Some recent buildings, such as West Dorset and Homerton, are beautiful and functional, and cost-effective. They also provide an environment conducive to healing, which fits happily into the locality. It can be done.

Reference Material:

The following books are available from the British Health Care Arts Centre:-

P. Coles Art in the NHS (1983) DHSS
P. Coles The Arts in a Health District (1985) DHSS
L. Moss Art and Healthcare (1988) DHSS
M. Miles Art for public places — critical essays (1989) WSA Press

J. Greene Brightening the Long Days — Hospital Title Pictures (1987) is available from the Tiles and Architectural Ceramics Society.

R. S. Ulrich View Through a Window may Influence Recovery from Surgery (1983) was published in Science, Vol 224.

A video on art in hospitals commissioned by the King Edwards Hospital Fund for London, with accompanying booklet by Lesley Greene, is also available from the Centre (price £15 video + book).

Estate Management

by

C. Davies Dip Arch, RIBA
Assistant Director, Dept of Health, London

I am grateful to Congress for this opportunity of sharing with your some thoughts on Estate Management. May I make clear at the start that you have asked for my personal views, they are therefore not necessarily those of the Department of Health, York University, The College of Estate Management or the Chartered Institute of Building.

The function of Estate Management has suffered for far too long from being ill-defined. Although this state of affairs is hardly the stuff of tragedy, it is nonetheless important because a more complete understanding applied throughout both private and public sectors would bring considerable National benefits. An enhanced interpretation would emphasise the proactive, creative and comprehensive. It would also highlight the consumer, the business, value for money, fast track, decisions analysis, quality and take a wider view of costs and benefits which looks well beyond the immediate.

Recently, in reviewing a 'State of the Art' survey of the quality of asset management in the UK*, the Financial Times concluded that the whole subject constituted a management blind-spot. Nothing less than such an assessment would begin to explain the condition of the national physical infrastructure, its general inefficiency and poor quality. Compared with Financial and Manpower management on organisation's estate ie its physical assets, facilities and working spaces etc — constitutes the one subsystem in which the average General Manager appears to be ill at ease. This usually results in a narrow, cautious approach. At other times ignorance is bliss and a 'macho' inspired rush to demonstrate virility and obtain cheap brownie points and quick profits results in the longer term loss of substantial benefit both in terms of financial and environmental quality.

Is this state of affairs that surprising considering that the subject is rarely addressed in management training and education? Just learning on the job, which is what most managers do, is not a satisfactory substitute, afterall each 'job' is so different and can just as easily distort ones experience. But shaping the future estate and sustaining it at an appropriate level of quality is too important to be left solely to professionals. In any case they are usually brought in to do specific jobs with little opportunity to shape the overview. The institutional structure largely inherited from our Victorian forefathers offers little comfort either. Architects, surveyors, engineers and more recently buildings each focus on one aspect of the subject. If one adopts the brick wall analogy, then the gaps are often larger in extent than what is solid, its purpose is ill defined, foundations poor and sometimes nonexistent and held together by weight of numbers rather than the presence of a bonding agent. As in all else the whole is greater than the sum of its parts. Thus even those who profess great expertise in estate management as moulded by tradition and as enshrined in the established training and professional institutions too often pass on to management an incomplete and distorted picture of the function.

Many believe the very title itself has come to be a limiting factor. Some believe it is no more than a rather grand and fashionable substitute title for building and engineering maintenance. It is often stated that General Managers in theNHS and in both public and private sectors, too often dismiss correspondence if it carries a heading which includes the work 'estate' or even worse 'works' believing that the subject has nothing to do with them and is all a matter of nuts and bolts and trivial detail. Estmancode, the NHS manual of 'good practice' published in 1972 has not helped much either because it quickly became weighed down with techical detail. The image and much of the content was counter productive. One could smell the oil and paint as the bulky document was opened. Dockets for plumbers and the turning circles of mowing machines are no doubt useful, but hardly the stuff of strategic management. This was a pity because Estmancode contained first class relevant management material. Hopefully the new image introduced in Estatecode will hit the right note both in presentation and content as will the training initiatives which are being organised in parallel.

It is also the case that estate management has a history of being bad news in that the function always seems to demand more and more money. Estate management is so often seen to be a reactive and negative acitivity. Investment in maintenance, however crucial, is not that visible to the patient or customer whereas money spent on other things seems to bring much more immediate obvious and visual benefit. Our timescales are different. The reality however is that proactive and creative estate management is as likely to release resources, and thus allow things to be expanded and developed, as it is to absorb resources. It should and must be good news. It enables desirable changes to take place. This idea lies at the heart of most of the initiatives that have been developed in the NHS over the last seven years and which are now hopefully becoming embedded in the culture of a service which aims as much at efficiency as it does in delivering health care. So what is estate management that we, particularly managers, planners, providers and purchasers, should be mindful of it?

Before seeking to give a definition, I would offer a comment on other competing titles that are gaining in popularity eg facilities management, asset management, property management etc. Look these words up in the dictionary and you will notice that they are largely interchangeable. But their proponents believe that one or other has a psychological advantage and for that reason have the edge. It is argued that the manager's attention is more likely to be caught by the word 'facilities' (particularly if he is American), assets and property than it is by estate or works, so the sooner we change the better, leaving the substance as it is, but changing the packaging. Afterall, we all know how important a title is in conveying an image. Those old enough to remember will recall how the BBC listening fitures shot up to 500% when the programme called 'Chamber Music at 10' was retitled 'Music in Miniature', or 'White Rain' was substituted for Dandruff Repellent Spray in ladies shampoo.

To substitute Facilities for Estate is seen therefore as a legitimate, indeed highly desirable and urgent case of image enhancement. It also detaches the subject from the fatal grasp of the traditional works orientated operator. For all that I am presently neutral on the subject seeing the advantage and disadvantage in whatever title is used. I have to acknowledge, however that the term 'Facilities Management' is becoming increasingly acceptable both here and overseas particularly the USA. The tide of opinion is therefore flowing strongly in that direction. There is one area however where I believe the facilities manager or planner can legitimately claim a hitherto unique input. It has to do with proactive space and equipment management.

LA GESTION DU DOMAINE

L'auteur offre une definition de la Gestion du Domaine qu'il discute dans toutes ces aspects et en particulier sur ayant trait au Service de Santé Britannique.

Businesses are increasingly aware that this area is one which is vital to the financial health and image of their business. Traditionally if the function is undertaken at all it fits very closely in with strategic and operational management. We need to acknowledge the pioneering efforts of the Facility Manager. He, at least got stuck in to space planning while others watched from the side lines. But to proceed if for no other reason other than familiarity, perhaps continuity and possibly nostalgia, and only for the purposes of this paper, I will stick to the title estate management. In which case I offer for your consideration the following:-

> estate management is the continuous process which optimises the value of an organisations physical assets within appropriate timescales; creating and sustaining an effective, efficient, safe and quality environment at acceptable cost.

Now before turning our attention to a brief consideration of a few key words in this definition, a few general comments. Congress will note that I have tried to bring together in that admittedly long winded definition two aspects of estate management that have previously lived in separate compartments. The first half addresses an area which has only recently become prominent in the Health Service. It is much more familiar to the city business whose investment is in property rather than gilts or shares. Property is held for no reason other than its investment value. In this environment buildings are designed not only to accommodate a given function but to also provide investment profit at the appropriate time. Although this is very much a secondary issue as far as health buildings are concerned it should be a factor in siting a project. How many hospital sites in the UK are substantially reduced in value, particularly important when the function needs to be relocated, simply because this factor was never on the agenda.

At the same time it is surprising how little attention has previously been given to improving the utilisation of assets — probably the most important factor in holding down revenue costs. This aspect of estate management not only provides the most important bridging point between the two halves of the definition, property overheads and revenue costs and their close interrelationship with asset utilisation runs vertically influencing both the macro and micro areas of decision making. It effects both the strategic and operational.

The second half of the definition is much more familiar to the NHS and Public Sector. But it often fails to see that the greatest benefits can only come from a carefully managed balance between the two aspects and with emphasis given to Utilisation. Estate management then draws into one activity the architect, engineer, surveyor, valuer, economist, accountant, manager, planner, lawyer, specialists in IT, decision analysis, nurse, doctor, etc, etc. Because it is fully concerned with creating a quality environment, it is neutral as to how this is to be achieved. Such an objective may require new buildings, upgrading, refurbishment or improved maintenance. Dogma as to which of these is preferred is not allowed to cast the deciding vote. The right decision emerges from a close local assessment of the various key factors, after having taken all serious possibilities into account within the well-known framework of option appraisal.

But where can this comprehensive understanding with all the necessary technical and management skills come from? The classic answer is from a properly constituted multi-disciplinary team. In my view the ideal management team which embraced the factors inherent in the definition would require some new players who are not traditionally part of the exercise. We know we can assemble the orchestra but from what source and with what background do we select the conductor? Should we be looking for a specialist conductor or is this the role of the General Manager? Bear in mind we are looking at the continuous function of managing the existing estate and not a project with a start and finishing date. In this context the specialist conductor is difficult to define because of our inheritance and very limited training opportunities.

We have inherited from our Victorian forefathers a number of professional institutes internationally eminent in their own fields, but locked into delivering a fragmented pattern of service as far as estate management is concerned. However, there are encouraging signs that Authorities are becoming increasingly and painfully aware of this management blind spot and the Training Institutions are beginning to respond. For example the CIOB have instituted a major new initiative in this area, Strathclyde University are offering an MSc in Facilities Management and are expanding into a Consultancy Service. We are likely to see the emergence of an Institute of Facilities Management this year as part of the Strathclyde initiative. York University is setting up a Centre of Asset Management in collaboration with the Manchester Business School and so on. Engineers and Architects, although they have a vital part to play are presently conspicuous by their absence. Your 12th IFHE Congress should be particularly interesting if you decide to return to this subject on that occasion.

Some further comment on the key words in the definition may be helpful in conveying the notion of comprehensiveness.

Estate

Embraces all internal and external physical assets in the ownership of the organisation ie land, buildings, all externals, plant and services, equipment, furniture and furnishings. It also includes the space between and around assets, including associated comfort conditions (climate, lighting, warmth, ventilation, noise etc). Apart from a very wide range of health buildings including industrial, training, officers, clinics etc the SoS for Health is also the owner of a considerable residential estate.

Continuous Process

It needs to be stressed that the function is an ongoing systematic activity, the opposite of ad hoc and piece meal. Although it is guided by a methodology it is not mechanistic. It needs to be driven or orchestrated. It requires clear direction and carefully considered monitoring. Interactive Resource Modelling provides the context for decision making.

Optimises

Finding just that optimum level for all resources and services to operate at their corporate best involves an understanding of how balances are achieved which are in the best interests of the organisation and its customers. There is no real benefit in forcing the estate resource to maximise if as a consequence other resources are then forced to operate at sub-optimum levels. But identifying just where that optimum point is at any point in time not easy to determine on its own. An interactive resource model has been created as a way of determining where that point lay. The model will need to be replaced by one which explores the provider/purchaser environment.

Value

The two definitions apply. The functional, convenience, amenity, physical and location value of an asset needs to be expressed in a way that enables its continuing importance to be judged against its financial worth. The financial valuation of all physical assets is now a fundamental part of the capital charging initiative in the NHS. The NHS will no longer be a 'free good'. Although extremely useful I doubt whether Capital Charging will be the panacea that some expect it to be. If it were the ultimate answer then asset management performance in the Private Sector would be far better than the Reading Report described.

Creates

There are two aspects viz: achieving the appropriate physical environment and sustaining that environment once it has been achieved. The first aspect is covered fairly comprehensively by estatecode, indeed it is what the so called seven steps are all about. Sustaining the environment requires very different skills. The factors involved standard setting, monitoring, auditing, feedback systems, budgeting, investing, contracts, and organisational standards.

Efficient

In estate terms this involves optimising the number of sites from which the service is delivered and holding no more space or land or equipment than is required to deliver the Service. Assessing an estate's utilisation with a view to achieving through rationalisation its maximum potential is important both in terms of capital and revenue expenditure. Just as crucial is energy performance and convenience in the movement of traffic, patients and staff.

Safe

Involves understanding, achieving, maintaining and monitoring statutory standards in and around health buildings. It also involves assessing risk and associated costs in a wide range of areas that have physical, control and organisational requirements. Most areas of risk involve all three to a greater or lesser extent depending on the nature of the hazard and our understanding of it. The key areas are as follows:-

(a) fire — largely covered by fire code
(b) legionnaires — covered by Code of Practice
(c) the handling, storage and distribution of substances hazardous to health
(d) the control of cross-infection
(e) sterilisation
(f) health and safety at work acts
(g) the various food storage, preparation and cooking regulations
(h) asbestos removal and other hazardous dusts
(i) electrical safety regulations, lifts and mechanical devices later temperature controls
(j) medical gases
(k) health hazards in pathology and mortuary departments

Quality Environment

This represents the ultimate goal. So what is it and can it be defined? Can it be measured? Maybe the quality environment is more describable, measurable and susceptible to measurement than we have thought possible. As a contribution to the debate I propose quality has the following elements. A quality environment will:-

(a) be clean, not only have surfaces and details to be selected so as to facilitate a state of cleanliness but minimum standards are continuously achieved and monitored
(b) in appropriate areas be maintained in a sterile condition
(c) be secure, that is surveillance of equipment and property will be sufficient to deter acts of theft and violence
(d) ensure that space is adequate for the function and is conveniently located
(e) the function is adequately equipped
(f) ensure that assets are maintained in good physical condition particularly those that are visible by patients, staff and the public and that critical life saving facilities are given the highest priority reducing the possibility of failure to an absolute minimum
(g) ensure that appropriate areas are comfortable, humane, restful, cheerful and that the whole building both externally and internally reflects the visual image of a caring, efficient and humane organisation
(h) ensure that adeqate lighting, heating and ventilation conditions are provided wherever staff, patients and visitors are located
(i) ensure that noise pollution is carefully controlled
(j) ensure that the management of waste and its movement is carefully organised so as to reduce it to its minimum and safest levels this also includes effluent and other emissions
(k) ensure that all spaces, but particularly access points, toilets, corridors, lifts, staircases etc are designed to take into account the needs of the handicapped
(l) ensure that carparking is adequate for visitors, patients and staff and convenient to entrances

Acceptable Cost

This will involve the process of estimating both capital and revenue costs of creating and sustaining the environment described above. Techniques for estimating capital costs are well established. Much less so is the whole area of life cycle costing and in particular its revenue component. Acceptable brings in the notion of priorities, choices between competing bids, relating estate demands to all other demands for scarce resources. It includes estate investment programming and careful analysis and the monitoring of costs through the information system.

Each of the aspects mentioned above need to be developed to the point where they are closely defined and where possible measured. The cost and benefits of improving a standard can them be compared with its relative importance across the board. At this point experience causes one to hesitate. All big monolithic systems are doomed to fail, it is a law which has in my experience remained inviolate. Furthermore any way forward which creates or enlarges bureaucracy, as measured by more people or paper, and the associated mechanistic and form filling approach must be resisted on principle because it is self-defeating. The way ahead therefore for estate management is to achieve the first ie real quality and efficiency without falling foul of the second.

* Reading University Publications

Contract Labour in Hospital Maintenance

by

E. P. Smithers
Engineering Manager,
Eastern Suburbs Geriatric Centre,
Victoria, Australia

Engineering Maintenance — The Case For and Against Contract Labour

Introduction

This paper projects the view that hospital maintenance can be deliberately structured to use contractors to strongly support a basic small in-house team. A number of aspects are treated to give this projection.

The basis of the projection is an Australian two hospital complex of 188 beds and day hospitals.

It is believed that the principles will provide useful thought for other countries also.

1. What Size Should the In-House Team Be?

The hospital engineer may think it should be bigger than it is — but in the view of the hospital authority or Health Department, a tight restraint applies to approvals for labour numbers. This restraint usually dictates the numbers in the case of newer hospitals. Older hospitals have an in-house labour team which is the result of initial establishment, worked over by many factors both internal and external over the years.

One thing is fairly sure. If the engineer thinks that on resigation or retirement in the team they can tighten up or reduce numbers — the first obstacle would be the appropriate union — at least in Australia.

We could debate the way that a reduction to an ideal team size should be established, without fixing the problem. Rather let me suggest a ground rule.

The team should be no bigger than is needed to handle the urgent work immediately and the non urgent work over an acceptable time frame.

Tied in with this is the availability or non availability of the appropriate trade within the team.

In any case, the fundamental guide should be that the work load must always keep all the team busy all the time and not in 'artificial work'.

With this philosophy of course, any overload periods or peak demand periods can cause a delay in 'normal' work completion time until the peak is past.

In exceptional times, say the settling down of a newly established 30 bed wing, a 'temporary employee' may be added to the team if funds allow.

In my own hospital, we have approval for a larger team than we employ. Thus the funds are arguably available for such a rarity.

It reasonable to expect the hospital to support the occasional use of temporary labour if we run a tight ship. We ensure as much as possible that we employ people on the basis of total flexibility of use within their competence.

Further stimulation on the question of labour philosophy, albeit on the basis of hospital in-house staffing, is well handled by Hy. A. Beshad[1] in an article 'Staffing and Productivity Assessment of the Engineering Department'.

2. What Should the Composition of a 'Small' Team Be?

'Small' obviously relates to a hospital size. A 40 bed hospital probably has a part-time handyman. A 200 bed hospital probably has a group which may be:-

1 carpenter/joiner
1 handyman
1 junior or apprentice
1 engineer

A 600 bed hospital probably has multiples of the above with electrical, biomedical, instrument and plumbing beside.

40 Bed	*200 Bed*	*600 Bed*
X	XXX	XXXXX
	X	XXXX
		XXX

You will notice that the smaller hospital lacks in trade cover, for example, no electrician, no plumber, no electronics technicians.

3. How Do We Handle the Demand for Services (Trade) That We Don't Employ?

It is useful for me to tell you a little of my own hospital as a background to this paper.

Eastern Suburbs Geriatric Centre, my employer, is a publicly funded hospital complex with two campuses.

One campus is quite old and is 44 bed with a day hospital. The other is up to five years old and comprises 144 beds plus two day hospitals. The hospitals are for geriatric rehabilitation and straight nursing care.

We make contact with reasonable sized specialist firms who supply the trades we need. For example, a plumbing firm or an electrical firm.

MAIN D'OEUVRE EMPLOYEE PAR CONTRATS — SERVICES DE MAINTENANCE DES HOPITAUX

L'utilisation de main d'oeuvre supplémentaire par contract constitue un trait commun à de nombreuses organisations. Cependant, il est normalement admis que la main d'oeuvre interne satisfait les besoins généraux de maintenance et d'entretien. Les contrats concernent alors les travaux exceptionnels: réfection des circuits électriques, étude et construction des bâtiments, révision générale de la plomberie, pour ne mnommer que les plus fréquents.

Cet article étudie les avantages offerts par l'utilisation de la main d'oeuvre interne, et les compare à l'utilisation exclusive ou majoritaire de main d'oeuvre par contrat dans le domaine de la maintenance. Les sujets étudiés comptent les services professionnels dans certains domaines spécifiques tels que le génie civil, électrique, ou la construction par exemple, mais aussi les services plus commerciaux comme l'électricité, la plomberie, l'air conditionné ou l'entretien électronique.

Il s'agit également de tenir compte de toutes les données par repport à la taille des hôpitaux concernés.

Les services par contrat comportent d'autres aspects tels que l'aide apportée, contre rémunération, par un grand hôpital spécialisé à de plus petits établissements voisins.

La disponibilité jour et nuit et 7 jours sur 7 de la main d'oeuvre par contract est également traitée par rapport à celle des services internes. Les activités syndicales des deux différents systèmes sont également prises en considération.

Et enfin, quelques hôpitaux de Victoria (Australie) sont passés en revue. Bien que cet article repose, de par les aspects pratiques ou d'opinion, sur la situation qui prévaut en Australie, les questions d'ordre général devraient être d'un intérêt international.

The firms need to be a reasonable size — say employing 30 or more people so that they have the back up to *always* be able to service our need — urgent or otherwise. A small firm, say four people, is not able to do this.

It can be argued that the larger firm has more expensive labour because of overheads, I have found this to be a minimal difference and the gains overrule anyhow.

Even if we thus establish a good relationship with a firm or firms in terms of their supply and service to us, it is worthwhile having them submit each year, a labour rate to be maintained for the year.

This is part of an 'honesty' system, since they do not know how many firms are asked to quote. Further, you may require their invoicing to be detailed to suit your personal auditing. These are further advantages over the usual in house recording, at least in the smaller hospital.

An interesting part of this contracting is the service to motor vehicles. Because of associated external health care areas and internal assessment teams, we have a fleet of 25 vehicles which are cared for by the Engineering Department.

Quotations are sought annually from suppliers to service these vehicles. Service includes pick up and delivery (free) with a labour rate. Service is done three monthly on a date basis.

Our hospital has neither the space nor the equipment for modern servicing and we would in any case only use a mechanic on a 15% time utilisation for the above vehicles.

A 1985 article in 'Hospitals'[2] talks of an increase in the use of Contract labour, noting among others, hospitals of 100-200 beds. The article covers an increase in the use of contractors from 11.5 to 19.1 percent because of encouraging results.

4. Advantages and Disadvantages of Contract Labour on Maintenance

Advantages of Maintenance Contract Labour

(a) Someone available 24 hours × 7 days.
(b) Labour is well versed in their trade covering commercial, industrial and hospital needs and is generally thus more competent or industry wise.
(c) You employ efficiently for the needed hours only.
(d) Record of all work by the trade over a long period is available for research if necessary.
(e) Clear total costing of the trade is easily available.
(f) You are more sure of having work done to the up to date methods and regulations.
(g) You are more likely, within the resources of a commercial organisation, to have the expertise and equipment required for the particular job at the time — eg: straight simple repair or installation or trouble shooting.
(h) Where a particular job requires two persons, the contractor supplies both, thus avoiding further depletion of your own work force.
(i) Where you would alternately employ one tradesperson — you avoid the potential prima donna syndrome.

Disadvantages

(a) You don't build up in house expertise.
(b) You don't create a departmental 'empire'!
(c) You have reduced personnel on site at any time for those instant, many persons, tasks.
(d) You still need to provide on site supervision.
(e) Perhaps there is the risk in times of tight financial policies that a new annual contract will not be signed whereas on site labour would continue.

5. Selling Our Services

A further aspect of use of contractors is for a hospital to contract or sell its services outside. At our hospital, we have established a reasonable service in manufacturing and selling handrails for patient home use. The handrails are made for patients of other hospitals as well as our own and for some home maintenance operations.

It seems that there is a ready market for large hospitals who employ a large range of specialist trades and technicians to advertise their availability and contract out to other hospitals. Of course liability insurance by the contracting hospital becomes a necessary issue, the more sensitive the contract area.

An Arkansas hospital[3] has been reported favourably in this contracting area, having started with establishing their own department to deal with their own needs in the bio-medical electronic area. They report that they cut $450,000 in service contracts with third party companies.

Obviously, their needs justified significant employment which they then contracted out to other hospitals.

6. What are the Guidelines for Employing Your Team Under the Concept of this Paper?

It would be illogical to employ a $20,000 pa tradesman when expenditure on electrical services on a contract basis was $20,000, since this implies that up to $10,000 was materials.

Further, if our expenditure was $40,000, then we would just be able to fill the time of an employed electrician.

We would dispense with the contractor, but how would we handle the out of hours problems, the rest days, the annual and sick leave.

It seems that the pivotal employment point is not to employ until we would need one and a half tradesmen to satisfy our needs as a minimum. Thus, when we employ, we would still use our contractor and keep their 'expertise', interest and service.

We make it quite clear at in house employment, that:-

(1) we expect the trade to do all they can to service the hospital in the available time, using contractors as a last resort; and
(2) we employ on the basis of multi-skilling and thus each engineering person is required to assist the others and in fact, as abilities exist, to work in other trade areas as time and demand allow and require.

The average 'handy' person who is a tradesman is generally able to apply inherent skills in other areas than their own trade.

Historically in Australia there has been significant demarcation among the unions. This is now breaking down and 'multi-skilling' is, we hope, a mark of the future.

Of course there are statutory restraints. A plumber or any other unlicensed trade may not work in electrical circuits (over 50 volts). He could, if trained, skilled and willing, repair a nurse call system at 24 volts. Again, there are plumbing installation restrictions. However, carpentry, joinery, tiling, plastering are not restrained by statute and these areas cover a multitude of maintenance requirements.

On the basis of the above then, a 'small' skilled flexible team can keep the hospital maintained for the most part, with considerable personal job satisfaction.

Those of you from larger hospitals may say:-

(1) union pressure is potentially greater the larger the team, thus restraining employment/contract flexibilities, and there may be more than one union; and
(2) we need to employ not one electrician, plumber, electronics technician, but several of each.

This is accepted, but the premise remains that whoever we employ must be kept totally busy, not half employed, thus still allowing the concept of contractors in maintenance to be effective.

It is known that at least one large hospital in Victoria essentially handles the painting by contract with a minimum employed 'in house' painting group. Here, of course, there is a multi year cycling contract to keep the appearance standard up continuously.

We ourselves employ a large contractor to service our mechanical services (air conditioning). This firm employs refrigeration mechanics, both electrical and mechanical.

7. Professional Services

The first approach is can we handle the work 'inside'.

If we judge that we do not have the expertise, then a professional may need to be engaged.

Typically, in my own case as a mechanical engineer, I recently had a necessary task involving civil works. My judgement was that I did not have the necessary expertise and neither did my team to execute the work.

The result was that a Civil Engineer and a recommended builder skilled in this type of task were used.

This section of my paper is rather obvious, but I have included it in view of the increasing professional litigation which is becoming more widespread.

The Health Department Victoria Australia protects hospital staff in the matter of general legal claims but should the matter become a criminal offence — that is someone is injured or killed as a result — as it is viewed — of professional negligence, the engineer effectively stands alone if sued.

It is thus important to ensure that correct competent professionals are used and that they understand their responsibility as necessary.

This again then, is a case for use of contractors in maintenance.

8. Desirable Concepts When Using Contractors

We should obviously use a responsible firm who will ensure their people are clean of work practice and personal habits and will be courteous and tactful with our total hospital staff. The firm's own supervision, keen to keep our business, will in my experience, ensure this.

We should make sure we have the necessary clear drawings and written procedures as well as adequate knowledge among our own staff, to ensure contractors are clearly instructed and helped to give us an effective solution.

If we only use our own staff, they notoriously or usefully — depending on your viewpoint — sometimes fly by the seat of their pants with intuitive local knowledge, *in areas where they lack expertise* or training or qualifications. Injury may also result to both personnel and plant.

Indeed, it is a good discipline to document our systems.

When making our initial agreement with the firms it is desirable to write to them, confirming labour rates, expected performance and service requirements.

9. Economic Factors

In endeavouring to evaluate economic aspects, two basic approaches are possible.

First, we can adopt an approach that will cause the results to at least lean our way or tend to prove our case, conveniently neglecting factors which are unhelpful, perhaps even unexplained.

Alternately, we can endeavour to quote all our known knowledge however it shows up our argument.

I have endeavoured to do the latter.

Table 1 shows a comparison of five Victorian hospitals ranging in size from large, although not the largest, to moderate. The types of hospitals represented are non-surgical rehabilitation/nursing home to full surgical general nursing. Also a specialist infectious diseases hospital is included.

The aim of the tabulation is to observe the following:-

(1) The percentage that total maintenance costs are of total hospital expenditure.

TABLE 1

VICTORIA AUSTRALIA PUBLIC HOSPITAL MAINTENANCE COSTINGS
JULY 1988 TO JUNE 1989 IN MILLIONS OF $ AUST

HOSP	BEDS	TOT HOSP EXPEND.	TOT MTCE EXPEND.	TOT MTCE % OF TOT HOSPITAL	HOSP MTCE LABOUR AS % OF TOT. HOSPITAL	HOSP MTCE LABOUR AS % OF MTCE	HOSPITAL FUNCTION
A	104	10.8	0.346	3.2	2.1	65	Geriatric rehabilitation non surgical. Large Day Hospitals. Mainly new construction.
B	320	47.5	1.790	3.8	1.3	36	General surgical hospital. Moderate age building.
C	436	21.2	0.948	4.5	2.2	49	106 Hostel, 52 Rehab. 279 Nursing Home 2 Day Hospitals, 4 Day Centres. Moderate age building.
D	150	32.2	2.222	6.9	3.3	48	Specialist infectious diseases, quarantine, laboratories, rehab. & nursing. 22 hectares of gardens
E	253	12.5	0.526	4.2	2.6	61	Rehabilitation and nursing home.

Nominal Conversions $1 Aust. = 0.50 = fr. 4.7^4 = DM 1.39 = Lire 1023 = Tesetas 88.96 = US$0.78

This ranges from 3.2 to 6.9 reflecting the differences in hospital uses.

It should be noted that maintenance costs in the table do not include fuel, light and power, but only maintenance labour and contract services and maintenance purchases.

The lowest, A, at 3.2% is a new hospital of straight rehabilitation type where the policy is definite by strong use of contract maintenance services.

The second lowest (B) also has a strong contract service policy. The other hospitals endeavour to use in house labour as much as possible.

(2) Hospital maintenance labour costs as a percentage of total hospital expenditure is also tabulated. The lowest at 1.3 is the hospital just referred to (B) — a general nursing and surgical large hospital with the strong contract involvement in maintenance.

Hospital A, is the second lowest in this rating at 2.1, indicating perhaps that the contract usage is minimal — or of course that in house labour numbers are too many! Seeing it is the author's hospital I don't think so.

The author's hospital, spending AUS$346,000 on maintenance in the year ended June 1989, spent out of this amount, the following amounts on contract maintenance and minor construction:-

	$	%
Plumbing	7,500	2
Electrics	13,300	4
Mechanical Services	20,000	6
Vehicle Servicing	10,000	3

Obviously none of these tasks would justify employing a trade in any area, further noting that materials can be 30 to 50% of these charges.

For your information, the average maintenance person's wage would be of the order of AUS$18,200 per annum.

10. CONCLUSION

I hope that the presentation has at very least, caused you to relook at your own maintenance procedures in terms of manning, to see if you can effect economies at the same time as using an external labour and equipment force to supplement your own.

References

(1) The Australian Hospital Engineer June 1989, Page 13.

(2) Hospitals — 16th September 1985, Page 73.

(3) Hospitals — 16th September 1985, Page 92.

Third Party Maintenance of Medical Equipment

by
W. Alexander
IAL Medical Services Division
Aeradio House, Southall, Middlesex UB2 5NJ

Introduction

Medical Equipment has been through a period of rapid development. As technology has advanced, treatment has become more dependent on equipment and in addition, safety requirements have become increasingly stringent. Along with the technical developments, we are also seeing industrial changes. Some of these changes are obvious, for example the increasingly international market place, mergers taking place between companies and acquisitions of one company by another. The recent rationalisation in the X-ray equipment industry provides an example.

Some of those changes are, however, not so obvious and one area in particular which we will discuss in this paper is the after sales service of equipment and the development of third party maintenance. The adoption of third party maintenance might be seen as a new departure for medical equipment in the UK. But it is already a well established arrangement for other types of high technology equipment (eg computers and aircraft) and also for medical equipment internationally. The difference is probably because the UK is unique in that it has a National Health Service (NHS) which dominates the market and is not a commercial organisation. However, major changes are afoot, and as the NHS becomes more commercial as a result of the measures proposed by the British Government, we expect to see some of the more fundamental forces assert themselves.

Before proceeding further, we must define a bit more closely what is meant by third party maintenance and put it into context by comparing it with alternative methods.

Third party maintenance comprises maintenance by someone other than the supplier or user of the equipment. The essence of this is, that because the third party is independent of the supplier, he can be available to service a variety of different makes of equipment, and because he is not the user he can provide the service to many different customers.

The traditional methods are for the maintenance to be carried out by either the user or the supplier (ie the first or second parties). Virtually all suppliers of medical equipment have a service organisation which can provide routine maintenance and a breakdown repair service. Clearly, they have an interest in ensuring that equipment continues to function properly in use, as well as supplying the equipment in the first place. This method of procuring maintenance is used almost exclusively by the private health sector and also very extensively by the UK National Health Service. In 1986/87, the latest year for which figures are available, the NHS spent £40m on medical equipment maintenance contracts, the vast majority of which would have been with manufacturers or their agents. This expenditure has been growing at 15% pa.

The alternative traditional method, which is also used extensively by the NHS, is to have an in-house maintenance team. The size of the team may be very small, say two or three people or could be much larger, up to 30 people. The level of expertise and scope of work can also vary from first line maintenance on a limited range, to in-depth cover of a wide range of equipment. However, the most complex equipment is still usually maintained by the supplier.

In the two sections below, we examine the factors which favour the further development of third party maintenance and those which mitigate against it. The information and understanding used in the arguments which follow have been gained from providing such a service in the market.

Factors in Favour of Third Party Maintenance

In this section we identify those factors which favour the further development of third party maintenance for medical equipment. They are discussed under the following headings:-

- Total Equipment Management
- Competition for Maintenance Contracts
- Dedication to Service
- Resource Effectiveness
- Delegation of Employment Problems

Total Equipment Management

A proper maintenance service does not include just the maintenance itself, but also, as pointed out in HEI 98, the management and control of maintenance. This is part of a climate in which users are increasingly conscious of their liabilities which could arise in the case of equipment failure. The termination of the NHS immunity for negligence and the changes in the Health and Safety at Work rules together with a tightening up of their application are all part of this climate.

By its very nature, third party maintenance will comprise different types of equipment supplied by various manufacturers. The number of items covered can run into thousands and it is very important to keep track of the maintenance requirements for each item and the work that has actually been done on it, both routine and breakdowns. Thus it should be possible to access the records of any one item from one central point. Steadily greater emphasis is being placed on this feature of traceability.

LA MAINTENANCE ET L'INDUSTRIE DES SOINS DE SANTE EN EVOLUTION

Les équipements médicaux sont passés par une phase de développement rapide. A mesure que progresse la technologie, les traitements dépendent de plus en plus des équipements disponibles et la problème des garanties de sécurité est de plus en plus aigü. Les développements techniques s'accompagnent de nombreux changements dans le domaine industriel; certains étant tout à fait évidents, par exempl l'internationalisation des marchés, les regroupements entre entre-prises et l'absorption d'une entreprise par une autre, ainsi la récente rationalisation des services d'équipements en radiographie, par exemple.

D'autres évolutions, en revanche, sont plus subtiles. Prenons par exemple ici le domaine des services après-vente des équipements et le développement de la maintenance par un service tiers. Ce système est déjà bien établi dans d'autres domaines de haute technologie (l'aviation ou l'informatique par exemple) ainsi que dans certains autres pays dans le domaine qui nous concerne. Ce qui rend le Royaume-Uni unique, c'est la position privilégiée du National Health Service, qui domine le marché et qui n'est pas une organisation commerciale. Toutefois, certains changements commencent à s'esquisser, le NHS se 'commercialise', conformément aux diverses mesures adoptées par le gouvernement britannique, et nous pouvons ainsi nous attendre à voir surgir de nouvelles forces de marché.

Cet article offre unt définition de ce qu'on appelle maintenance effectuée par un tiers, puis compare cette méthode à d'autres dispositions pratiquées, et enfin en identifie les avantages.

Computer systems provide an obvious facility for managing maintenance on this scale, but they are no panacea. Signatures may still be required on job dockets to verify the work that has been done, and this tends to mean storing a considerable volume of paper.

Equally, it is very difficult to find off-the-shelf packages which fit the requirement exactly and are sufficiently user friendly. It is our experience that existing maintenance packages are geared to fixed installations in one building or site and lack flexibility particularly in the reporting facilities. They require extensive tailoring to fit the requirements of a third party maintainer, and the most cost effective solution may well be to write special purpose applications using existing database packages.

For the computer systems and other aspects of control, a third party maintainer can provide the overall view which is vital for the management of the complete equipment inventory. This is clearly impossible for any manufacturer, and, while theoretically possible for an in-house team, they often have difficulty getting access to adquate resources.

Competition for Maintenance Contracts

Medical equipment is complex and expected to last a long time and, therefore, the maintenance costs will be a very substantial proportion of the whole life costs of ownership. Clearly, manufacturers would accept that customers are entitled to exercise competitive tendering when purchasing new equipment. However, once purchased, if equipment can only be maintained by the supplier, all competition for maintenance has been stifled. But as the National Health Service becomes more commercial, we can also expect it to become more competitive.

Third party maintenance provides an opportunity to bring competition into this area of work, not just on price but also on the way the service is delivered. There are many features which can be varied in a maintenance contract, for example the response times in the event of a breakdown, whether spares are included in a fixed price or charged separately or whether all breakdowns are included or not.

Thus the customer can take advantage of the competitive environment by setting out the features of the service he wants and then judging which service organisation meets them best and provides the best value for money. This may very well not be the cheapest option. A high quality maintenance service can reduce breakdowns and thereby increase utilisation of the equipment and related hospital facilities, for example operating theatres or X-ray rooms.

Dedication to Service

Most manufacturers and suppliers are very well aware that if they do not provide a good after-sales service, they will earn an adverse reputation and sales of the equipment itself will suffer. Typically, these companies have well established service departments, with trained engineers available on call, a supply of spare parts and training facilities.

However, the motives for providing the service are mixed and connected with the objective of selling the equipment. The emphasis will vary between different companies, some may almost regard the original equipment sales as a loss leader and seek their profit from the subsequent service and spares revenue, whereas others may take the opposite approach and find the service aspect an unfortunate burden, and in which case it will be treated as a 'Cinderella' part of the organisation.

A third party service organisation is not encumbered with such external considerations. It must, by its very nature, be an organisation dedicated purely to service, with a reputation that stands or falls on the quality and value for money which that service provides. To meet this requirement, it must be independent of the supply or manufacture of equipment.

Resource Effectiveness

There are many resources required to provide a sound maintenance service. These include tools, test equipment, workshops, spare parts and technical information. But the key resource is people. Qualified engineers are in short supply and it is vital that they are used as effectively as possible. In particular, they should be spending as much time as possible with their hands on the equipment or in direct contact with users or customers.

Having both a number of customers and a range of equipment allows the maximum opportunity for deploying resources effectively. In particular, uneconomic travelling to service just one item of equipment can be minimised, but at the same time, engineers have the back-up of a substantial organisation. It could be said that these are internal issues which need not affect the customer. But, if the service organisation is managed effectively and can take advantage of these opportunities, it should result in a more cost effective service.

Delegation of Employment Problems

One of the key reasons why private hospitals very rarely employ their own medical engineering staff is the extra complication that would be entailed. Even the NHS, which does employ its own staff, can find considerable difficulty in attracting suitably qualified and experienced staff. The qualifications and experience required are very specialised and there is a surprisingly small pool of suitable people in the whole of the UK.

It follows that employing engineers is also a specialised field in itself. It is important to have knowledge of the employment structure in the industry, and to be able to evaluate the suitability of previous experience and qualifications, for example, the emphasis of particular courses or the particular types of equipment worked on.

Factors Inhibiting Third Party Maintenance

After this catalogue of overwhelming advantages in favour of third party maintenance, it is hard to see why all users of medical equipment are not falling over themselves to sign up. There is certainly a lot of interest in the concept, but it is still in its early stages and there must be good reason for this caution. We have identified possible reasons under the headings:-

- Danger of a Radical Approach
- Fears over Technical Expertise
- Lack of Co-operation from Manufacturers
- Isolation of Manufacturers from Users

Danger of a Radical Approach

As mentioned above, the concept of third party maintenance is still in its infancy in the UK and potential users are naturally cautious about making a change in the way they organise their maintenance. This caution is strengthened by the life-critical nature of much medical equipment. No one is going to change hastily from an existing system which often works perfectly well, to another system which might appear to have only marginal benefits.

However, as was pointed out in the Introduction, third party maintenance is a well established method for other kinds of high technology equipment. Motor cars are one example where 30 years ago most maintenance and all spare parts were provided through a network of field distributors. Since then, the market for maintenance and particularly spare parts has become much more open. Commercial aircraft are another case in point, where the manufacturer does not normally provide a regular maintenance function. It is done by specialist maintenance companies. Compared with medical equipment, motor cars and aircraft are just as critically dependent on good maintenance, they are potentially just as life threatening, and, particularly in the case of aircraft, they involve just as much advanced technology.

Equally, it should be recognised that viewed with an international perspective, third party maintenance is also widely accepted for medical equipment. For example, in Germany, there are at least two active and well established companies providing this service.

Fears over Technical Expertise

The sources of information and technical understanding of any item of equipment must be the manufacturers. They will have developed the equipment in the first place and seen it through its teething problems. They should then be keeping track of its performnce in service and produce modifications as necessary. The engineers, will work only on a particular make of equipment and will, therefore, gain an in-depth knowledge of its faults and how to repair them.

No third party maintenance organisation, servicing a variety of equipment from perhaps 50 manufacturers, can hope to gain such a detailed understanding of each item. However, with well qualified engineers, and support from the manufacturer, a very high level of competence is perfectly practical. In many cases it is possible and worth while for a third party maintenance orgaisation to send its engineers on training courses organised by the manufacturers.

The level of expertise that can be expected will include a complete planned preventive maintenance schedule and a repair capability that can deal with perhaps 80% or 90% of faults. But that still leaves a small number of faults where only the manufacturer or his UK agent, will have the necessary expertise or facilities to effect a repair.

Lack of Co-operation from Manufacturers

The previous section drew attention to the support that was necessary from the manufacturers. However, some of them are not exactly encouraging third party maintenance because it is in competition with a section of their business. But the vast majority of them accept third party maintenance organisations and some even state it as part of their policy that they will co-operate.

At the end of the line, it is the customer and the user who must be satisfied, and most manufacturers see that if those customers wish to contract their maintenance to another company, it is in their long term interests to co-operate.

However, there is a small minority of manufacturers, or their UK agents, who are resisting. This can take the form of general evasion to outright refusal. The key resources required are manuals, spares and access to training courses, and there are companies who are refusing to supply some or all of them. Clearly, this stance prevents a third party maintainer from providing the quality and breadth of service that he would wish to provide.

One of the reasons for non co-operation is the question of liability, which is attracting steadily more attention and concern. The manufacturers see themselves as potentially being held liable for a servicing error which would be out of their control, but which would reflect on their equipment. Clearly, if there is a servicing error, the maintenance company would be liable, and, therefore, they must be adequately covered by insurance. That leaves a possible cause for concern, that there could be a dispute between the servicing company and the supplier as to whether a fault was a service fault or inherent in the equipment.

We believe that manufacturers and suppliers who refuse to co-operate are restricting competition. Providing that their genuine concerns over safety and liability can be met, there is no legitimate reason why they should not supply a third party maintenance company with spares and manuals.

The Office of Fair Trading has made an announcement that it welcomed the decision of one manufacturer to supply independent third party service companies with spare parts and manuals, provided they meet suitable standards of skill and servicing practice. As a result of this company's decision the Director General of the Office of Fair Trading decided not to take further action under the Competition Act.

Isolation of Manufacturers from Users

Our final point also concerns co-operation between the supplier and maintainer. If all maintenance were to be carried out by a service company, the manufacturers would cease to gain first hand knowledge of how their equipment was performing in the field. At the moment, third party maintenance is only a tiny fraction of the market and while we think that it will become a substantial part, it will never become the total. There will always be a mix of work carried out by both types of organisations; thus manufacturers are not in any real danger of losing contact with the performance of their equipment in service.

But, the value of both sides keeping in contact must be stressed. The service company will encounter problems in the field and it is essential that they should feel free to discuss these openly and honestly with the manufacturer. Equally, the manufacturer should be open with service companies, and let them know of general problems, developments in applications and modifications.

Conclusion

We have seen that there are identifiable benefits from adopting third party maintenance for medical equipment, but that there are also some considerable difficulties on the way. The concept is still proving itself for medical equipment in the UK, but we believe that commercial forces will reinforce the trend towards more competition and hence more third party maintenance. None of us must lose sight of the fact that it is the customer who decides what he wants and if the customer requires third party maintenance, then it is in all parties' interests to provide it.

Modernising Health Care Buildings

by

Derek H. Jones
Director
International Hospital Services CC
PO Box 38986, Booysens, 2016
Johannesburg, South Africa

Introduction

The modernisation of any existing building causes great inconvenience to those in occupation. This is even more so in the case of a Health Care Building.

Patients and consequently staff cannot be moved from the building during the work since there is usually a critical shortage of patient beds. This therefore means that areas are temporarily closed, patients and staff relocated elsewhere in the building, whilst the work is carried out. This results in staff frustration and inconvenience to patients and visitors. As a result planners, engineers and contractors must be aware of this and plan for minimum interference during the contract period.

The maintaining of services throughout the building whilst work is carried out is essential, and is an additional cost factor.

The Need to Modernise

It is a well known fact that medical science has developed at a considerable pace in the past 10-15 years. Since most buildings are older than this they can no longer provide the facilities required for this new and improved technology.

The Effect Upon Hospital Services

Any modernisation or upgrading has a major effect on the services in a hospital. It invariably means additional air conditioning and ventilation loads which therefore affect the electrical power requirements.

The older hospitals were not equipped for computerisation, usually this has been added during its lifetime, however in a modernisation programme this is improved upon and added to.

In South Africa we find that a modernisation programme invariably increases the bed capacity, whilst additional facilities such as Magnetic Resonance are included, and the reception/administration areas are also upgraded.

The effect of this on the electrical system results in a need for increased power supplies. Since the original supply was normally of a minimum size, this results in the supply authority having to bring in heavier cables, which means a new sub station having to be built and the main distribution systems upgraded throughout the clinic, despite the extensive use of low energy sources for lighting etc.

In our upgrading programmes the lighting is given particular attention since this can add to the patient and visitors sense of well being. By increasing lighting levels with correct implementation of low energy sources of light ie low voltage units, it is possible to do this without adding greatly to the power consumption.

Corridor lighting may be replaced by single tube 36 watt continuous fluorescent fittings, placed to one side of corridor. This system has several advantages. Firstly, by placing the lights to the side of the corridor they do not cause discomfort to patients being wheeled on beds through corridors as in the case of centrally located units which cause intermittent bright and dark patches as the patient is moved. Secondly, by arranging switching circuits to the fittings, it is possible to control the level of light for various times of the day, ie every fourth tube on. We usually incorporate an emergency circuit which is connected to the standby generator, this circuit is left on continuously which provides a low level of light during daylight hours and an adequate low level at night to allow staff and patient movement through corridors to wards, toilets, kitchen etc.

Wards

The trend is towards a composite bedhead unit, which contains all the patient services. General ward lighting is by means of a fluorescent in the top of the bedhead unit which allows light to wash the wall and ceiling, whilst a small fluorescent is used for reading. The night light is also incorporated in the unit for each bed.

Gases, power outlets and nurse call radio systems are all included making for a neat compact unit, with all services easily accessible for patient and staff use and for maintenance.

Evaluation has proved that although the cost of the unit appears to be high, when the installation cost of all the various services installed in the conventional manner are taken into account, the bedhead system is comparable and certainly more convenient, particularly when there is more than one bed against a wall, ie multiple bed wards.

Many hospitals are now providing television outlets in their wards. This means a complete new installation not only of TV aerial cables, but amplifiers, aerial systems etc.

Ward Facilities and Duty Stations

With the upgrading of a clinic it has been found that changes also take place to the common facilities for each ward area, including the sisters duty station.

Dealing first with the duty station, we experience changes to the nurse call system. This is replaced by a modern, smaller and more functional unit than previously installed. Facilities for emergency or crash call are connected direct to Intensive Care, and intercom to recovery and theatre sisters is normally added. Since most modern systems operate by means of a micro-processor, this requires rewiring for nurse call, intercom and radio. We also find during the upgrading process that more post office telephones are required and so provision has to be made for these. Computer terminals have not yet been required at duty stations in South Africa. Provision for their future installation is being made, since we feel that a computer linked message system for doctors use, to give instructions

RENOVATION D'UN DISPENSAIRE

La renovation de ce genre de bâtiment peu causer d'importants problémes aux projeteur ainsi qu à l'entrepreneur car les travaux sont en général exécutés alors que le bâtement continue à fonctionner.

Le document donne une bréve description sur le genre de travaux de modernisation, électricité conditionnement d'air, ventilation, gaz médicaux et système d'appel radio pour les infirmiéres pour les diffèrentes section de l'hopital.

Il étudie ques service seront affectés par les travaux.

Le document y compris les diapositives illustrent les améliorations apportées aux bâtiments par la renovation.

for patient care and prescriptions etc, as well as being linked to the patient nurse call system will be required in the near future. The provision of additional power outlet and data cable conduit at this stage is far less disruptive than trying to provide them in the future.

Other areas which are affected during upgrading are the ward kitchen and sluice rooms. The main changes to the ward kitchen is provision of small power outlets for refrigerators, kettles and microwave ovens, the latter being used to reheat food for patients who miss their meal due to absence from the ward for treatment etc. Further provision is made for heated food trolleys used to transport food from kitchen to ward. These need to be plugged into a power supply to keep them hot until staff have given out meals.

The main change being experienced to sluice rooms is the installation of automatic bedpan washers. These not only require an electrical power supply but also some changes to the layout of the room are necessary to accommodate them and of course the plumbing services are affected, both for water supply, and waste (sewage) piping.

Kitchen

It has been our experience that the kitchens are upgraded during a modernisation programme. This would entail either closing a kitchen partially, or completely and bringing meals from another outside source. Alternatively, if sufficient beds are closed during ward renovations, the kitchen may be reduced temporarily whilst alterations are carried out.

As the kitchens have usually reached the end of their useful life the equipment is changed. This results in replacing all services since electrical loads change. Plumbing, gas outlets and drain positions are in a different location due to a replanned layout designed to give maximum efficient use. An extract hood is added over the main cooking area. This hood sometimes contains a built in washing facility to remove grease from the filter system, this then requires a hotwater supply to the hood and a circulating pump together with its associated control system.

Lighting invariably undergoes a considerable change particularly due to the revised kitchen layout and to bring lighting levels up to standard, since most of the kitchens were illuminated by incandescent bowl fittings or bare tube fluorescent fittings.

Intensive Care Units

These are generally the most affected in any upgrading scheme. The original would have had less equipment for monitoring etc, than modern units, it is not unusual to see multi way adaptors or plug units in use because of the lack of power outlets.

The modernised ICU is now fitted with an overbed unit similar to those in the wards but without an uplight. Each bed is currently equipped with 12 power outlets which are spread over various circuits so that a fault cannot interfere with all the outlets. The power circuits are also connected via an isolating transformer of a 1:1 ratio and an earth monitoring system.

The bedhead will contain data cables and patient monitoring outlet points, as well as gas supplies which consist of oxygen, vacuum and medical air. The oxygen and vacuum being duplicated for each patient bed. A gas alarm panel which will indicate gas failure or low supply is then located at the ICU duty station.

The lighting is again improved and general lighting levels raised. Incandescent downliters controlled by dimmers fitted to the bedhead are installed over the patient chest position; these are used at night on low brightness as a night light for patient observation when the main lights are switched off. They are also used for examining patients since they are not affected by screening curtains when these are pulled.

Since the ICU is a closed area, air conditioning is required to maintain all year round patient comfort conditions. This is normally installed as a separate package unit with its own filtration system. This unit will be sited at some point convenient to the ICU or if small enough can be located above the ceiling in an adjacent corridor.

As there is always a separate isolation cubicle provided to the ICU this is provided with its own air extract system separate from the main ICU.

In some of the health care buildings there is provision for a maternity section. Here the changes take place in the Neo Natal area. These changes are generally the same as for the intensive care units, with once again a minimum of 12 power outlets per cot.

In all cases the intensive care unit and Neo Natal power supplies, together with the overbed or cot downliters and duty stations are connected to the emergency generator power source.

Operating Theatres

Most operating theatres in old buildings were provided with incandescent ceiling mounted bowl fittings which normally contained 2 × 60 watt lamps for general illumination. This was in addition to the operating lamp. The result was a very dim and gloomy atmosphere with a high contrast between the operating table and the remainder of the theatre. These lights are replaced with a fluorescent unit with suitable gasket sealing to allow for washing down. The fluorescent would contain either three or four tubes which are wired separately to a connector block. The purpose of this being that by means of a selector switch it is possible to vary the lighting level in the theatre by selecting one — two — three or all tubes to be illuminated in each fitting.

If sufficient funds are available a composite panel is installed in the theatre. This panel contains:-

- Lighting controls for general and operating table lights.
- Earth monitor alarm unit.
- 4 power outlet sockets.
- X-Ray viewing screen.
- Intercom system connected to theatre duty sister's station. (This is a hands off system.)
- Radio unit (recently a tape unit has been added in several hospitals in order that surgeons may listen to procedures whilst working).
- Gas outlet points.
- Swab count board.

All power outlets are replaced using double pole circuit breaker controlled outlets. These are connected via an earth monitor system to an isolating transformer similar to the ICU.

Since the old theatres were only usually provided with four power outlets it therefore becomes necessary to wire for additional outlets. The number of which varies according to the procedures carried out, but normally a minimum of 10 outlets are provided.

Radiology

Most X-Ray departments in the older buildings are small and contain generally obsolete equipment. The usual scope of the department involves the use of 'Buckie Tables' and check X-Ray machines. Some have added scanners for Computer Tomography.

Generally speaking the department is modernised and expanded, new equipment is installed, modern film processing used to replace old, and the doctors reporting and viewing area brought up to date. In some cases a Nuclear Magnetic Resonance Imaging installation is provided.

The installation of a CAT Scanner or NMR unit will create many problems for the engineers, as both machines require extensive air conditioning, not only for the computer equipment, but also for the control room and patient areas.

This has a very great effect on the electrical installation particularly when added to the energy requirement of the machine itself, the latter requiring some 60kVA. As these machines are computer dependant for their operation, it is necessary to ensure that a stable and constant power supply is provided. This is achieved by providing a UPS system backed up by the hospital standby generator. Several more problems arise, these being:-

Space has to be provided for the computer equipment, the air conditioning plant and the UPS system. The latter needs to be as close to the main incoming supply to the computer as possible to reduce voltage drop on the lines. Each of these rooms has to be provided with lighting and small power in addition to any major power requirement as in the case of the air conditioning plant.

The additional standby power requirements could be more than the generator spare capacity, which leaves two options open to overcome this problem. One being to replace the generator with a larger one or the alternative being to provide a second unit dedicated to this specific load. the second option is normally the most economic solution provided space is available.

The installation of new X-Ray equipment up until a few years ago meant cutting up floors to install cable ducts, however, with the use of fibre optic cables this has been reduced in the case of normal machines to a 20mm conduit between control point and the machine.

Lighting in the modernised X-Ray department is mostly confined to adding fluorescent lighting to improve the overall level of illumination, whilst retaining the incandescent lighting for specific functions, which is usually connected to a dimmer.

The doctors reporting and viewing room is being provided with conduits to allow for the future installation of monitor screens. These conduits will be used when the 'Optical Disk' system of picture storage and retrieval has been perfected.

Gas Service

Very little has changed over the years as far as medical gases are concerned, in the modernisation programme it has been found necessary to change gas outlets to make a particular installation standard, as most clinics had a mixture of different makes and types. New gas alarm panels connected back to the gas manifolds have been installed, and the manual change over for gas bottles has been replaced with an automatic shuttle system.

Conclusion

In this short paper I have tried to show the work involved in bringing a health care facility up to date. We must not however lose sight of the changes which are to come in health care and the equipment still under development, as well as the continual improvement of that which is already available, provision must therefore be made where possible for these developments in any modernisation programme.

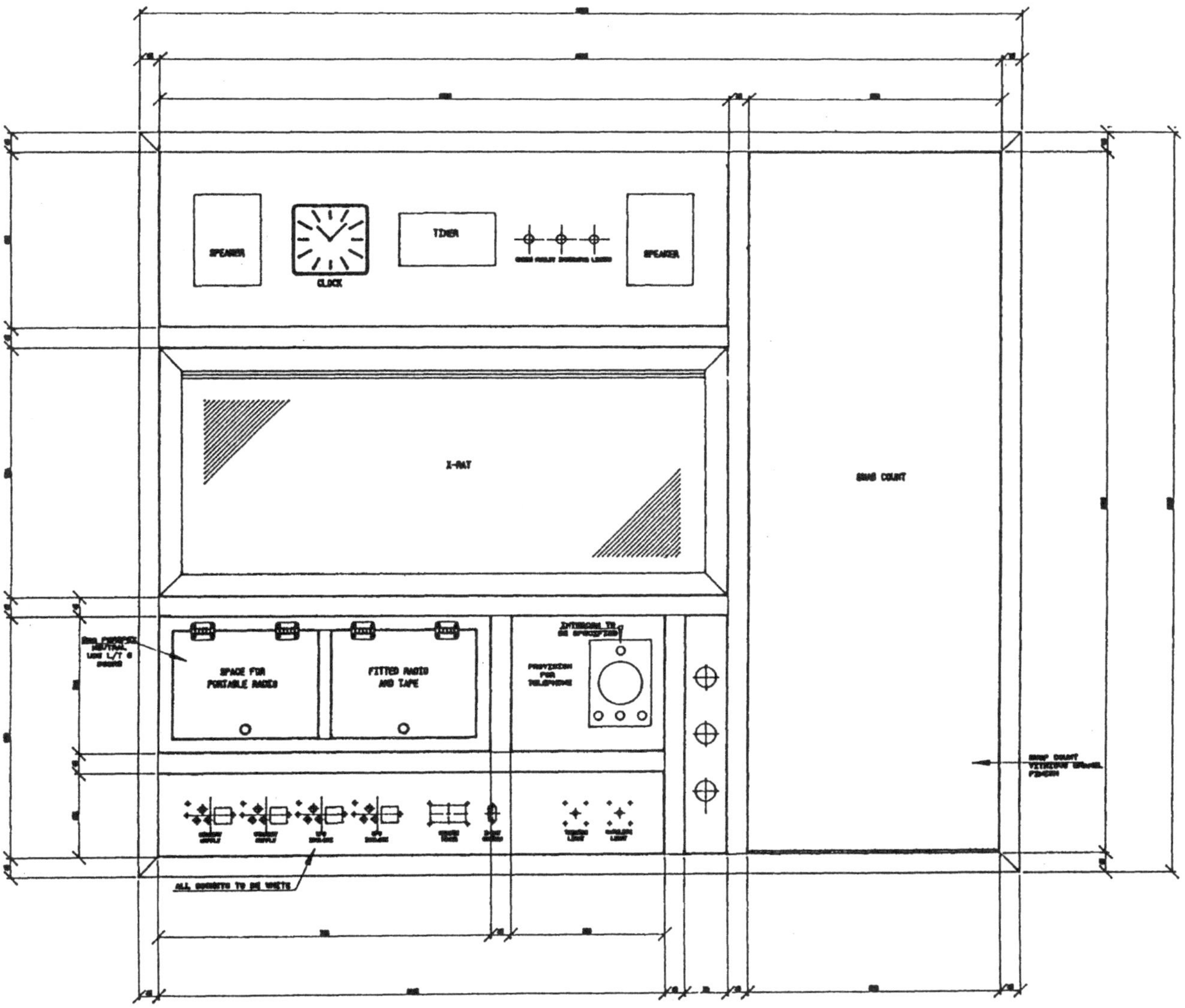

K12 Theatre Control Panel

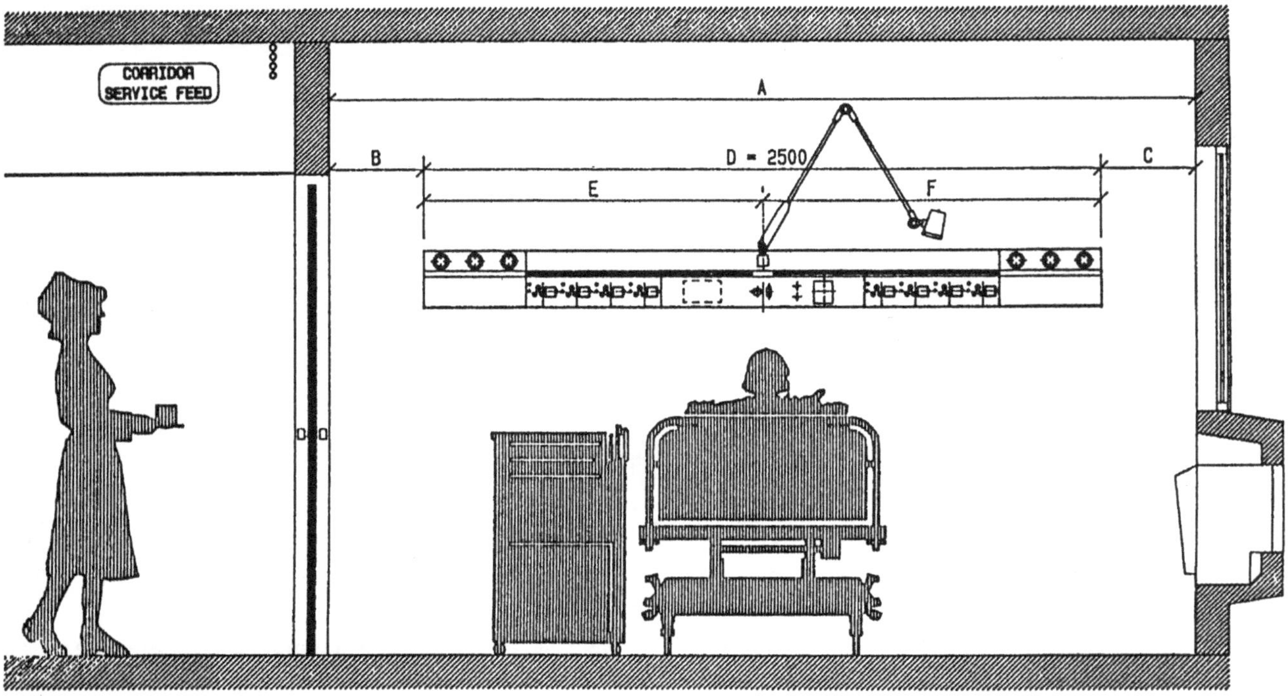

Typical One Bed Ward Layout

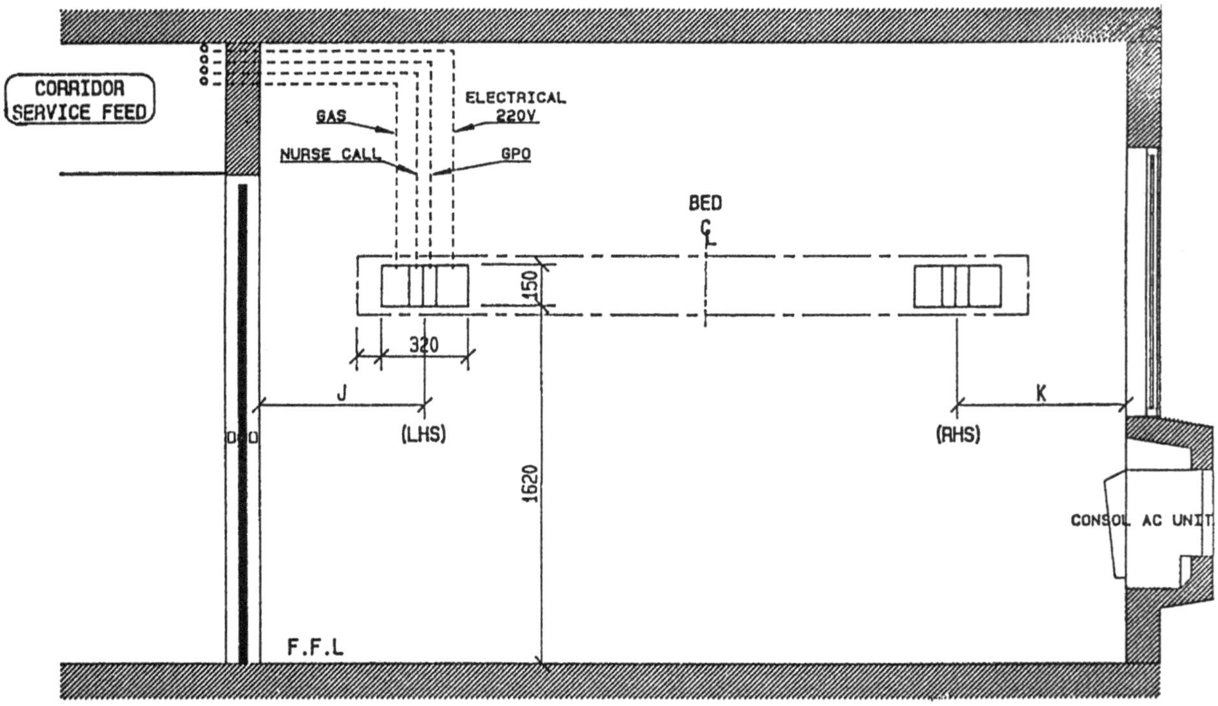

Typical Ward — Recessed Service Entry Box Mounting Left or Right Hand

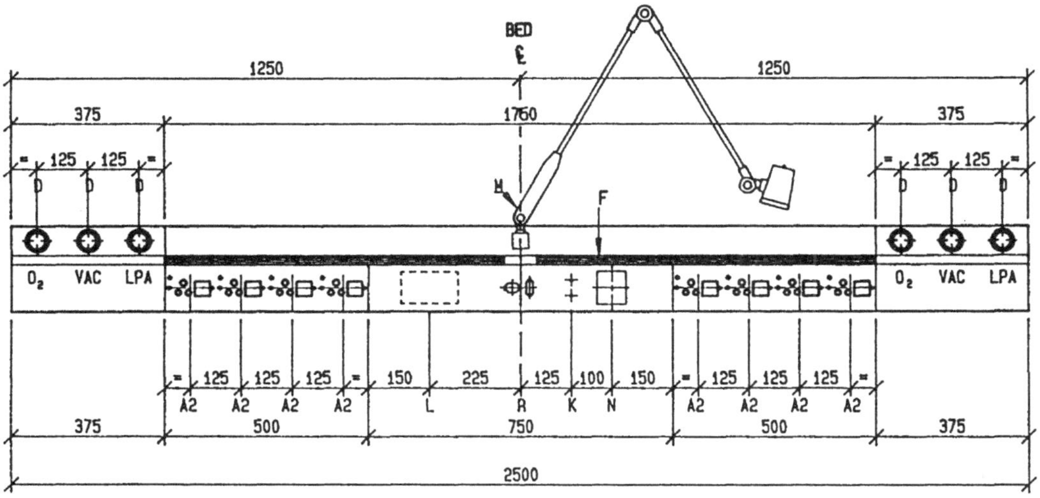

Type A — 1 Bed Module

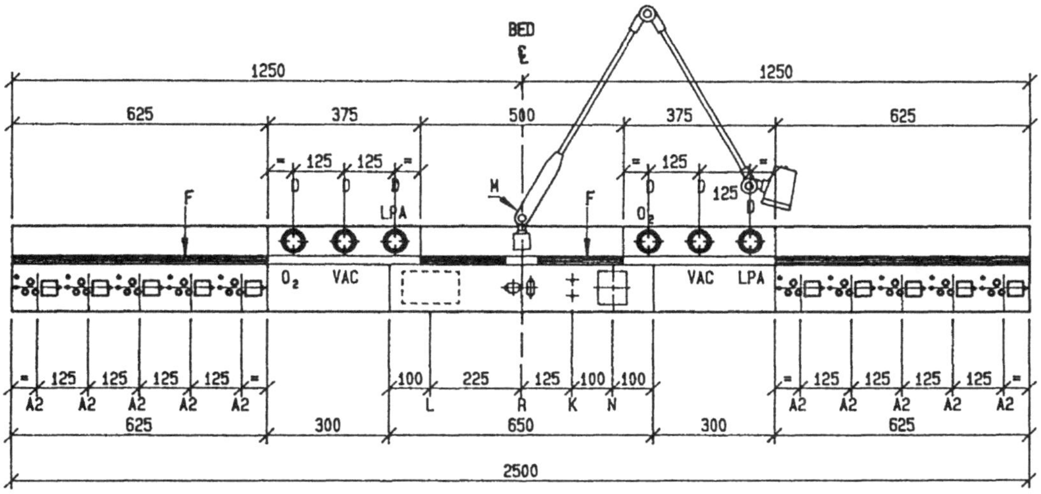

Type B — 1 Bed Module

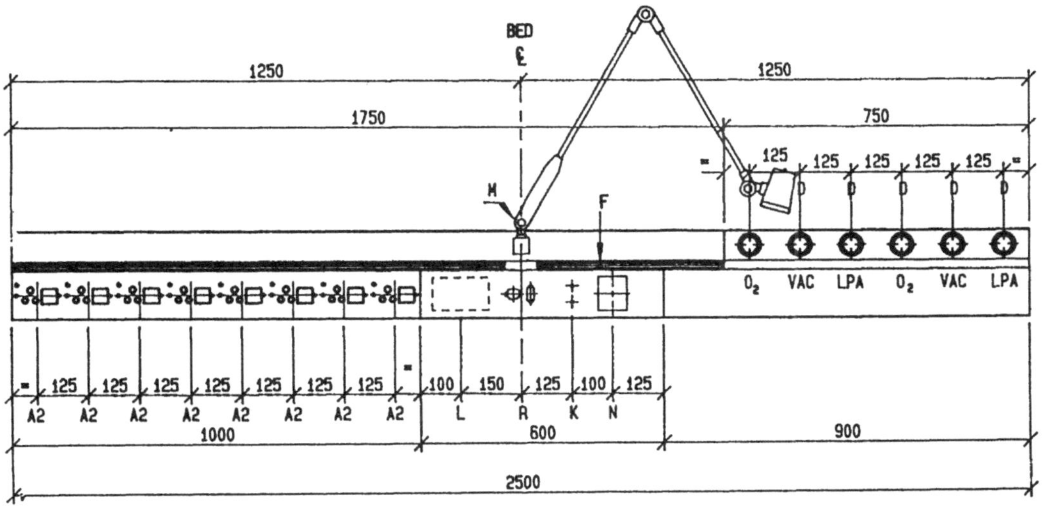

Type C — 1 Bed Module

Works Information Management System (WIMS)

by
David A. Butler FRICS
Assistant Director/Chief Surveyor
Department of Health

Introduction

The National Health Service Estate (NHS) in England is valued at over £20 billion, comprises some 2,000 hospitals and well in excess of 100,000 separate buildings.

The annual capital expenditure exceeds £1 billion and there are currently about 500 projects either in planning or under construction each costing over £1 million. The largest of these schemes is the Chelsea and Westminster Hospital project due for completion in 1992 at a cost of about £200 million.

Responsibility for the daily operation of this estate is devolved to hospitals or units through several management levels, eg Regional, District and Special Health Authorities.

The Department of Health and the NHS are aware of the importance of making the most effective and economic use of the estate by developing improved planning techniques and better management procedures.

The quality of decisions made by managers can only be as good as the information on which they are based.

The range of information for estate management is extensive covering building and engineering aspects and revenue and capital budgets. Traditionally much information has been derived from data collected for many different purposes, eg site surveys, labour performance records, asset registers, etc.

The various layers of management have differing information needs because the nature, range and depth of their decisions varies.

WIMS: The System

WIMS is the generic name for a computerised information system aimed at assisting estate management. The system has been under development since 1979. All the major aspects of works and estate management have been covered within the suite of programs which is designed to extend over both the long term development of services and the day-to-day works management activities.

WIMS 1

The system was initially developed for use on single-user micro computers with hardware independent versions following under other multi-user operating systems. Some of the latter developments were on database systems to allow greater flexibility in accessing data and producing ad hoc reports.

WIMS 2

In 1985 the development of a second generation of WIMS began. The philosophy and major requirement for the development was a much improved facility for the integration of data across applications both in the estate management area and with the requirements of other disciplines.

WIMS 2 APPLICATIONS

Identification of Estate Applications
The estate processes are:-

- Support Asset/Property Registers
- Schedule Maintenance Jobs
- Monitor Asset/Job Performance
- Monitor DEL/Labour Performance
- Support Maintenance Contract Management
- Purchase Estate Materials
- Monitor Energy Consumption
- Support Capital Project Management
- Support Capital Design
- Support Estate Rationalisation
- Reconcile Financial Information
- Support Capital Charges

All of these processes and their main associated information areas (except Capital Design) will be supported by WIMS 2 applications, as shown below.

WIMS2 Applications

Estate Process	*WIMS2 Applications*
Support Asset/Property Registers	AO/PL/RP
Schedule Maintenance Jobs	AO
Monitor Asset/Job Performance	AO
Monitor DEL Labour Performance	AO
Support Maintenance Contract Management	AO/FC
Purchase Estate Materials	FC
Monitor Energy Consumption	EM/FC
Support Capital Project Management	SP/CP/FC
Support Capital Design	—
Support Estate Rationalisation	SP/PL
Reconcile Financial Information	FC/AO
Support NHS Capital Charging	CAA

Key:
PL = Property and Land
AO = Asset Operational
FC = Financial Control
SP = Strategic Planning
CAA = Capital Asset Application
RP = Residential Property
EM = Energy Monitoring
CP = Capital Project Management

SYSTEMES DE GESTION DE L'INFORMATION BATIMENTS ET EQUIPMENTS

L'administration nationale de santé (the National Health Service) en Angleterre comprend environ 2 mille hôpitaux et nécessite une dépense annuelle du capital de plus d'un trillion de livres. C'est nécessaire d'avoir un système comprehensif de gestion pour ménager efficacement une proprieté si grande.

WIMS est un système technologique d'information, visé à aider la gestion de la proprieté. Tous les aspects importants de la gestion des travaux et de la proprieté sont contenus dans WIMS.

Les realisations d'usage courant de WIMS comprennent un programme qui a la facilité de soutenir un registre des bâtiments et du domaine et un programme régulier de fonctionnement; de permetre l'entretien bien concu; de completer efficacement des travaux prévus et le dépannage.

Il y a aussi une gestion financière qui permet le surveillance de tout ce qui a trait à la gestion de la proprieté, y compris les budgets et la planification soutenir des stratégies de rationalisation de la proprieté.

The current existing WIMS 2 applications are as follows.

I. Property and Land Applications

Outline of Functions

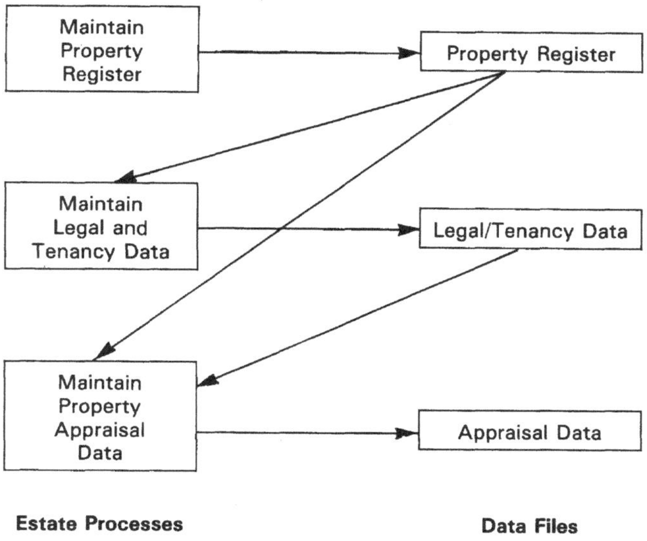

The Property and Land Application provides facilities for maintaining a comprehensive property and land register. It allows land and buildings to be split down into a five level hierarchy:-

- Site
- Land portion
- Building
- Building portion
- Functional space

Basic information is held at each level and each user is left to decide how to split down their estate in order to allow relevant details to be held at the appropriate level of the hierarchy.

The types of detail that may be held are split into two categories: the first, Legal/Tenancy, has the following topics:-

- Leasehold detail
- Legal requirements
- Occupancy detail
- Relevant authority detail
- Restrictions
- Rights
- Town Planning/Geological

The second, Appraisal, has:-

- Annual costs
- Energy performance
- Functional suitability
- Physical condition
- Statutory standards
- Utilisation
- Statistics

II. Asset Operational Application

This application deals, generally, with the day-to-day operations of Estate Management Departments. Three main facilities are provided:-

- Asset Register
- Work Planning and Processing
- Work History

In the Asset Register each asset is assigned a unique identifier and each asset record contains comprehensive inventory information including asset type, management unit and location descriptions.

In the Work Planning Section, details of the work that it is required to do on the assets are stored and scheduled. This work will include planned maintenance, requisition and breakdown work, work related to specific upgrade and other projects, and other tasks, all of which will be split between directly-employed and contract labour. Details of completed work are stored as history. The history information provides financial and technical management information, some of which may be used to assist in decisions regarding new asset purchases or modifications, closing the asset management loop.

Outline of Functions

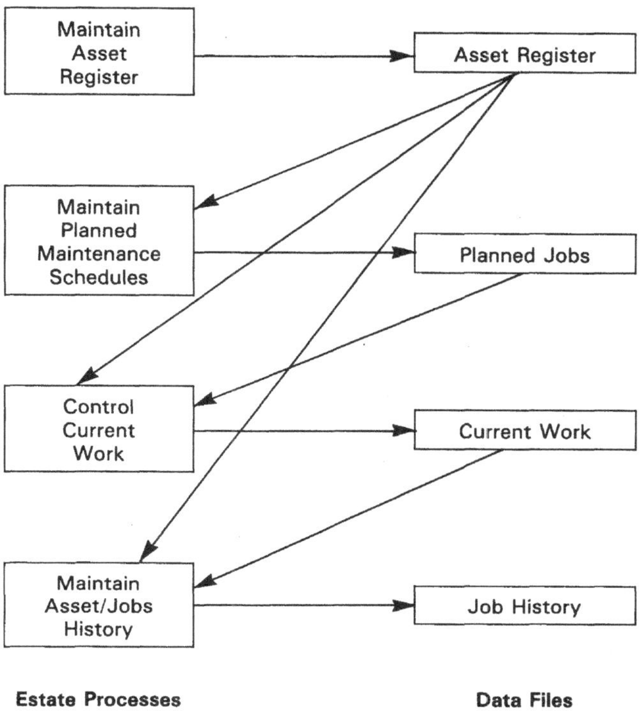

In the Asset Operational Application, the wide range of work that estate management departments have to handle is divided into two types: routine periodic inspection and maintenance jobs. These are both loosely described as 'planned maintenance' (PM) and 'one-off' jobs which may be requested by users and could be due to plant or equipment failures, or is work to be done on modification and other project work.

Work to be done may only be planned against a specific asset already created in the asset register, this is to ensure that any expenditure can be tracked back into a current work file.

The Current Work File (CWF) holds records of all jobs that are current, that is all PM jobs planned for a current week (or weeks) and all outstanding one-off (generally breakdown and requisition) jobs. These last are created directly into the CWF when requisitioned or reported.

Facilities are provided to enable the CWF to record details of the progress of a job and a 'reason for delay' code, both of which are intended to enable the estate department to provide users with information on the current status of work.

As notifications of completed work are received, by the return of dockets in the case of in-house work, and by a job completion note or invoice for contract work, the details are entered against the appropriate CWF record.

Various routines are available to update the CWF, the main update transfers all completed jobs to the history file, automatically deleting them from the CWF. There is also a routine to enable any unstarted job to be cancelled, in this case details of the cancelled job appear on a mandatory report.

III. Financial Control Application

Outline of Functions

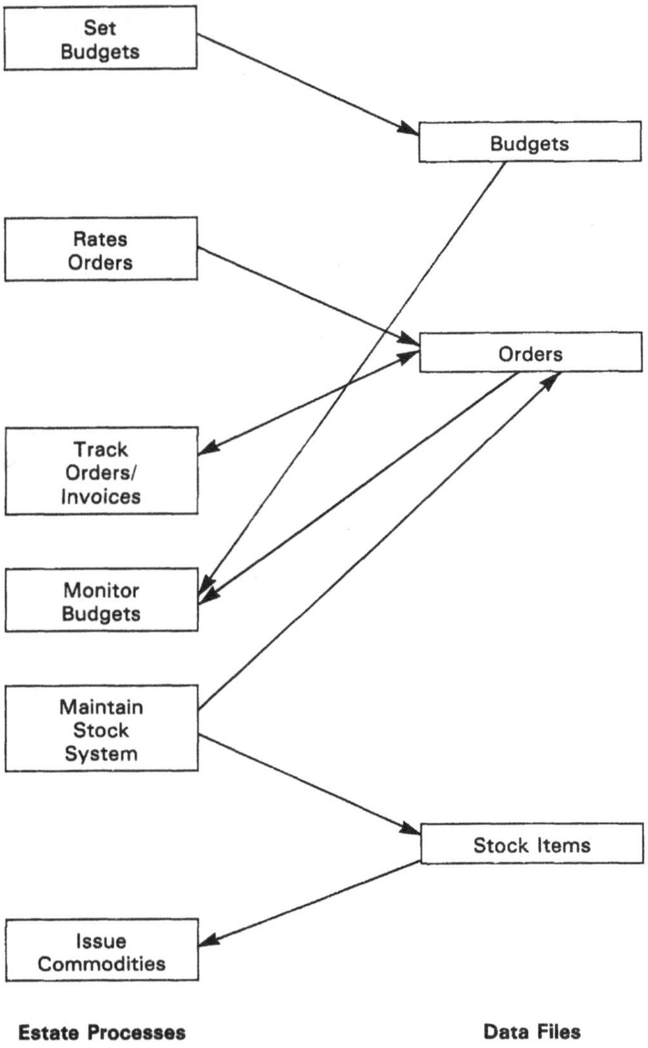

All records of completed work are transferred into a permanent history file. This history provides the basis for all areas of management information and standard reports are available for technical, financial and summary purposes.

Analysis for specific management purposes include reports of maintenance costs, by equipment type, so providing data for management budgeting and by building so, for example, that revenue costs may be taken into account during estate rationalisation.

The range of estate cost information may be divided into three categories:-

- DEL (directly employed labour) Costs
- Non-DEL (eg contract work) Costs
- Commodity (eg parts and material) Costs

The two prime capabilities of the Financial Control Application (FCA) are:-

- It allows an Estates Officer to maintain an overview of all estate finance matters on a day-to-day basis.
- Its output, in the form of total annual estate spending, should reconcile with the equivalent Finance Department figure (which may have originated from a Finance accounting system like SAS or IRIS).

This reconciliation will be conditional on the amount of control that an Estate Department has on the order and invoice processing of the two components, non-DEL labour and commodities, and on the differences of approach in the methods of calculating overheads by the Finance and Estate Departments.

There is a further capability that cost information (for services like non-DEL work and commodities) recorded as financial transactions in the FCA is transferable to the Asset Operational history so that the costs may be attributed to a specific asset or group of assets.

In the summary the FCA:-

- Allows budgets to be set up for various Estate activities.
- Allows orders for services and commodities to be made against the Budgets.
- Allows invoices for services and commodities to be charged against Orders.
- Works on an annual basis with reconciliation at (monthly) intervals with a facility for handling 'carry-overs' into another financial year.
- Includes a Stock Control (Stores) system.
- Logs all transactions with the various types of transactions that are only being allowed to privileged users.
- Interfaces with the WIMS 2 Asset Operational Application in order to transfer contract and, optionally, commodity costs to charge against assets in the Asset Operational Application.

IV. Strategic Planning Application

Outline of Functions

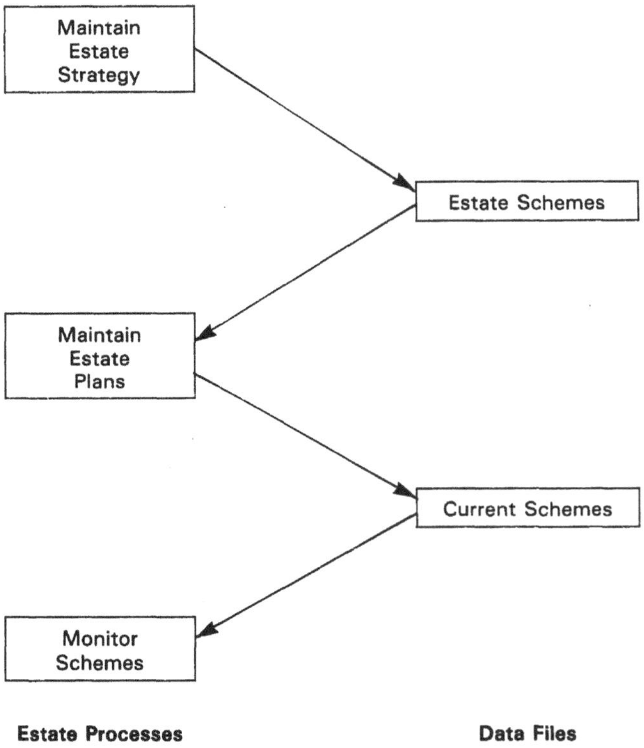

This application supports NHS estate rationalisation strategies which are intended to ensure that the NHS property and land holdings match current and foreseeable requirements. It includes facilities for modelling and for the strategic monitoring of a number of concurrent revenue and capital schemes in a Health Authority.

The SPA can make use of data held in the WIMS 2 Property and Land Application and enables broad details of future and current capital and revenue 'schemes' (and their component stages) to be recorded. The SPA can provide information on the consequence of estate expenditure on specific health departments and health functions.

V. Capital Asset Application

A recent change to the accounting arrangements of the Health Service requires that the cost of holding capital assets must be included in the charges for providing health care services.

Developed to meet the needs of the NHS Capital Charging initiative the Capital Asset Application (CAA) shares a common asset register with the Asset Operational Application although capital assets may only be input or amended via the CAA. Audit trails for financial asset information are provided by means of a transaction log. Two sets of reports are available, one for management purposes and the other provided to be used in conjunction with end-of-financial-period update routines.

VI. Future Development Plans

A number of programs are available in WIMS 1 or other separate systems which still need to be brought into the WIMS 2 system. These include the following.

Residential Properties. The requirement here is for an extension to the Property and Land Application which will hold the additional information which is relevant to tenants and residences, eg accommodation availability, tenant details, rent details. A link with the Financial Control Application would provide details of rent payments.

Energy Usage Monitoring. The requirement here is for an additional extension to the Property and Land Application to hold the details of energy targets and usage for buildings or sub-buildings for energy monitoring purposes. A link to the Financial Control Application would provide energy and utility cost data.

Capital Scheme Control. This application which currently exists under the Department of Health CONCISE system will include facilities for the approved contractors list with details of each contractor's capabilities and performance on past schemes and tenders, tender management to select a relevant sub-set of the approved contractors to invite to tender for schemes and scheme monitoring and control of both physical and financial aspects of each capital scheme.

Further extensions to these main areas may be required at a later date, for example, a further set of details in the Property and Land Application to cover Listed Buildings information.

Conclusion

WIMS offers an integrated estate management information system that has now developed well beyond the implication of its title that it is simply a works information system. It is subjected to continuous research and development in response to the demands of managers of estates anxious to make the best use of their estate resources both in the long term development of health care services and the day to day works management activities.

The various routines can be operated by the full range of staff in estates and works management, thus fully exploiting the interest and commitment of staff irrespective of the grade and background.

The range of current WIMS 2 application interactions is illustrated in the following diagram.

WIMS2 Application Interactions

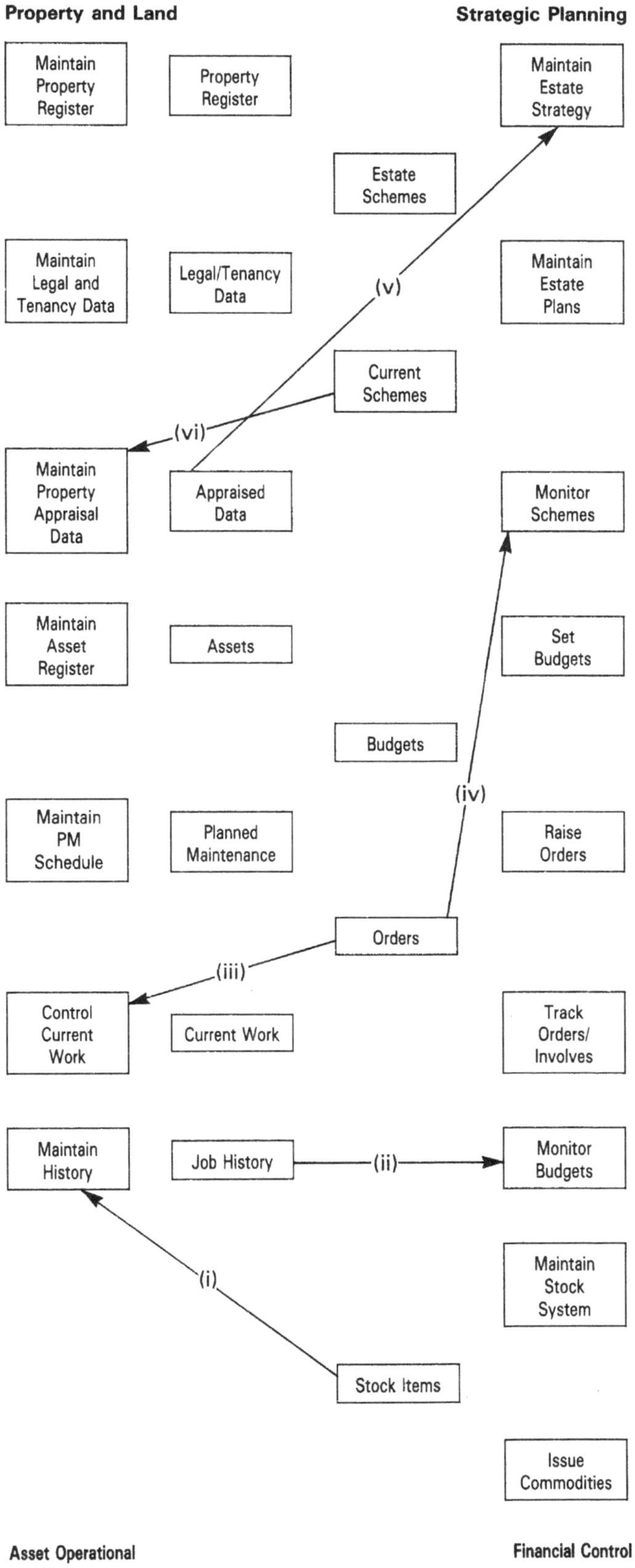

Facility Management in Health Care

by

W. van Blaricum
(graduate of the Technical University Delft)
Academic Hospital Rotterdam — Dijkzigt
Dr. Molewaterplein 40
3015 GD Rotterdam
The Netherlands

Description of the Dijkzigt Hospital

The Dijkzigt Hospital is a university hospital situated adjacent to the faculty of medicine of the Erasmus University of Rotterdam. The hospital complex is connected with the buildings of the faculty by way of footbridges.

The total gross floor area of 139.000m^2 includes space for the clinical departments, the out patient departments, the clinical laboratories and the administrative building. There are more than 12 different air conditioning systems with 104 air conditioning plants for conditioning the air for the clinical departments (950 beds, 10 intensive care units, 29 X-Ray rooms, one of which has a Magnetic Resonance Imaging and 21 operating theatres, one of which has a kidney stone lithotriptor), the air for the laboratories and the air for the out patient departments.

The hospital has 3,500 employees.

The hospital buildings, came into use between 29 to 9 years ago.

Keeping Buildings 'Up to Date'

One of the main tasks of facility management is to keep the building 'up to date', so that the board of directors can devote their full attention to their 'health care' task.

To achieve this goal, in Dijkzigt facility management is projected and achieved by:-

— reorganisation of buildings; eg between 1975 and 1978: the electric installation and the sewerage system were renewed and the air-conditioning installations on the nursing wards (commissioned in 1961) were installed;
— renovation of building; eg during 1983 and 1984 the laboratory building, commissioned in 1961, was renovated; only the reinforced concrete structure was left untouched, the remainder (inner walls, installations, windows, etc) were demolished and rebuilt;
— adjusting rooms to the demands of new medical apparatus, such as X-Ray scanners, a kidney stone lithotriptor, a Magnetic Resonance Imaging system, isolation wards for infectious patients and immunised patients, etc;
— maintenance; preventive, corrective and substitution, substitution comprises the replacement of an electric fan motor as well as the replacement of complete installations, in the case of reorganisation or renovation of a building.

Realised Costs per Year Maintaining Buildings Up to Date

— Preventive and corrective maintenance: 2% of the replacement value of the *installations*.
— Substitution maintenance (including reorganisation and renovation): 2,7% of the replacement value of the *installations*.
— Reorganisation (excluding partial replacement of installations), renovation, (excluding partial replacement of installations) and adjustments: 0,15% of the replacement value of the total *building*.

Table 1 shows the total replacement value of the buildings in Dutch florins, as well as, the replacement value of the installations in the buildings.

Total floor area in m2	Total value f. x 10^6 =	installations f. x 10^6	+ structure + f. x 10^6
48,000 m	f. 233.- =	102.-	+ 131.-
13,100 m	f. 59.5 =	23.5	+ 36.-
8,000 m	f. 28.5 =	6.5	+ 22.-
3,400 m	f. 10.5 =	1.5	+ 9.-
9,200 m	f. 27.0 =	2.-	+ 25.-
9,600 m	f. 32.5 =	6.5	+ 26.-
18,100 m	f. 108.- =	58.-	+ 50.-
2,600 m	f. 10.5 =	3.5	+ 7.-
18,100 m	f. 79.- =	29.-	+ 50.-
9,800 m	f. 45.5 =	19.5	+ 26.-
139,900 m	f. 634.- =	252.-	+ 382.-

Table 1: Replacement Values Dijkzigt-Buildings.

Facilities in and Around the Buildings

In the buildings users (patients, visitors and personnel) have to feel safe. To create that condition, the following measures are taken:-

Safety

— Intensive care units, operating rooms and special examination rooms are provided with an electrical patient safety installation to avoid electrocuting patients by very small currents (30mA) and very low voltage (10mV);
— the Dijkzigt complex has several emergency power plants with a total capacity of 75% of the peak demand (one of the emergency installations has been constructed as a combined heat power plant);
— the Dijkzigt complex has water tanks with a capacity of one day demand;
— the use of special building materials, curtains,

GESTION DES EQUIPEMENTS DANS LES SOINS DE SANTE

Depuis 1975, l'Hôpital Dijkzigt dispose d'un système de gestion des équipements de soins de santé. Pour ce faire, il a fallu élaborer, avant, un système de gestion des bâtiments. Beaucoup des activités liées à ces systèmes ont été automatisées au cours des dernières années. Il existe aussi en parallèle un système de gestion des bactéries. Toutes ces dispositions permettent aux responsables de disposer d'un très grand nombre d'informations, qui, une fois mises en contexte, donnent une ideée de la qualité des équipements et des services. Il est aussi possible de mesurer rapidement les coûts des opérations en cours et ainsi de pouvoir changer d'approche si nécessaire. Pour l'Hôpital de Dijkzigt, cela a permis en 1988, de réaliser des économies de 10% par rapport à 1977.

matresses, etc which are hardly or totally non-inflammable;
- the Dijkzigt complex has an automatic fire detection system, except for the clinical wards where nurses are on duty 24 hours a day;
- air conditioning installations, which create air pressure differences between operating rooms and the corridor, between safety rooms and the corridor; and
- tanks for nuclear waste etc.

Security

To minimise the criminal behaviour TV-cameras have been installed around the building complex and in the lifts of the main building. All the emergency exits have an electric lock, which will be opened automatically by an alarm of the fire detection installation. The doors in the corridors between the clinical buildings and the other buildings, also have an electric lock. These doors are locked after working hours (see sheet 1).

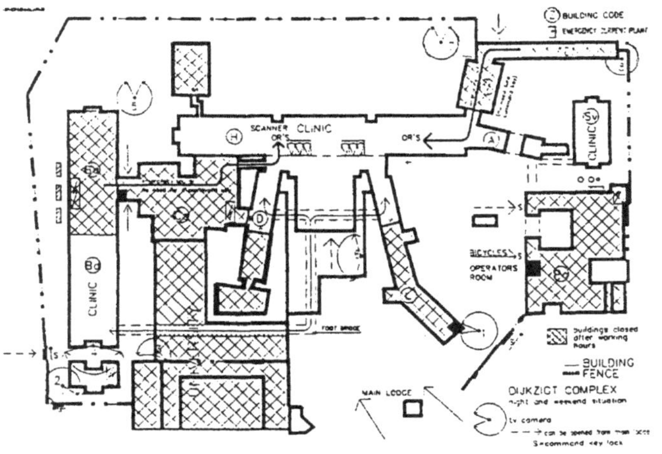

Sheet 1

After working hours it is necessary to have a key card, which is programmed to release the lock. The same card is also used to gain access to the parking facilities or to pay for ones lunch in the hospital restaurant. Each card has a world-wide unique code, like a gene passport.

Communications

Dijkzigt has a digital telephone exchange, which allows the use of one single line for text, data and voice simultaneously. A paging system (bleepers) for people who are frequently on the move is coupled to the exchange. This coupling enables every employee to use the internal telephones to initiate a call to a bleeper without the need of a telephone operator.

Various Facilities and Services

One of the many tasks of a facility manager is his responsibility to ensure, that buildings are kept clean, warm in winter and cool in summer. Meals have to be on the nursing wards at the right time and at the right temperature. Fresh linen has to reach the nursing wards in time. Dirty linen as well as rubbish, have to be removed. If they come from infectious patients they must be packed in special bags or barrels.

Building Management System

To be able to render all the above mentioned facilities and services 24 hours a day, every day of the year, one needs to set up a building management system (see sheet 2). Any automation, which is economically feasable, is implemented. The major advantage of an automatic system is the on line output of measurements in terms of graphs or tables.

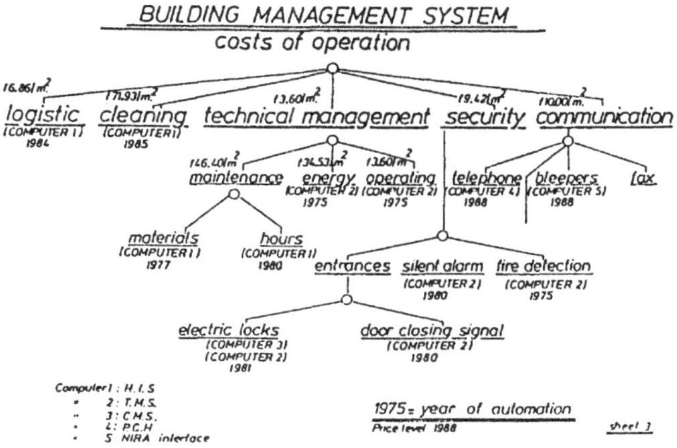

Sheet 2

Logistics

The lifts in the main building (13 floors) are operated by a micro-processor, which calculates the most economical use of the three liftcabins (by measuring speed, load, number of stops, etc). From all these data it is possible to produce a graph, showing how long it takes to answer a call within 10 secs, 20 secs, etc (see graph 1). So it evaluates

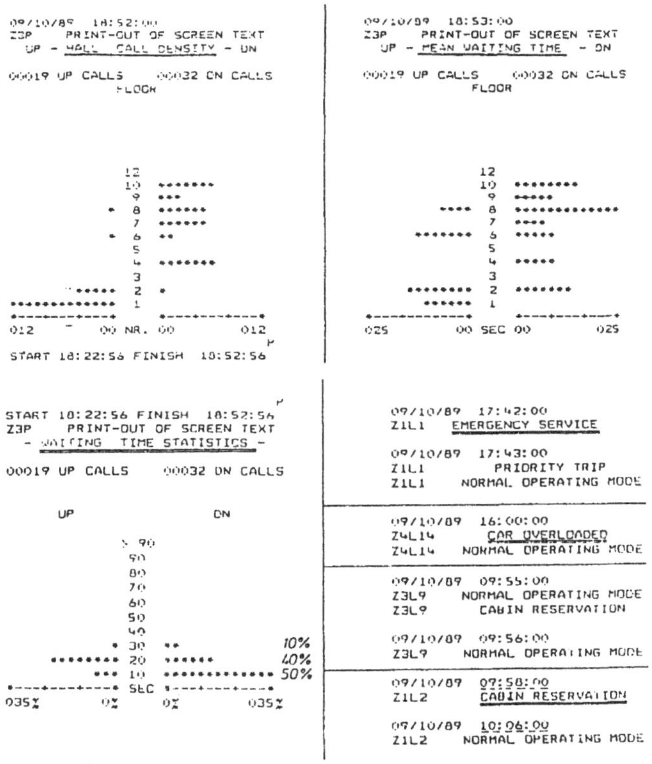

Graph 1

the *quality* of your lift transport (and whether the number of lifts is sufficient). It also shows the average waiting time on each floor or the number of up and down calls on each floor.

Since the introduction of micro-processor steering the complaints about waiting times have stopped. Since 1975 the lifts have also been coupled to computer 2, (with the technical management system). Since then complaints about long locking-up times in lifts, have come to an end.

Computer 1 (a very large computer system with the Hospital Information System) contains a programme which controls the storage of a large number of articles in the main-store, as well as in the sub-stores on the nursing wards. With this programme the costs of cleaning materials are reduced by 30%.

Cleaning

Since 1986 computer 1 also has a programme, which calculates the cleaning time of bedrooms, offices, operating theatres, examination rooms, toilets, etc. This programme has recently been coupled to a statistical programme, in order to measure fairly objectively the *quality* of the result of cleaning activities.

Graph 2 shows the development of cleaning costs since 1977. The dip in 1986 demonstrates the influence of a newly appointed head of the cleaning department, while the

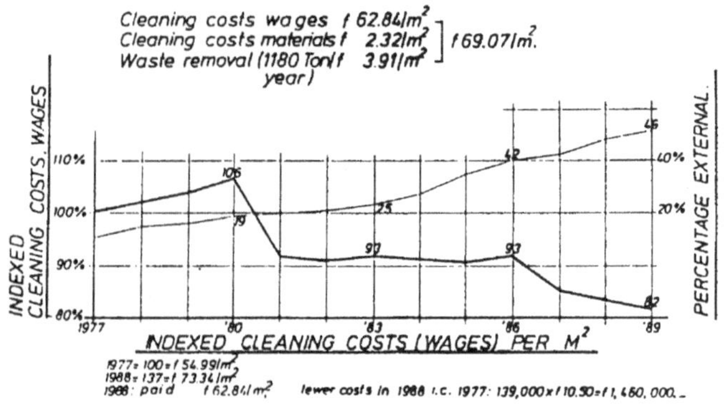

Graph 2

drop since 1986 has been caused by automation. Ever since the cleaning programme has been installed in computer 1, uniform quotations can be acquired and the control of own cleaning activities has much improved.

Bacteria Management System

To keep bacteria away from places, where they are unwanted under any circumstances, a bacteria management system can be established and again be computerised (see Sheet 3).

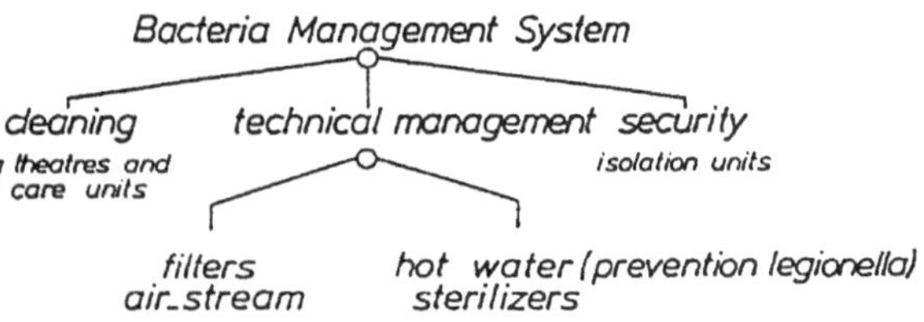

Sheet 3

The bacteria management system comprises the cleaning of operating rooms, intensive care units, isolation rooms on the basis of special protocols, which are laid down in the cleaning programme of computer 1. It includes an element of technical management; replacing filters in the air-conditioning installations, measuring the airsteam pattern in the operating rooms (the air around the operating table must be free of bacteria), keeping hot water free from legionella by heating the water sufficiently and by avoiding dead ends in the hot water system, the sterilisers (steam and gas) which are fitted out with micro-processors are connected to computer 2, by analysing the data the breakdowns are reduced to less than 0.3% of the number of processes. The safety aspect applies to the isolation rooms (normal isolation protects staff and visitors from infectious patients, reverse isolation protects immune patients from staff and visitors).

Technical Management

Maintenance: since 1977 the costs of materials, small repairs and contracts have been guarded by a programme in computer 1. Likewise the working hours of our own personnel are guarded by another programme in computer 1. As a result, nowadays we need 14% fewer hours for 20% more orders compared with 1980. The increase of orders is due to the extension of the floor area by 25%.

We perform preventive maintenance to avoid urgent break downs. So the number of urgent break downs over a certain period is a measure for the *quality* of the preventive maintenance.

Graph 3 shows the development of the number of urgent break downs and of the number of connections of air-conditioning installations, freezers, sterilisers, lifts, water treatment plants (reverse osmosis, softener etc) combined heat and power plant to computer 2, the technical management system computer.

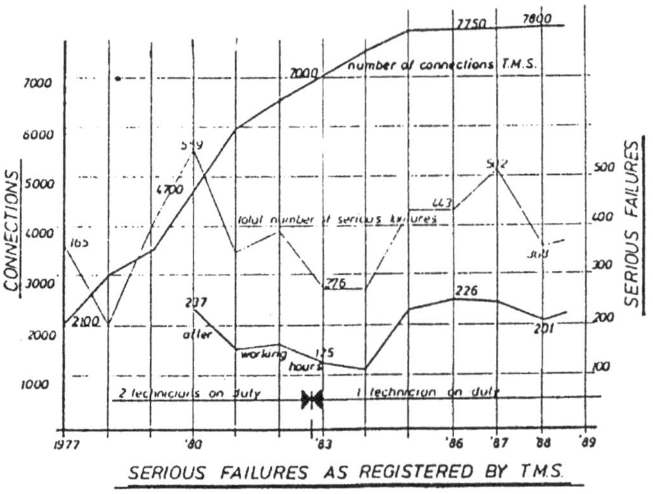

Graph 3

The rise in the number of urgent break downs in 1980 was due to the connection of a 12 year old air-conditioning installation to computer 2. After replacing some parts urgent break downs came down to a normal level. As the urgent break downs are recorded in black and white by computer 2, it was justified to reduce the watch from two to one technician, also with regard to the following facts: most of the urgent break downs occured during working hours and were caused by maintenance works and secondly most of the operations of the installations, plants, etc are executed by computer 2.

How we lowered the use of energy, you can read in the proceedings of the 9th International Congress of Hospital Engineering at Barcelona, Spain, page 565, 'Energy saving in existing Dutch buildings, measures and results'.

Graph 4 shows the investment in energy saving measures

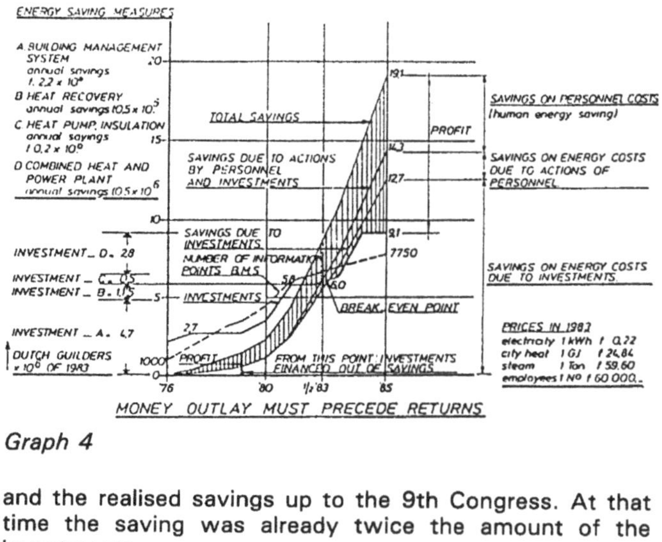

Graph 4

and the realised savings up to the 9th Congress. At that time the saving was already twice the amount of the investments.

Graph 5 shows the development of the m² floor area, the

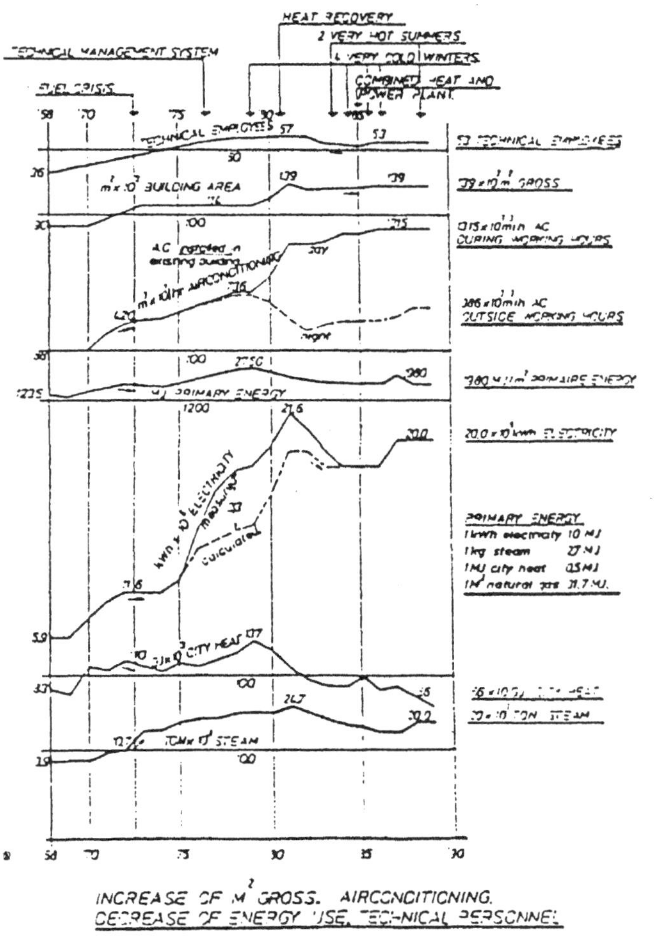

Graph 5

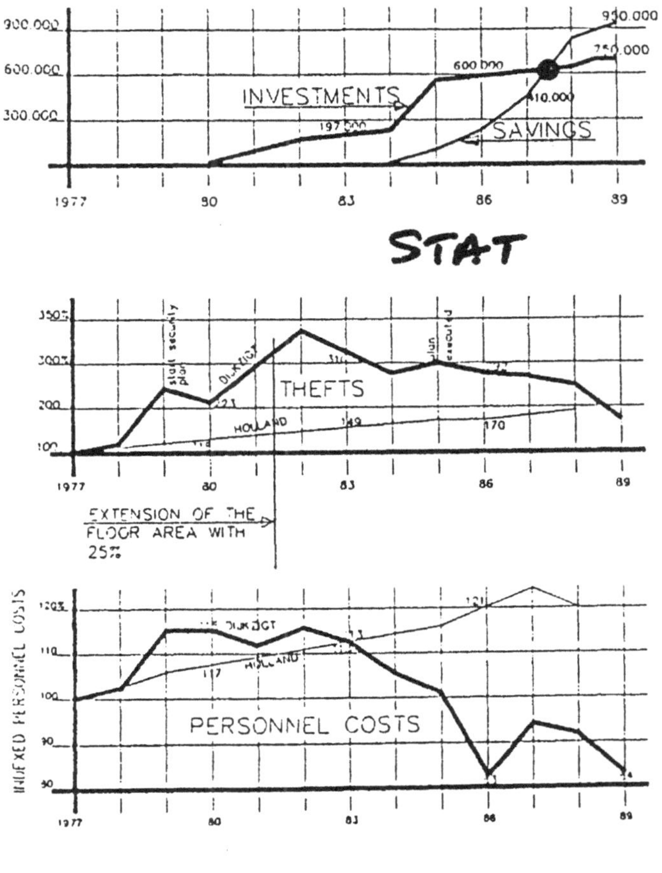

Graph 6

m^3 air, that are conditioned, the use of steam, city heating, electricity and primary energy.

The measure of the time, that the air-conditioning installations of the operation rooms are in full use, gives an interesting view on the actual working hours of these rooms and tells the management something about the actual number of rooms, needed.

Security

Graph 6 shows the investments and the savings, the development of the number of thefts and the development of personnel costs; the dip in 1983 is due to the closing of all the buildings after working hours, with the exception of the nursing wards and the first aid station.

As computer 3 registers the number of accesses, granted to a person at a certain door, but also to a separate parking facility, we can now see if that person rightfully makes use of that parking facility.

Communication

As mentioned before, our telephone exchange is a computer, so again a lot of data are available. This way we can measure the work load of the switchboards (see Graph 7) and so, in view of the work load we can determine whether the number of operators is sufficient.

We can measure the number of abandoned calls and the time, that all our incoming lines are busy. This says something about the quality of our attainability by phone.

To reduce the work load of the operators we have programmed the exchange in such a way, that a call for a phone, that is busy, is no longer connected to the switchboard. This is also cheaper for our customers.

Table 2 shows the number of abandoned calls and the average time before the calls were abandoned. You see the difference, earlier: fewer abandoned calls and a long average waiting time, later: up to 100% more abandoned calls (no switching to the operator), shorter average waiting time, so the third advantage is that our incoming lines are less occupied, so fewer lines are needed.

By using an interface between the telephone exchange and our paging system, we can measure the number of calls made to each bleeper. So we can actually measure whether the bleeper owners are mobile indeed, see Table 3. When the bleeper owner is not mobile, he has to hand in his bleeper. The result is, that for two years now there has been no increase of the number of bleepers.

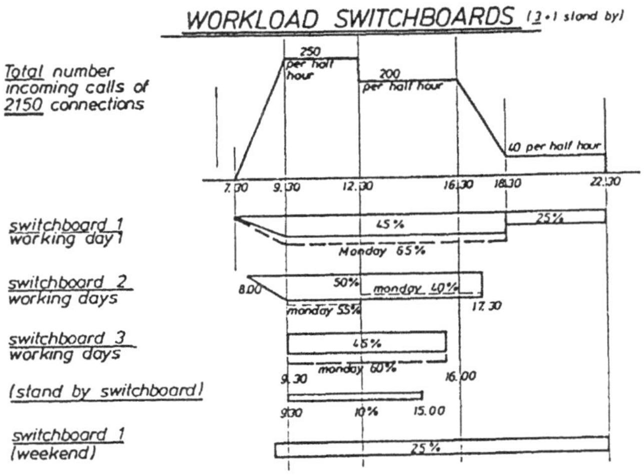

Graph 7

Financial Result

Table 4 shows the amount, that we paid less in 1988 in comparison with the costs in 1975/1977 as a result of introducing a building management system and automating a great deal of its activities since 1975.

Customer: Dijkzucht PCM Periode From: Monday July 4 1988
Daily Line Utilisation Report

Group Name: Incoming (1-48)

Line Identification	Number Offered Calls	Number Handled Calls	Average Duration Handled	Average Waiting Time (Sec)	Number Abandon Calls	Percent of Abandon	Average Wait Bef. Abandon	Number Outgoing Calls	Average Duration Outgoing
31 & 20	114	89	172.1	23.7	25	21.9	46.3	0	0.0
Total	5436	4031	197.0	21.4	1405	25.8	48.5	2	20.5

Customer: PCM Periode From: Monday October 16, 1989
Daily Line Utilisation Report Lines in this Group: 48

Group Name: Netlijnen In (1-48)

Line Identification	Number Offered Calls	Number Handled Calls	Average Duration Handled	Average Waiting Time (Sec)	Number Abandon Calls	Percent of Abandon	Average Wait Bef. Abandon	Number Outgoing Calls	Average Duration Outgoing
Total	7283	4405	195.0	17.3	2878	39.5	19.8	3	21961.0

Table 2

Measured between 14.11.88 14.30
and 22.11.88 3.30 ie nearly 3 days

Zoemer Nummer	Kosten-Olaats		dental oproepen
bleeper	*department*		*calls*
→ 5514	2300	= *CVCL*	448
→ 5547	1700	= *Radioloog*	550
5503	1550		200
6151	7100		193
5606	4000		148
5540	6200		141
5555	5100		135
5522	7100		130
5640	4000		127
5620	4000		125
5609	4000		124
5513	2200		119
8814	—	*no department*	1
7901	—	*means: wrong*	1
7902	—	*number dialled.*	1
5041	7500		0
5466	5300		0
4520	0349		0
4277	0349		0
5247	8000		0
5391	0331	*no call in 8 days*	0
5506	1550		0
5509	1550		0
5511	1650	*Conclusion*	0
5537	8000	*these employees*	0
5534	0000	*are not on the move.*	0
3914	0851		0
3700	0331		0
3641	0349		0
3526	1100		0
5658	5200		0
5022	5200		0
5677	5300		0
3400	0349		0
5035	7300		0
7831	6100		0

Table 3

Facility management
Result Building Management System.

	Paid in 1988	% of total.	less paid c.w 1975	Own person	Contrac-ting
Cleaning costs	f 10,300,000.-	24%	f 430,000.-	140	50%
Phone and guard costs (incl telephone costs)	f 2,700,000.-	6%	f 400,000.-	13	25%
Costs of energy (incl. operators, overhead, à f. 1,000,000.-)	f 5,800,000.-	22%	f 4,300,000.-	53	-
Maintenance-costs of installations	f 5,700,000.-	13%	f 255,000.-		60%
Maintenance-costs of buildings.	f 800,000.-	2%	f 190,000.-		
	f 25,300,000.-	67%	f 5,575.000.-	206	
Linen. (incl. replacement à f.780,000.-)	f 4,000,000.-	10%	(washing external)	12	85%
Costs of catering (incl. f.4,100,000.- costs of food)	f 9,100,000.-	23%	(dish external)	73	40%
	f 38,400,000.-	100%		291	

Table 4

Table 4

Sick Building Syndrome

Even if the facility management acquit themselves well of their tasks (clean building, well maintained air-conditioning installations, etc) the sick building syndrome, caused by psychological factors, can arise. People do not like to be ruled completely by a technical management computer. So, in our buildings sunshades are not regulated by a sensor, but can be operated by our employees (part of the necessary sunshade is realised on the outside by a fixed board). The lights are neither controlled by a sensor, but can be operated as well by our employees. On several places big temperatures and humidity meters are fixed on the wall, so that our employees can see whether it is too hot or too dry.

Finally

The arrival of micro-processors has made it possible for a facility manager to measure the quality of the facilities and services, in an economic way, so that he is able in quite a comfortable way at less costs to keep his building healthy and up to date and the inhabitants content.

What Future for Old Hospitals?

by
Prof Eduardo Caetano
Lisbon, Portugal

What is an Old Hospital

The future of old hospitals is a matter of concern to Portugal because there are still some very old hospitals working in the country, specially in the cities of Lisbon and Oporto.

Portugal is a 850 years old European nation: in the middle century the country possessed over 500 hospitals being nearly all of very small size. By the end of that century, King John the Second replaced many small hospitals by some centralised large hospitals principally in Lisbon, Coimbra, Oporto, Evora and other towns.

Portuguese navigators built over 60 hospitals in Africa, India (The 'Hospital de El-Rei' in Goa could receive up to 1,500 patients in the 16th century!), China (Macao), Ethiopia, etc, and about 300 in Brasil. All hospitals could be identified by some similar building characteristics.

Since the word 'old' in abstract has a very broad meaning, it is advisable to systematise old hospital buildings according to pre-arranged periods of time. Consequently four categories are suggested: new, modern, old and ancient (or antique) hospitals.

For the purposes of this paper, new hospitals are those built since the beginning of the 70's; modern hospitals may be considered those built since the 20's; the time period for the old hospitals category may start about the middle of the 18th century; and ancient hospitals will be those built or established before the middle of the 18th century.

Of course, other criteria could be set. For example, the old hospitals period is rather difficult to establish: it could be divided into three subcategories (very old, old and freshly old hospitals, for example) in order that a finer and better classification of hospitals be achieved as far as time is concerned.

Although theoretically an old hospital in certain conditions can function as a modern one, in practice it is extremely difficult to make an old hospital perform in obedience to modern technology. In reality, modern technology imposes many requirements that our engineering ancestors didn't dream of obviously.

An old hospital can be renovated by remodelling the building, installing engineering services and equipping it with the most recent medical devices; nevertheless, the basic design can not be radically altered, otherwise it would not be an old hospital but a modern hospital inside an old envelope!

The Origin of Very Old Hospitals

Some ancient and old hospital buildings were designed and built purposely to be hospitals as, for example:-

(a) The 200-bed Omnia Sanctorum Hospital (All Saints Hospital), in Lisbon, that replaced dozens of very small 7-bed hospitals; the building from 1492 was unfortunately destroyed by the terrible 1775 Lisbon earthquake and the hospital moved into the Convento de Santo Antao (St Anthon Convent School) where it is still working.

(b) In the Hospital Distrital De Évora there are some remains yet of the original 340-bed Hospital do Espírito Santo (Holy Ghost Hospital) inaugurated in 1495 which replaced 12 small hospitals one of which, the Hospital de Jerusalem for pilgrims, was born in 1143, according to some historians.

(c) The Hospital Thermal Da Rainha D. Leonor (Queen Eleonora Thermal Hospital), at Caldas da Rainha, was the first thermal hospital in the world built as such! The original capacity was 100-bed, in 1485. Since then many alterations were introduced but the old thermal pool and the chapel are from origin.

(d) The Hospital De Sao Marcos (St Mark Hospital), at Braga, was inaugurated in 1508, demolished later and replaced by another building in 1770 to which was added a beautiful building about the same age.

(e) It was an English architect, John Carr, who designed the Hospital De Santo António (St Anthony Hospital), built in Oporto 210 years ago and still working; it is a beautiful sample of hospital architecture well preserved (it was built with hard granite!).

A good deal of old hospitals had origin in convents and monasteries and a few in noble houses and places. Some are working yet. For example, the rural Hospital De Santo André (St Andrew Hospital) at Montemor was born as a St Andrew Inn for pilgrims in 1354; later, in 1460 became a Hospital-Inn and finally a Hospital in 1531 that was demolished and replaced by the existing building in 1748.

In general the transformation into hospitals was done peacefully but in a few cases it was by force as it happened in Lisbon immediately after the 1755 earthquake that killed about 50,000 persons. According to legend the monks had to leave in a hurry.

Most probably the conversion was not difficult: convents and monasteries had the facilities needed for hospitals then: small and large rooms, kitchen, refectory, stores and even a small infirmary with a pharmacy eg the Convent of Mafra.

Of course, the hospital technology of two centuries ago was incipient in comparison with that of the beginning of the 20th century. So, it can reasonably be presumed that, then, the needs of hospital facilities are very few: a hospital was mainly a special boarding house where patients could sleep, eat and rest and, also, be observed and treated. The specific medical facilities needed for diagnosis and treatment were very few rooms: a consultation room, a surgical room mainly for amputations and a pharmacy.

Until 1960 most Portuguese hospitals belonged to the Misericordias, religious instructions from the Middle Age. therefore there was a religious influence in hospitals, specially outside Lisbon and Coimbra (the 13th century university town). That influence was rather strong through several centuries but started to diminish in the beginning of the 20th century and finally came to an end in April 1974 with the 'carnation' revolution!

QUEL FUTUR POUR LES VIEUX HÔPITAUX?

Les anciens et vieux hôpitaux qui restent encore doivent être préservés et sauvés parce qu'ils sont un témoignage historique très important de l'évolution de la santé et de la technologie hospitalière pendant beaucoup de siècles. En plus, ils sont beaux!

Bien que les bâtiments de ces hôpitaux ne soient pas convenables pour les activités hospitalières de haute technologie, ils peuvent être utilisés pour bibliothèques; musées; instalations d'enseignement; de la direction et administration; et, parfois comme hôpitaux de jour ou centres de santé.

Les anciens et vieux hôpitaux doivent être sauvés aussi parce qu'ils sont un patrimoine des villes et des nations et un héritage de l'humanité.

Characteristics of Old Hospitals

Portuguese old and ancient hospitals are physically characterised by being mostly small in size and short in height; by having line, T, cross or square shapes with inside or adjacent courts or gardens; and by following the monobloc pattern with a main central corridor or a lateral (most common) corridor overlooking the courts or gardens. They were built with thick walls, small windows and roofs with tiles discharging the rain-water directly to the earth. Usually old hospitals have a good thermal balance and a satisfactory noise level because of the thickness of the walls, the small aperture of the windows and the type of materials used (bad transmission coefficients).

Functional characteristics are very poor, eg, functional flexibility, according to the needs of a modern hospital because the programming needs were, then, very few and the design matched these needs.

The small size of most old and ancient hospitals does not permit to obtain the level of efficiency that is expected from hospitals today. Although, nowadays, the trend is to reduce the hospitalisation (or the number of in-patient beds) due to a much shorter average length of patient stay than some years ago, nevertheless, there still is a minimum that shall not be surpassed in order to be efficient.

Characteristically there is a big reduction of beds (50% to 60%) when an old hospital is renovated.

Old and ancient hospitals present many safety problems, such as: an easy biocontamination, fire hazards, no defence against earthquakes, very poor vertical circulation and a potential dangerous emergency exists in case of a general panic or when everybody has to abandon the hospital very quickly. Lisbon and the southern part of Portugal are located in an Atlantic fault zone that passes through the Azores to Gibraltar, Naples, etc.

Maintenance of old and ancient hospitals is both a headache and a challenge: a headache because repairs or works are usually more expensive than budgeted and take more time to be executed than forecasted; and a challenge, for the reason that one never knows what will happen when a work or even a repair is started. Nevertheless even if the cost of maintaining an old hospital alive is somewhat above the cost-effective rule that the administrators so cherish, it shall be protected at least for the sake of spiritual values.

Difficulty of Adaptation to Modern Technology

Taking into consideration both some shortcoming inherent to old hospitals and an ever increasing technological hospital, is there any room for old hospitals in the future? The answer is: hardly, if the idea is to transform an old hospital into a new autonomous one.

It is very, very difficult, almost impossible, to make an old hospital function as efficiently as a new one without losing its antiqueness and spending too much money. Even if all the inside disappears and just the outside walls and roof are kept, an old hospital can surely be ameliorated but it will always suffer from the implications of an important condition: the constraint provoked by the 'envelope' where the renovation will be made. It won't ever be a 'correct' solution!

Is a thorough renovation and adaptation to modern technology advisable, as far as the binomial cost-benefit is concerned? The answer is: no, for most old hospitals. That's why a good deal of old hospitals are considered both an economical burden and a technical headache! However that does not imply that one should agree with their destruction or abandon because they can still play a useful role; the challenge is to get the most out of them in a complementary basis. Considering the most old hospitals are adaptable to many tasks within the hospital or health area, an adequate renovation may be recommended in certain circumstances as, for example, within the framework of a Master Plan. However, the renovation must always obey a compulsory condition: the old hospital shall not lose its character!

Although at first sight the logical conclusion seems to be: get rid of old hospitals to avoid trouble, engineers and architects should fight to preserve and keep them. There is no incoherence with this position when other values than just pure materialistic values are taken into consideration.

What Fate for Old Hospitals?

Often old hospitals are located in fine sites inside the cities, frequently downtown, and some even possess large areas of terrain. For example, the ancient Hospital de S.Jośe (St Joseph Hospital) in downtown Lisbon has a 51,000 sq m terrain. Some still get gardens and few trees. As a rule, space is small or practically non-existent.

As a consequence of the city growth and the dislocation of part of the housing to periphery, now most old hospitals are within tertiary zones (commerce, services and housing).

Some old hospitals, such as the Hospital Santo António in Oporto and the Hospital Sao José in Lisbon play an important role in the hospital structures of there cities.

It's amazing that today the poorer hospitals, in respect of building facilities, comfort and safety, are located in Portugal's most important cities (Lisbon and Oporto)! The reason is that they are ancient and very old hospitals and the upgrading has been relatively scanty. However, outside those cities, the country is satisfactorily covered by modern hospitals, principally those of the district type.

A choice of four alternatives is the most common fate for old hospitals in big cities: the sale; the replacement by new ones; the renovation; and the preservation.

(a) The scale for housing developments has been a permanent fate for many years although theoretical! Politicians enjoy speaking about it. However, there is no known single case of an old hospital having had this destiny since the beginning of this century.

About 20 years ago it was decided to sell the seven hospitals (five ancient and two old) belonging to the Lisbon Civil Hospitals Group. The idea was that the money from the sale would permit to build new hospitals to replace those. Contractors and real estate eople from different countries (USA, Canada, Germany, UK, etc) came to Lisbon. Firstly they were full of enthusiasm, euphoric, but after investigating a little locally, they disappeared and never returned. Why? Because the Municipality of Lisbon would take almost 80% of the land for streets, parking, social facilities, etc, leaving to them approximately 20% of the purchase only as useful area; besides, they could not build above a small number of stories. Furthermore they had to wait until new hospitals were built to receive patients and replace the old hospitals! Of course the business didn't interest them . . . and so the seven old hospitals were saved.

Again, today, there is a renewed appetite for old hospital terrains from more aggressive real estate people. Can old hospitals survive?

Shall the centre of big cities be empty of hospitals? Knowing that those hospitals are subjected to several shortcomings such as pollution, noise, vibration, lack of green protection zones and lack of parking space, shall they be removed from the centre? That is the question! The answer is that people who live or work in the centre of a big city shall have hospital support right there. In fact it is almost axiomatic that hospitals shall be sited where people exist.

(b) The replacement of an old hospital by a new one in the same place has seldom happened in Portugal during the last decades. It is a difficult task to do when the hospital continues in function, alive, due to many shortcomings such as: dust and biocontamination; noise and vibrations; functional disruption; long period of time to do the works; and high costs.

A process of improving the job is to 'break' the hospital

into several blocs and start the replacement bloc by bloc according to a Master Plan that integrates both the physical and functional aspects.

A simpler solution, although it has been rarely used, calls for provisional facilities to where patients, personel and equipment are transferred and from where they go back to the new building when it is ready.

Another easier way is to build the new hospital in the same site but not in the same place; this solution did happen several times.

(c) The renovation of old hospitals usually covers remodellings and or extensions.

This fate has taken place for many years and it is still a valid solution whenever the remodellings and or extensions are made according to a full Master Plan.

Vertical extensions are usually dearer and provoke much more trouble than horizontal extensions, as it occurred recently for example in the Hospital de Leiria.

(f) The preservation of most old hospitals should be enforced. After all they can be easily adapted to receive cultural, administrative and other hospital activities such as libraries, teaching facilities, archieves, museums, etc, as well as other health services or institutions eg homes for the elderly or health centres.

Often the hospital directorate and administration quarters can be located in old hospitals in a well dignified manner.

Sometimes it is not difficult to install a day hospital in an old hospital building when the ground floor is large enough and the main corridor is sufficiently wide.

Whatever the fate, old hospitals shall not be abandoned neither deserted. On the contrary, they shall be preserved and saved. The strategy used by some to let an old hospital decay or rot in order to press the Ministry to replace it by a new one shall be avoided. In most cases there is no replacement so that patients and personnel will take the consequences. For example, there are plans and programmes for new hospitals in Lisbon snce 20 years ago; however, the cost is so high that their construction has been postponed several times . . .

All things considered, the correct solution points out that it is worth keeping most old hospitals as examples of hospital and health architecture and that proper tenants shall be provided on the assumption that they are adaptable to many tasks within the health area.

What Has Been Happening?

Unfortunately, until about 25 years ago, some 'predators' destroyed or mutilated quite a large number of beautiful old hospital buildings mainly partly but in a few cases totally! What annoys mostly is the fact that they did it thinking that they were doing a fine piece of management. When somebody complained, they just didn't understand the reason for the protest and comments such as: 'we had such a nice vacant space here!' and 'we decided to get some profit from a non productive building' could be heard.

Why the abandonment and destruction of old hospitals? There are two main reasons: ignorance and lack of sensibility, as the following examples illustrate:-

(a) the old Hospital de S.Isidoro (St Isidore Hospital) at Caldas da Rainha, an interesting sample of hospital architecture was abandoned and is a ruin;

(b) a lovely large ward of the very old Hospital de Faro was spoiled when an intermediate floor was built!; and

(c) part of the very old Hospital do Espirito Santo at Evora was destroyed to build a new surgical bloc on the same site; fortunately, the other half was saved just in time!

Of course, it requires sensibility to beauty to admire and defend old hospitals: it is our duty to defend and preserve them according to the original design whenever possible.

For many years old hospitals had been 'suffering' minor or major renovations including remodellings and or small or big extensions. Sometimes the remodellings have benefited the old buildings specially when they have not spoiled their original character. It was what happened, eg, to Hospital S.José in Lisbon and to Hospital D. Manuel Aguiar at Leiria.

We all must be alert against a special subtle tactic used by some 'smart' persons: they just let old hospitals rot. For example, when they forget about maintenance letting old hospitals decay and die! When blamed for loss they candidly respond with the chronic lack of funds! It is rather Machiavellian since doing so they can hardly be accused of the destruction of old hospitals . . .

In principle, the remaining old hospitals must be preserved and cared for because they are both a patrimony of a nation and an heritage of mankind. They may not be technologically suitable but most are beautiful indeed!

To Save old Hospitals

Sometimes the preservation of old hospitals seems to rely on Master Plans dealing with one or more hospitals. In-fact old hospitals can usually play an important role within the general hospital structure, according to the rule: services needing higher technology will be incorporated in new buildings and simpler services in the old buildings.

Let ancient and very old hospitals live because they represent and document periods of the history of health; they give a great amount of information about design, materials, function and technology; they are a live document of the hospital evolution through the ages; they help to study the treatment of diseases; they are priceless witnesses of the history of mankind; and they are beautiful. Therefore, it is urgent to save old hospitals from the materialistic wave of real estate business so aggressive and wide spread nowadays.

Often it is an act of courage to protect an old hospital in order to avoid its destruction because it is necessary to fight against persons, prejudices and economic values. We, engineers and architects, deeply related to hospitals, must struggle hard to preserve old hospitals. Going further, it can be said that it is the duty of all those who work in or for hospitals, either engineers and architects or administrators, doctors, nurses and technicians to defend, protect, and save old hospitals.

Besides the historical, architectural and engineering values, an old hospital remains as a symbol of the noble struggle against disease and suffering and death in the course of time.

Fire Safety in Health Care Premises

by

D. W. Luscombe
Department of Health
Euston Tower, London

Firecode

Fire Safety and Control in NHS Health Care Premises centres around the Department of Health's Firecode suite of documents. This suite was launched in 1987 under the Departments' Health Circular HC(87)24 and copies of the documents, the Health Technical Memoranda and Fire Practice Notes, are available from HMSO. Documents published at that time were:-

(1) Firecode: Policy and Principles
(2) Firecode: Fire Precautions in New Hospitals (HTM81)
(3) Firecode: Assessing Fire Risk in Existing Hospital Wards (HTM86)
(4) Firecode: Directory of Fire Documents
(5) Firecode: FPN 1 — Laundries
(6) Firecode: FPN 2 — Storage of Flammable Liquids
(7) Firecode: FPN 3 — Escape Bed Lifts

Amongst the absentees at the November 1987 launch were three titles that have very recently been completed and printed. They are:-

Nucleus Fire Precautions Recommendations
HTM 82 — Alarm and Detection Systems
and
HTM87 — Textiles and Furniture

Further HTMs and FPNs are in various stages of preparation and a FPN on kitchens will emerge shortly.

After an initial issue of this guidance to the NHS the sales to consultants etc via HMSO continues at a brisk pace. The best seller is HTM86 — Assessing Fire Risk in Existing Hospital Wards, with around 3,000 copies at the end of last year.

Following the issue of PL/CE(89)2 of December 1989 entitled 'Fire Precautions in Health Buildings — Commercial Enterprises on Health Service Premises' a further Fire Practice Note (FPN 7) on the same subject is now in preparation.

Also under consideration at the present time is a proposed draft for a re-issue of HTM 83 — General Fire Precautions. Future work on Fire Practice Notes includes a new FPN 4 on Central Processing Units (Cook-Chill factories); FPN 5 on Boiler Houses and Incinerator Rooms and FPN 6 on Laboratories.

The 'Action' paragraph of HC(87)24 which launched Firecode sets out Authorities responsibilities relating to fire precautions and in this respect the message is particularly germane to this paper. In view of this relevance and the influence this message has had on the direction of subsequent fire matters work in the Department it is felt that a re-statement here of paragraph 9 of HC(87)24 would be appropriate.

> 'Health Authorities are asked to ensure that all statutory requirements relating to fire precautions are scrupulously observed and that the fire precaution specified by the Secretary of State, which are now set out in Chapter 3 of Firecode: "Policy and Principles", continue to be observed and that the fire precautions specified by the RHAs are asked to monitor DHAs' observance of this guidance; RHAs will be accountable to the Department for the application of this guidance to premises for which they are responsible and for their monitoring of DHA's performance. General Managers are asked to bring the contents of Firecode to the attention of all Nominated Officers (Fire) and to other staff as may be necessary and appropriate.'

When considering the likely target or audience for Firecode recognition should be acknowledged of the fire statistics provided each year by the Home Office. These statistics show an average of about one incident per annum for each of the hospitals in the NHS. Of the fires attended only about 25 extended beyond the room of origin.

It should be noted that the statistics do not include the smaller incidents which are sometimes referred to as the waste paper basket fires which are quickly extinguished by vigilant nursing staff or patients and which do not therefore result in a call to the local brigade. All fires in the Health Service are cause for concern and initiatives such as Firecode are aimed at reducing the national averages. Whilst on the subject of statistics it is worth bearing in mind the results of surveys about the cause of fires in hospitals. Clearly the main culprit is smoking. Smoking is not only bad for your health but statistically it can be demonstrated that it is bad for hospital building, patients and staff.

In summary it will be seen that Firecode recommends: fire risk separation; compartmentation; structural measures; choice of safe textiles and furnishings; alarm provision and evacuation procedures.

Low Rise Plus Progressive Horizontal Evacuation

In addition to Firecode a further control exercised by the Department regarding fire risk in health care buildings is enshrined in the major policy message found in HTM 81 — 'Fire Precautions in New Hospitals' and the 'Nucleus Fire Precautions Recommendations' documents. In both cases the emphasis is on the policy of adopting low rise developments. Coupled with the low rise philosophy is the concept of progressive horizontal evacuation of patients between compartments and sub-compartments. Also included in this concept is the provision of a clearly defined hospital street which will form the main route of ingress and egress for staff, patients, visitors, supplies and services and which should be constructed as a compartment.

PREVENTION DES INCENDIES EN MILIEU HOSPITALIER

Cet article décrit les activités du Département de la Santé dans le domaine de la prévention des incendies en milieu hospitalier.

Le document relatif aux Recommendations en vue de la Prévention des incendies (Firecode et Nucleus) y est cité. Les travaux du groupe de recherche (National Fire Policy Advisory Group) et du groupe de travail sur la législation concernant les bâtiments (Building Legislation Working Group) y figurent également et sont discutés.

L'article compare en outre les systèmes d'alerte actuellement disponibles aux développements Nucleus. Il est fait mention en particulier de magasins, de centres commerciaux, et de foyers dans les établissements hospitaliers.

Tout en établissant des mesures de base essentielles telles que la séparation des risques, la compartimentation etc, l'article n'oublie pas le rôle des responsables dans la prévention ni l'utilité d'un contrôle constant des niveaux de formation et de participation des personnels.

Il est question aussi du rôle de moniteur du Département et de sa participation telle qu'elle est envisagée pour le futur développement de recommandations dans ce domaine.

Health Service Estate Journal

A further valuable initiative that has recently been the subject of development by the Department is the Health Service Estate Journal. This journal is published quarterly by HMSO on behalf of the Estates Directorate of the Department of Health. It contains news, features and comment on a wide variety of estate matters and is increasingly being seen as an appropriate vehicle for disseminating information on Fire topics. It is of interest to those concerned with the estate and supplying goods, including services, plant and machinery. Contributions come from the Department of Health, the NHS and private industry. Enquiries or proposed contributions should be addressed to the Editor at the Department of Health, Room 619, Euston Tower, London NW1 3DN. Tel: 01-388 1188 Ext 3240.

National Fire Policy Advisory Group

When thinking of the problems of Fire Safety and Control in Health Care Premises reference is inevitably made to the National Fire Policy Advisory Group (NFPAG). This Group meets three times per annum with the 'chair' being provided by the Department of Health. It has a membership of seven Department Officers, nine NHS Members and one each from the Department of the Environment Building Regulations Division, Home Office Fire Services Inspectorate, Fire Research Station, Scotland, Wales, Northern Ireland and the Association of County Councils. The main thrust of the Group over the last few years has naturally been towards the completion and early publication of the full Firecode suite of documents. Clearly this Group provides links with other Government Departments and bodies who have major policy interests in fire safety. The Group is very widely based with a significiant NHS multi-disciplinary membership which includes District Fire Officer representation. The brief for the Group is 'to review, consider and co-ordinate all aspects of fire precautions and fire prevention in relation to all health and personal social service buildings, to formulate policy and issue guidance as appropriate'. From this brief it can be seen that the Group will be the prime mover in the preparation of Firecode guidance documents. Amongst other things the Group considers appropriate research topics. Current subjects under way or under consideration include:-

(a) Sprinklers for life safety where following earlier work new initiatives are currently being taken through one of the NFPAG sub-groups.

(b) Reliability of fire detectors coupled with automatic fire detection systems. Here again following earlier work consideration is being given through NFPAG to further research activity.

(c) Surface spread of flame. This work follows consultation with the Home Office Fire Services Inspectorate and London Regional Transport Authority.

Mention should be made at this point of another Department of Health/NHS multi-disciplinary group that meets three times per annum with the 'chair' being provided by the Department. This Group — the Building Legislation Working Group — whilst not having a direct brief on fire matters does from time to time direct matters of concern to NFPAG. BLWG members have recently proposed an interest about the possibility of work on the problems associated with surface spread of flame on built-up paint surfaces. This initiative has been taken up by NFPAG and as mentioned above research work is being considered in this area. Additionally one of the NHS members of the BLWG has lead a small team in producing an illustrated guide to HTM 81. Although not produced as one of the mainstream Firecode documents it has been well received by the Department and others in the Health Service who see it as a useful addition to HTM 81 — 'Fire Precautions in New Hospitals'.

Age and Condition of the Existing Building Stock

When considering fire safety and control in health premises attention will also inevitably focus on the age and state of the building stock. The NHS estate includes a wide and disparate range of building types including our Victorian heritage, large 60s style macro-block buildings to the more recent cost effective low rise (and inherently more safe) Nucleus buildings. (See Firecode — Nucleus Fire Precautions Recommendations published in June 1989 which is a revised and updated version superseding the first edition published in February 1979). The space within these buildings includes complex laboratories, 24 hour manned ward accommodation, day time facilities such as outpatient departments, offices, kitchen blocks, workshops etc. Additionally, hospital staff, patients and visitors represent the range of personal characteristics displayed by the population at large. Hence some patients smoke, staff may carelessly dispose of smoking materials and pyromania is just as likely to occur in a hospital as it is on our local common. Hospital fire precautions guidance has to be sufficiently comprehensive and yet flexible to address all these issues and yet respond to new developments and change. Any upgrading required for fire precautions in the older hospitals will be discharged in accordance with the Home Office draft guide to Fire Precautions in Hospitals, which applies to existing premises. When considering the increasing stock of new building, attention will focus on such recent developments in Architecture as the use of Atria. Also the growing tendency in health care buildings to introduce shops and shopping malls in new design (see PL/CE(89)2 of December 1989 entitled 'Fire Precautions in Health Buildings — Commercial Enterprises on Health Services Premises' and the forthcoming Fire Practice Note No 7). These new developments in hospital design which will also include new materials, textiles and furnishings as well as sprinklers and fire detection technology will of course receive careful consideration by NFPAG. There also has to be a constant awarness in the Health Service of the high proportion of non-ambulant hospital patients and demands that would necessarily fall on staff if these patients had to be evacuated in the event of fire (see Firecode: FPN 3 — Escape Bed Lifts). Staff training is essential in this area so that everyone knows what is expected of them when an emergency arises. Another new dimension in health buildings and one that is found increasingly in other areas is that of vandalism. Such problems, whilst relatively minor in terms of financial loss, do divert valuable resources that would otherwise be available for direct patient care and safety.

Role of Management in Fire Precautions

Finally and at the risk of repetition it should be said that fire precautions in the Health Service are not simply a matter of risk separation, compartmentation, structural precautions and control measures but are more fundamental, requiring an awareness of potential risk, continuing assessment and response to the risks. Essentially fire precautions are a matter of management and in this respect the nomination of a senior officer responsible for Fire coupled with observance of Firecode is of paramount importance. The nominated senior officer responsible for fire matters should be supported, where appropriate, by Fire Safety and Specialist Fire Prevention Officers. Key factors in the management strategy will be: risk assessment; analysis of risk; implementation of practical precautionary measures; staffing implementation and maintaining staff awareness.

The Department's responsibility in this area of hospital safety has resulted in the direction of resources for the preparation of Firecode. Although, like the Home Office draft guide, Firecode guidance is non-statutory, the Secretary of State has directed that it should be applied.

It follows that training and staffing levels contribute to safety in hospitals. The ultimate life saving measure is evacuation. The policy in Firecode is progressive horizontal and vertical movement of patients away from the fire. Patients will need to be evacuated stage by stage to safer areas as the scope for local containment reduces. Staff will be present in 24 hour patient occupied areas and will be familiar with the layout of the building and be aware of the communication system. Training and practice drills will be essential to maintain the level of competence. Where the staff turnover is high, or where agency staff are employed, management has the additional responsibility of ensuring that new and part-time staff are equally capable of responding to a fire — additional effort will be necessary in such cases. In essence fire precautions strategy could be expressed as: avoidance; rapid detection; effective containment; control and extinguish and progressive horizontal and vertical movement.

In summarising the management involvement in Fire Safety in Health Care premises the following three key action areas have been identified:-

(1) The implementation of fire safety policies locally with the Fire Safety Officer taking an initiative to participate fully in the risk assessment, introduction of improvements and the training of staff.

(2) The monitoring of the implementation of Firecode. (In the same way that the Department monitors Regions, seeking assurances regarding appropriate systems and procedures for fire precautions so Regions will be monitoring Districts compliance with the requirements of Firecode guidance. See also paragraph 9 of the Departments Health Circular HC(87)24 of November 1987).

(3) A firm commitment to the DH/NHS reporting procedure, thus ensuring that incident data can be reviewed, analysed and utilised for the further development of guidance (see particularly paragraphs 3.14 and 3.15 of Firecode — Policy and Principles).

A Review of Current Practice for Fire Alarm Detection Systems in UK NHS Hospitals

by
S. M. K. Platt, Dip EE CEng MIEE
Department of Health
Euston Tower, London

Introduction

The provision of effective fire detection and alarm systems in hospitals is a vital component of the overall fire safety strategy which is necessary to portect patients, staff, visitors and property from fire. In the United Kingdom, the Department of Health's guidance document Health Technical Memorandum No. 82 (HTM 82), provides the general principles and technical guidance for those persons in the National Health Service who have responsibility for the design, specification, installation, commissioning, testing, operation and maintenance of fire alarm systems in hospitals. It is intended that the document should be read in conjunction with the associated British Standard Code of Practice (BS 5839: Part 1: 1988) and other relevant sections of the Department's Firecode suite of documents.

The guidance within HTM 82 applies to all new premises covered by the Department's Firecode document Health Technical Memorandum No. 81 (Fire Precautions in new hospitals) and those 'Nucleus' hospitals covered by the special Nucleus Fire Precautions Recommendations. HTM 82 also applies to existing hospitals where fire detection and alarm systems are being renewed or undergoing major upgrading.

Full compliance with HTM 82 will satisfy the requirements of the UK Home Office's Draft Guide to Fire Precautions in Hospitals with respect to fire detection and alarm systems.

The Relationship of HTM 82 with the BS Code and Why the HTM is Needed

The British Standard Institution's Code of Prctice in its various forms has been with us now for some 25 years. Similarly there have been several forerunners to the 1989 edition of HTM 82. In 1956 early guidance was promulgated to the National Health Service in the form of a Circular (HM (56) 36 and this was replaced in the late 1960's by HTM 16 (Fire Precautions), which included more specific information about fire detection and alarm systems. The first edition of HTM 82, published in 1982, was identified with the 1989 version of BS 5839; Part 1 which brought in special requirements for life safety, a topic of particular interest with respect to health care buildings. It is therefore appropriate that these two documents should remain closely in step.

The BS Code of Practice quite properly deals with fire alarm systems in general. It gives comprehensive guidance which is suitable for a range of premises under various forms of occupation. Therefore although much in the Code is also relevant to hospitals, in some instances the full requirements of the Code are not appropriate to the needs of health care buildings, and in others, some enhancement may become necessary. That is why the Department, in consultation with the Home Office, found it necessary to produce HTM 82.

The Department's recent revision of HTM 82 became necessary to take account of the changes introduced by the 1988 publication of BS 5839: Part 1. However it would be wrong to assume that the new HTM bears little resemblance to its predecessor. In fact a considerable part of the original document has been carried forward such that the 1989 edition has mainly undergone changes of emphasis to:-

- keep abreast of advances in technology;
- align it with the current BS Code; and
- promulgate some of the Department's work which examined the reliability of various methods for communicating with the Fire Brigade.

If it is to be effective in a hospital, a fire alarm system must:-

- in normal circumstances permit efficient, undisturbed operation of health care functions;
- limit disturbance during a fire situation;
- reflect any special operational and safety policies; and
- integrate successfully with other components of the fire safety strategy.

In many premises the primary function of the fire detection and alarm system is to initiate evacuation of the building and to complete it in the shortest time possible. In hospitals, however, it is usually neither desirable, necessary, nor practicable to attempt a full evacuation.

Therefore, the main functions of a hospital system may be summarised. They are to:-

- detect and give prompt warning to fire (preferably only to staff);
- indicate the location of the fire (and thus the spaces to be evacuated);
- establish an alarm call to the fire brigade; and
- actuate other associated parts of the fire safety system (eg release door hold-open devices).

HTM 82, in conjunction with the other documents of the Firecode suite, takes account of these factors.

An Overview of Some Significant Changes Incorporated Within the New HTM 82

The internal format of the new edition will be easily recognised by readers of the previous version as, like its

SIRENES D'INCENDIE — SYSTEMES DE DETECTION DISPOSITIONS ACTUELLES DANS LES HOPITAUX DU SECTEUR PUBLIC EN GRANDE-BRETAGNE

Cet article repose sur les recommendations principales énoncées dans le nouveau document Firecode (UK), Memorandum Technique de Santé 82. De nombreuses comparaisons sont établies avec le Code de Pratique (Normes Britanniques) actuel qui y est associé (BS 5839: Part 1: 1988).

Les raisons pour lesquelles il a été nécessaire de réviser le MTS et de l'ajouter comme supplément au Code (Normes Britanniques) sont passées en revue. L'article se réfère à quelques domaines spécifiques et étudie les circonstances dans lesquelles les dispositions contenues dans le Code (NB) ne sont pas applicables aux bâtiments de santé sans certaines modifications. La conclusion souligne l'importance de la fiabilité lorsqu'il s'agit de choisir des méthodes de communications d'alarme aux casernes de pompiers.

predecessor, it is written to follow the content of the new BS Code in a logical style, for ease of comparison.

Some examples of the more significant changes to be noticed in the revised HTM are as follows:-

- a much expanded section dealing with the provision of communication between hospitals and the fire brigade;
- two new appendices describing and comparing some of the automatic communication methods available;
- more information on addressable alarm systems with a new appendix explaining their properties and virtues; and
- a new appendix intended as a briefing checklist to augment the requirements of the BS Code for purposes of planning and consultation.

A Brief Review of Some Points of Significance Within the Revised HTM

Before consideraing these in turn, however, it may be of use to recall some important elements forming the Department of Health's overall fire safety strategy for hospitals.

Medical and nursing needs of patients in a typical 28-bed acute nursing section require that a minimum of two nurses are on duty at all times. The Department's fire precautions recommendations agreed with Home Office are based on the assumption that that standard will be met.

The mobility of patients may be classified in terms such as 'bedfast', 'wheelchair-bound', 'assisted-ambulant' and 'ambulant'. Typically at any one time we may expect that some 14 of the 28 patients will be bedfast, six will be wheelchair-bound and eight assisted-ambulant or ambulant.

Three fire conditions are recognised when evacuation may become necessary:-

- Extreme emergency — immediate threat to life safety from fire or toxic fumes.
- Emergency — no immediate threat but where one may occur soon from fire spread.
- Precautionary — no immediate threat but where fire has occurred in nearby or adjacent accommodation.

In the design of modern UK hospitals a widely used concept, that of progressive evacuation, in which there are as the main horizontal and vertical escape route. This vital link connects hospital departments with fire escape exits and protected lift enclosures. It also provides a recognised firefighting platform for the brigade.

The basic strategy for fire evacuation fulfils a further concept, that a progressive evacuation, in which there are three main stages:-

- horizontal evacuation from the fire compartment to an adjoining compartment;
- horizontal evacuation of the entire fire compartment to a more distant fire compartment on the same floor; and
- vertical evacuation to outside of the building, moving from upper floors via stairways, or by the use of the special escape bedlifts meeting the requirements of Firecode's Fire Practice Note No. 3 in the case of bedfast patients.

To facilitate progressive horizontal evacuation every storey must be divided into at least two connected fire compartments with at least two fire escape exits. When certain criteria are breached (eg wards with excessive numbers of patients or excessive area), then fire compartments are further divided into fire subcompartments to produce smaller fire and smoke tight cells. The maximum permitted travel distances over escape routes are carefully regulated, both for alternative and single directions of travel. High fire risk and high fire load departments are separated from patient areas or are specially protected.

Having now established the basis for the Department of Health's hospital fire safety strategy we can now resume consideration of some important additions and alterations embodied within the revised HTM 82 and make comparisons with the 1988 BS Code.

Choice of System Type

The BS Code of Practice introduced a method for classifying fire alarm systems suitable for installation in a range of premises. Systems were classified in terms of the type of system and the extent of the protection each could provide for property or life. Systems may be specified as:-

Type P	—	automatic detection systems intended for the protection of property which may be further sub-divided into:
Type P1	—	systems installed throughout the protected building;
Type P2	—	systems installed only in defined parts of the protected building;
Type L	—	automatic detection systems intended for the protection of life which may be further sub-divided into:
Type L1	—	systems installed throughout the protected building
Type L2	—	systems installed only in parts of the protected building; Type L2 systems should normally include the coverage required of a Type L3 system;
Type L3	—	systems installed only for the protection of escape routes; and
Type M	—	manual alarm systems (with no further sub-division).

The 'L3' system adoped in the BS Code is based on the principle that at least escape routes should be protected with an automatic detection system. As we have noted already, the Department's Firecode guidance starts from the basis that alternative means of escape are provided and that most patients are under constant supervision. In addition any identified fire hazard rooms are provided with fire resisting enclosures and automatic detection. Those patient areas not having continuous nursing attention are required to be fully protected by fire detectors.

The effect of this policy, in terms of the BS Code, is that hospital departments have L2 and L1 systems, except that escape routes themselves are not necessarily provided with automatic detection. This is because they are intended to be fire sterile areas and as circulation/communication routes they should be in use continuously. However, to cater for infrequent use during silent hours and to comply with Building Regulations, in cases where fire resisting doors are held open with automatic devices, some corridor protection may be prudent or necessary.

Appendix H of the BS Code deals with smoke alarms (self-contained or single-stage fire detectors) for use in domestic residences. These detectors are sometimes proposed for hospitals on grounds of cheapness. The Department's HTM 82 refers to their limitations and advises against their use except for very occasional short-term periods where a staffed area may be temporarily without cover from the main system.

Fire Alarm Warnings

The warning system within a hospital must form an important part of the progressive evacuation strategy referred to earlier and it must minimise disturbance and distress to patients and staff. The evacuation policy presupposes that it is the staff who should be alerted to the occurrence of a fire so that they may perform the safety duties for which they have received prior and regular training. The warning method should be chosen to fit these criteria.

Appendix 4 of HTM 82 provides guidance about the acoustic characteristics and siting of sounders for audible alarms in patient areas. Electronic sounders having adjustable outputs in preference to bells are recommended. A two-stage alarm should be provided giving an evacuation signal within the fire zone and, initially, only an alerting signal in other zones, where staff need to be brought to a higher state of readiness as part of the fire safety routine. In addition to any visual alarms required in accordance with the BS Code it will be necessary to provide visual warning signals in those parts of hospitals where audible warnings are unacceptable, for example in operating theatres and intensive therapy units.

The use of alpha-numeric displays to provide more informative fire warnings at suitable locations, such as nurses stations, is likely to become more widespread with the introduction of more advanced systems.

Control and Indicating Equipment and Fire Zones

New fire alarm control and indicating equipment installed within UK NHS hospitals should meet the requirements of BS 5839: Part 4: 1988. The Department expects that the panels of modern microprocessor-based systems should be no more difficult to use in a fire emergency than those of conventional systems.

In general, hospitals should be arranged into fire alarm zones to accord with the principles of the BS Code. Where hospital fire compartments are divided into sub-compartments to accord with the fire design strategy, a zone should be made conterminous with a single sub-compartment. In large hospitals it may be convenient to group a number of zones to form Sectors as allowed by the BS Code.

Alarm sounders must be grouped to agree with evacuation zones and their signals arranged to match the requirements of the particular evacuation strategy.

Ideally door hold-open devices should be controlled on individual or zonal bases. In practice doors bounding a number of alarm zones may meed to be released in response to an alarm from any of the zones.

False Alarms

The BS Code lists a number of common causes of false alarms all of which are equally applicable to UK hospital installations. Such alarms are highly disruptive to hospital routines and cause an unnecessary waste of scarce resources. They also result in an embarrassing attendance of the fire brigade. Indeed some UK fire authorities are already threatening to recover the costs of false alarm call-outs from health authorities.

The BS Code provides for the use of transmission delay units which are special devices for automatically delaying the transmission of fire alarms to the brigade. They may be used in circumstances where there are high incidences of false alarms where these cannot be reduced by other methods. However Transmission delay units are not recommended for UK hospitals because they may cause search routines to become less thorough leading to the possibility of serious incidents. Such units contribute nothing to solving the problems experienced by hospital staff from false alarms.

Some research work has been undertaken by the Department in co-operation with others on one addressable fire alarm system using analogue detectors. The results from this work indicate that such an arrangement appears to produce fewer false alarms than would be expected with conventional systems. This result is welcome and is one reason why such systems are now recommended to authorities for installation in new hospitals and in those hospitals undergoing major refurbishment.

Manual Call Points

As mentioned earlier, vigilant nursing and other staff are normally present who, with the necessary training, can act promptly in a fire emergency. Very often such staff may detect fire in advance of the automatic devices. Thus the provision of suitably located manual call points can save valuable time in initiating an alarm and obtaining help. In recognition of this advantage HTM 82 recommends that call points are provided in wards at nurses' stations and along escape routes, as required by the BS Code.

Communications with the Fire Brigade and Other Off-Site Organisations

Section 3 of the HTM 82 deals with this important topic and is considerably more informative than its predecessor. This is because it takes account of technological advances and because it contains the results of some Department of Health sponsored research into the reliability of various communication methods between hospitals and fire brigades.

The principles of communication recommended between UK hospitals and brigades would probably be considered as excessive in other fields where protection of property, rather than life, appears as the predominant issue. However the HTM 82 guidance assumes that fires at hospitals pose a serious threat to their many non-ambulant occupants and is framed accordingly.

HTM 82 defines two methods for calling the fire brigade, known as Primary and Secondary Methods.

The Primary Method involves a designated person contacting the brigade by voice communication using either the UK public '999' emergency telephone system or, if available, by means of a direct telephone link. To allow for a possible failure of the Primary Method a Secondary Method should normally be provided. This will result in two calls being received by brigade control.

Where the Primary Method of communication can be considered as having high reliability, as specified by the HTM, the Secondary Method may also be by manual means or occasionally omitted altogether. However in many instances primary methods will be supplemented by automatic secondary methods connected either directly or indirectly to brigade control. The last method may be often via a commercially operated remote manned centre (RMC). Sometimes the RMC may be located at another health service facility, such as an ambulance control centre.

The various methods of communication are compared extensively in Appendix 3 of the HTM and include the use of ambulance service radio networks. Digital Communicators (Digicom) and 999-autodiallers are also reviewed, in Appendix 3A.

The UK Department of Health arranged a study of fire alarm communication methods and their associated brigade response times. Some of the main conclusions of the study are worthy of closer attention.

The study was concerned with establishing the availability of service via remote manned centres using different signalling methods, with their overall response times, and making comparisons. The circuits studied were from a statistically significant sample of protected premises to fire brigade controls, and involved timed trials carried out from 60 separate premises in 1987, each premises being tested twice.

Two methods of fire alarm transmission were compared with that of using the '999' Public Switched Telephone Network, viz direct (dedicated) circuits and digital communicators (also via the PSTM). The results are shown in Figure 1 as cumulative plots.

It is seen that the transmission times for alarms via central stations using dedicated channels closely matches that for calls via the '999' PSTN service, with an expectation that some 90% of calls would reach the brigade within 60 seconds and 98.5% within 90 seconds.

By comparison digital communicators ('digicom') are seen to be markedly inferior. Only about 70% of such calls succeeded at first attempt and the method appears to be slow and unreliable when compared with the other two methods. In the trials, however, the 'digicom' systems passed over PSTN trunk circuits which were routed through a number of switching centres. Appendix 3A of HTM 82 recognises that where 'digicom' circuits remain within the same local PSTN network significant improvements in performance may be possible.

The UK Home Office has taken a close interest in the outcome of the study and has since proposed the establishment of performance criteria for the transmission of fire alarms from systems protecting life-risk premises, using circuits routed via central stations.

Conclusion

The intention of this paper has been to provide an appreciation of the UK Department of Health's current recommendations for automatic fire alarm systems for use in its NHS hospitals. The principal recommendations of the recently revised HTM 82 have been used as the vehicle for achieving this aim, and comparisons made between it and the current BS Code of Practice. Some essential differences in philosophy when applying the BS Code to health service premises have been highlighted.

Health Technical Memorandum 82 forms one element of the Department of Health's Firecode suite to which further documents are to be added. Firecode documents may be purchased in the UK from HMSO Bookshops at prices ranging from approximately £3.00 to £7.00. A list of available documents is shown in the Firecode publicity handout.

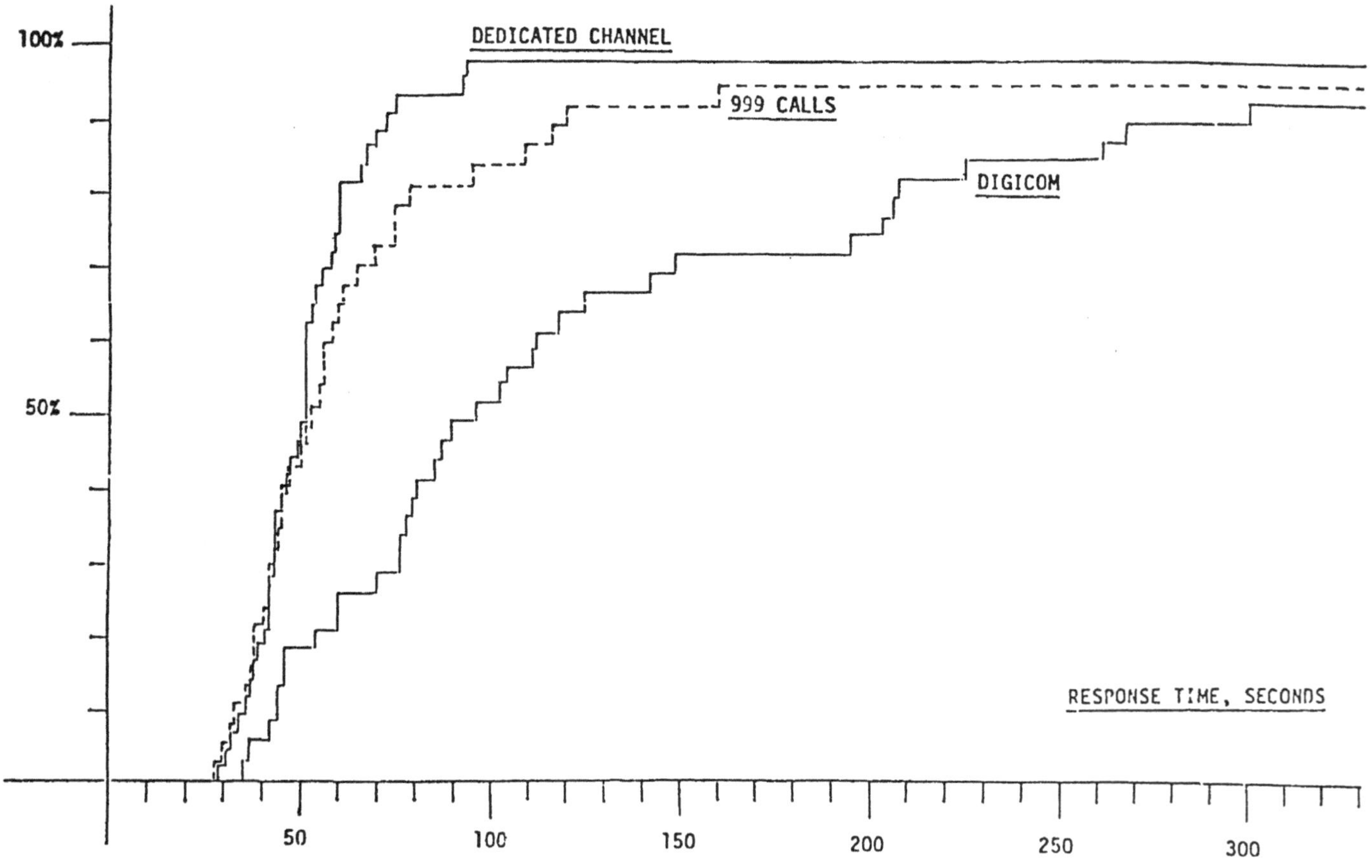

Cumulative Response Curves

Reproduced by permission of DHSS

Fire Safety Evaluation System for Canadian Hospitals Phase I Report

by

Ralph J. Bartlett, PEng
R. J. Bartlett Engineering Ltd
102 Queen Street
Fredericton, New Brunswick, Canada
(Tel: (506) 459 3070)

1. Introduction

This paper is presented with permission from the Institutional and Professional Services Division, Health Services and Promotion Branch, Health and Welfare Canada.

Fire safety evaluation or grading systems are used throughout the world as a means of determining levels of fire protection in buildings. Insurance interests have used such methods for decades dealing mostly with items related to risks and building protection..

In the past 15 years, evaluation systems have been developed to address life (fire) safety concerns in buildings. With the onset of higher technology, building regulations have changed over the years to address 'better' methods for providing adequate fire safety in buildings. This has caused a variation of the levels of fire safety in buildings. Older buildings tend to have lower levels of fire safety protection compared with buildings constructed under the criteria of later building regulations. Many of the evaluation systems have been developed to address these variations. To a large extent, the evaluation systems are used to determine options for improving fire safety without having to rehabilitate buildings to meet current building regulations. This concept has proven itself effective and, based on this, Health and Welfare Canada commissioned a study to investigate the possibility of developing an evaluation system for use in Canadian hospitals. This paper is a summary of Phase I of the commissioned study.

The main objectives of Phase I were to study existing evaluation systems pertaining to hospitals throughout the world, to study the impact of National Building Code of Canada requirements for hospitals, and to prepare a framework for developing an evaluation system for hospitals in Canada based on Canadian standards.

Since the development and implementation of a fire safety evaluation system in the US in the 1970's, many hospitals in Canada have been evaluated using the US method. This has proven satisfactory, however, global acceptance of the US evaluation system has never occurred. The US FSES is based on life safety criteria in the National Fire Protection Association Standard, NFPA 101.

This paper shows that the concepts behind the US evaluation system are good, however, the level of safety basis of NFPA 101 is different than the level of safety basis for the National Building Code of Canada 1985.

This paper addresses other evaluation systems that have been developed that are, or may be, applicable to hospitals. An extensive literature search was conducted, the results of which are reported in Section 2.

This paper describes the study team's recommended approach for developing an evaluation system for hospitals in Canada. A framework of the proposed method is presented along with a methodology for testing the proposed method for use in Canada.

2. Literature Review

The following activities were conducted as part of the effort to identify existing evaluation systems that are applicable to hospitals. Automated literature searches were conducted on two occasions at the Fire Research Information Service Library at the National Institute of Standards and Technology (NIST) (formerly National Bureau of Standards, NBS) in Gaithersburg, Maryland. Meetings were conducted with Mssrs. Nelson, Shibe and Gross at NIST to obtain insight on the US FSES system as well as to assist in identifying efforts in other countries. Contact was made with Dr Eric Marchant, University of Edinburgh, Scotland, to determine the status of the approach formulated by Marchant as well as to identify any relevant activities in Europe or in other Commonwealth nations. Contact was made with Dr Vaughn Beck, Australia, to determine the applicability of his evaluation technique to hospitals.

As a result of these activities, four credible evaluation systems were identified for use in hospitals. They are as follows:

SYSTEME D'EVALUATION DE LA SECURITE EN CAS D'INCENDIE APPLIQUE AUX HOPITAUX DU CANADA. RAPPORT DE LA PHASE I

Les systèmes d'évaluation de la sécurité en cas d'incendie sont utilisés à travers le monde comme un moyen de déterminer le niveau de protection des édifices en cas d'incendie. Afin de défendre leurs intérêts, les compagnies d'assurance ont utilisé ces méthodes depuis plusieurs dizaines d'années pour la plupart des cas impliquant les risques ou la protection des édifices.

Durant les quinze dernières années, des systèmes d'évaluation ont été développés en ce qui concerne la sécurité des vies humaines dans les édifices (en cas d'incendie). Avec l'avènement de nouvelles technologies, la règlementation de la construction a évolué de pair afin de répondre à de 'meilleures' méthodes de protection qui fourniront une sécurité adéquate en cas d'incendie dans les édifices. Ceci a causé une variation des niveaux de sécurité en cas d'incendie dans les édifices. Les constructions plus anciennes offrent des niveaux de sécurité et de protection moindre par rapport à celles construites selon les critères de règlementations plus récentes. Plusieurs systèmes de d'évaluation ont été développés en tenant compte de ces variations. Les systèmes d'évaluation sont utilisés en grande partie pour établir des options pour l'amélioration de la sécurité en cas d'incendie, sans toutefois aller jusqu'à rencontrer le niveau de la règlementation actuelle. Ce concept s'est avéré efficace et, basé là-dessus, Santé et Bien-être Canada commanda une étude pour examiner la possibilité de développer un système d'évaluation à l'usage des hôpitaux canadiens. Ce rapport est un sommaire de la Phase I de cette étude.

Les objectifs principaux de la phase I étaient d'étudier les systèmes d'évaluation existants pour les hôpitaux à travers le monde, d'étudier l'impact des exigences du Code national du bâtiment du Canada sur les hôpitaux, et de préparer un cadre de travail pour le développement d'un système d'évaluation, pour les hôpitaux de Canada, basé sur des standards canadiens.

Ce rapport traite de systemes d'évaluation qui ont été développés internationalement et qui sont, ou peuvent être, appliqués aux hôpitaux. Les résultats d'une recherche approfondie de la littérature est présentée dans ce rapport.

Ce rapport décrit l'approche du groupe d'étude pour le développement d'un systéme d'évaluation pour les hôpitaux du Canada; un systéme d'évaluation pour les hôpitaux du Canada; et enfin une méthodologie pour tester la méthode proposée à l'usage du Canada.

US Fire Safety Evaluation System — This method was developed using a Delphi approach co-ordinated by staff members at the Center for Fire Research, NIST. The intent of the method is to provide a means of comparison of the level of fire safety existent in a facility with that required by NFPA 101. The Delphi group assigned point values of occupant characteristics and building features based on 'professional judgment'. The method, now included in NFPA 101M, is used throughout the US and parts of Canada as an approved method of examining code equivalency and also as part of the accreditation process. Extensive experience has been obtained with the method, with several papers available documenting the experiences relative to validity and ease of use.

As part of the literature review, the project team compiled a report detailing all aspects of the US FSES. That report also compares the US FSES with the UK method.

UK — Firecode: Assessing Fire Risk in Existing Hospital Wards — This method was also developed using a Delphi approach, directed by Dr Eric Marchant. In this case, the method was based on a draft version of the Fire Precautions Act, 1987. This method was developed after a prior investigation indicated that the US FSES was inappropriate for British hospitals. The major deficiencies in the FSES were attributed to the following:-

(a) The level of safety prescribed in NFPA 101 is substantially different from that prescribed in British standards.

(b) The design features of British hospitals are substantially different from US hospitals due to age differencs and operational characteristics. Often, British hospitals are very old structures, eg 19th century. In addition, and perhaps more importantly, apparently the large open wards frequently encountered in British hospitals are due to desired operational characteristics of the facility as prescribed by the British health care profession. The lack of compartmentation resulted in the British hospitals receiving highly negative ratings on the basis of the US FSES. The open ward concept differs markedly from the well-compartmented wards typically found in US and Canadian hospitals, especially those constructed in the last 20 years. This major difference in hospital design philosophy may have been a major consideration in determining the US FSES to be inappropriate.

As part of the literature review, the project team compiled a report detailing all aspects of the UK method. That report also compares the UK method with the US FSES.

Australia — Dr Vaughn Beck has developed a probabilistic method of evaluating the risk associated with office occupancies under the jurisdiction of the Australian building codes against the risk deemed to be acceptable under a given code. Recently, this method was purchased by the National Research Council of Canada and adapted to apartment buildings within the National Building Code of Canada jurisdiction.

Presently, this method cannot evaluate the risk associated with hospital occupanices. However, it may be adapted to do so with comparatively minor input being required.

The method is based on the comparison of two fire safety systems and the probability of losses associated with each. One system is the building code, while the other is the building under review. The method does not give absolute risk factors, but compares the two systems.

Beck's method contains two major evaluation sections: one associated with the spread of fire and smoke, the other with the response and movement of people. The evaluation of fire growth throughout buildings and individual compartments determines the probability of fire and smoke spread from one area to another. It calculates both fire and smoke spread under sprinklered and nonsprinklered conditions. It takes into account features such as available or induced smoke ventilation and interconnected floor spaces.

The response and movement of people is probabilistically evaluated in accordance with the occupants' levels of mobility, alertness and building geometrey.

France — The French have developed a method of evaluating health care facilities. The method, in a general sense, is based on the fundamental philosophy behind the US FSES method in that the same life safety parameters are being reviewed. This method, however, also contains a high risk probability coefficient drawn out of standard insurance company risk evaluation methods and formulas. The method appears to contain formulas which give erroneous results. In following through the calculations within the paper on hypothetical but realistic situations, results were obtained indicating that a 30 bed hospital ward can be completely evacuated by means of stairs in under three minutes. This timely evacuation is improbable.

A copy of the French evaluation system was received and translated by the project team. It appears that the French system is a cross between the US FSES and the Australian approaches with a relatively simplistic presentation.

Others — Mention has been made of a method developed by Gretener specifically for health care facilities (Switzerland). This reported method may be confused with the French system, as no information or references to a separate method by Gretener have been found.

Some individuals contacted at NIST believe that a Japanese system may exist. No information or references to a Japanese system for health care facilities were found. A Japanese system does exist for dwellings and again could have led to misdirected speculation of the existence of a system for health care facilities.

Dr Marchant was confident that no other systems applicable to hospitals existed in Europe other than the French and UK systems. He also indicated that he did not know of any systems being developed in South America, Asia or Africa.

In summary, based on the literature search for evaluation systems used to evaluate the level of fire safety in health care facilities, there appear to be four credible methods in existence. These four are the ones developed in Australia, France, United Kingdom and the United States.

3. Description of Proposed Evaluation System

3.1 General

The evaluation system that is proposed is, to some extent, based on the framework of the US FSES. The Canadian Hospital Fire Safety Evaluation System (CHFSES) will incorporate the main structure of the US FSES; ie risk assessment, containment safety criteria, extinguishment safety criteria, people movement safety criteria, and general safety.

Unlike the British method, which provides one general evaluation result, the CHFSES will present results under four categories:-

(1) Compartmentation
(2) Fire Safety Systems
(3) Egress Systems
(4) General Safety

Unlike all of the other evaluation methods, the CHFSES will reflect the level of life safety accepted in Canada, based on National Building Code of Canada 1985 (NBC) requirements.

3.2 Code Comparison NFPA 101 1988 ● – ★ NBC 1985

Since the US FSES is based on the requirements of NFPA 101 and the CHFSES will be based on the requirements of the NBC, a comparison of NFPA 101 and the NBC was conducted to determine the validity and applicability of the US FSES to the hospitals regulated under the NBC. This comparison analysis considered requirements pertaining to new hospitals.

It is clear that the two documents are based on similar fire safety principles in some instances and different fire safety principles in others. As an example, NFPA 101 relies on human detection of fires whereas the NBC requires automatic smoke detection in all patient sleeping rooms and corridors serving these rooms.

NFPA 101 is a model document that does not address all the fire safety requirements that are addressed in the NBC. Many fire safety components, such as standpipe and hose systems, are not regulated under NFPA 101. Instead, locally adopted regulations are used to supplement NFPA 101 to cover areas omitted. As a result, the US FSES does not address water supplies and fire fighting elements of a building.

The CHFSES, in addition to addressing all requirements in the NBC, has been developed such that the end user should only require an understanding of the fire safety requirements in the NBC and its referenced standards.

4. Framework for CHFSES

4.1 General

The framework for the CHFSES is presented under the following section headings. The information is presented in general terms. It is intended that the information provide a general understanding of the framework.

4.2 Hospital Information

Hospitals are evaluated on a per zone basis (eg patient ward). Before each zone is identified, a general survey of the hospital must be conducted. Information on fire departments, water supply, building maintenance, building age, building construction, etc has to be determined.

4.3 Occupancy Risk Parameters

The evaluation will require information on the 'people' aspect of the surveyed fire zone. Factors such as patient profiles (age, mobility, population), zone location (with respect to grade), and hospital staffing (staff/patient ratios) are determined.

4.4 New or Existing Building Factor

The General Safety aspect of the building is largely affected by the fact that the hospital is new or existing. Other evaluation systems express factors that essentially lower the level of fire safety expected for existing buildings. This reflects a higher risk level which is deemed to be appropriate.

4.5 Safety Parameters

The evaluation will require information on factors affecting fire safety. The building and fire zones will be described under sections in the following categories. Associated integer point ratings are assigned to each category.

Construction — Categories similar to NBC Section 3.2.2 (structural fire protection) are listed. The evaluator need only inspect the existing structure/drawings to select an evaluation number.

Interior Finish — Flame spread ratings are determined by comparing wall and ceiling materials with a list appended to the CHFSES. Correlating points are assigned.

Corridor Walls — The evaluator will inspect the corridor walls to determine if they constitute a fire separation, and, if so, will determine the fire resistance rating inherent in the walls. Points are given depending on the wall construction.

Corridor Doors — The evaluator will inspect the doors along the corridor. A determination of the door contribution to compartmentation will be made.

Zone Dimensions — Each fire zone is inspected to determine zone size and location of exits.

Vertical Openings — Shafts, service spaces etc, that penetrate horizontal fire separations will be inspected. Interconnected floor openings will be determined along with protected openings.

Hazardous Areas — Areas in the hospital that contain potential fire hazards (eg fuel-fired appliances) are identified and considered in the evaluation. A list of potential fire hazards will be appended to the CHFSES.

Smoke Control — Methods for controlling the movement of smoke will be determined. Smoke shafts, openable windows, mechanically assisted duct systems and zone smoke barriers are some of the control methods recognised by the CHFSES.

Egress — General egress routes will be identified and inspected to determined possible egress options. These may range from multiple direct exits to single stair exits.

Detection and Alarm Systems — The evaluator is required to consider factors such as the presence of manual pull stations, fire department connections, and automatic detection.

The effects of early warning smoke detection and alarm systems are addressed in the CHFSES in terms of its impact on fire safety.

Automatic Sprinklers — The evaluator has to consider the factor of sprinklering. The highest points possible in the CHFSES is given to complete sprinkler protection.

Sprinkler protection is becoming a more prevalent means for providing fire safety in existing hospitals in lieu of improving structural fire protection and/or compartmentation. The positive and negative aspects of this approach have been analysed and are reflected in the CHFSES.

4.6 Individual Safety Evaluations

The points derived from the safety parameter section (4.5) will be carried to a table where their impact on the four basic safety categories will be tabulated. The four categories include:-

(1) Compartmentation;
(2) Fire Safety Systems;
(3) Egress Systems; and
(4) General Safety.

4.7 Mandatory Safety Requirements

The CHFSES has a table indicating the levels of fire safety that are mandatory for the first three categories described in Section 4.6 (compartmentation, fire safety systems and egress).

This table identifies mandatory numbers based on evaluated fire zone location and whether the building is new or existing.

4.8 Results

The CHFSES has a final table intended to provide the user with simple equations to determine whether the inspected fire zone has a point rating greater than or equal to the mandatory number requirements.

4.9 Additional Requirements

This section includes a number of fire safety components that are considered to be necessary. These items, such as emergency lighting, emergency generators and fire safety plans are considered mandatory.

5. Proposed Method for Testing the CHFSES

The CHFSES will be tested through a combination of computer analysis and field testing at existing hospitals.

5.1 Computer Analyses

R. J. Bartlett Engineering Ltd, has written a software program that will model all possible hospital construction configurations recognised by the NBC. Newly constructed hospitals (assumed) will be modelled to ensure that the CHFSES will accept all hospital designs fitting the minimum requirements of the NBC.

In addition, computer programs will be used to model fire growth, compartmentation, smoke spread, automatic detector response times and egress. This information will be used to support the development of some of the assigned point ratings in the CHFSES.

5.2 Field Tests

Several hospitals across Canada will be selected for field testing. The hospitals will be inspected and the results will be analysed with the CHFSES.

5.3 Modifications

The results from the computer analysis and the field tests will be studied and any necessary changes to the CHFSES will be made.

6. Summary

This paper presents the Canadian Hospital Fire Safety Evaluation System (CHFSES) as a framework based on the project team's analysis.

The CHFSES will be vigorously tested to ensure that the final product is unquestionably an effective fire safety evaluation system for hospitals in Canada.

The CHFSES will be a dynamic system that can easily be modified to reflect changes in the National Building Code of Canada.

Constructing A Hospital Around A Hospital

by
Robert Edge
Director, Project Management
Peterborough Civic Hospital
Peterborough, Ontario, Candan K9J 7C6

Peterborough Cibic Hospital is a 434-bed active care facility with a floor area, before construction, of 294,000 sq ft, which includes the three temporary combustible construction annexes, which are shown at these points: (Item A: Plot Plan of Peterborough Civic Hospital).

The lined areas show a 90,000 sq ft addition, and a renovation in this area of the north wing of a further 14,000 sq ft is to be done at the end of the project. The new building is free-standing and is built up against the existing structure on these three major elevations.

Hospital Departments such as Laboratory, Nutrition Services, and the existing Emergency/Admitting Department have major involvement with the construction area. CSR and Linen Services will also be disrupted by the construction of various phases.

The addition is being constructed to house a new and greatly expanded Emergency Department, together with Admitting services on the first floor, an expanded Supply, Processing and Distribution basement. Also included in the basement are lockers rooms with washrooms, etc, for almost 1,000 female staff. In the shelled-in floor above the first floor, a future project will be formulated to house expanded Operating Rooms, a Recovery Room and an Intensive Care unit. In the third floor area below the mechanical room, only a partial floor is being constructed at this time, and will house a new computer services department for the hospital. The fourth floor of the tower at the west side of the building will be for mechanical services. The structure is designed so that both of these floors may be expanded at some time in the future to house new hospital departments. During the preparation of working drawings, it was recognised that complete new electrical services and communication services would be necessary to support a project of this size. In order to get a start on this part of the project, we formed a small pre-construction phase of the job. Plans were drawn up for underground duct banks, the relocation of some parking facilities and roadways, and this project was started in the fall with the expectations that we would begin construction the following spring. Due to the length of the approval process with our Ministry of Health, the ductbanks were in place almost two years before we actually started progress, however, it was a big advantage to have the underground services and roadways finished before we actually started into the major project.

The construction process will close off this small door into the old Emergency by the west side. When we realised that construction was imminent and began to survey the changes that would be necessary to access the building, it was discovered that almost all patients for Emergency, many patients coming in for admission, most physicians, and a considerable number of our staff used this one small mandoor for access to the hospital. It was also known of course that this would be one of the first doors which would be closed off by the construction. Following this thought process further, it was decided that the construction project would close off most of the accesses that physicians and patients, even visitors, using when coming to the Hospital for Emergency or Outpatient Services. Our first steps therefore were to make sure that physicians and staff understood that there would have to be some major changes made to their method of ingress-egress to the building. Parking facilities were expanded, signage was installed on a temporary basis to get patients and staff to change their parking habits. Some staff and physicians would now be using a basement corridor to access the hospital through which they had never walked before. In order to facilitate this type of entrance to the building, we found it necessary to produce signage such as is depicted by this logo of the hard hat. Lines were painted down corridor walls in a bright colour so people could follow the lines, so to speak, from the entrance door to the elevator. The hard hat logo was used in publication, and in signage to alert people to the fact that changes were being made as a result of the construction project. Various barriers and fences were erected and moved from time to time to route people around areas where construction was changing, sometimes on a daily basis.

Maps such as theses (Item B) were sent out to various organisations who used the hospital, showing the route they would use in accessing parking areas and entrances to the building. The Fire Department was provided with this map (Item C) to show the construction site and indicate their route to access the area in the event of a fire, either on the site or in the Hospital. As changes were made to the driveways around the building, the Fire Daprtment was regularly notified and they often made routine calls with a pumper crew on duty at the time to keep an eye on what was going on at the hospital so they would be familiar with the different changes in roadways, etc. This Fire Plan with the accompanying instructions was devised in consultation with the City Fire Department, the Hospital Fire Safety Officer and the contractor to make sure that in the event of a fire on the construction site, prompt notice of course would be supplied to the Fire Department and also that fire department response would not be made under the impression that they were dealing with a hospital fire if in fact the fire was on the construction site. The fire protection for the existing building became an issue during the planning, design, and working drawing stage of the project. At that time, we put some money into the project budget so we would be able to maintain fire separations between the construction and the existing building as the situation changed during the project. This is a sketch (Item D) of the method we chose to fireproof windows and other openings in the existing building to keep the fire separation between the site and the building in a suitable condition. In some cases, it was found necessary to make openings into the existing building where corridors to new construction would eventually be made. At these exits, we provided temporary doors, which had been taken off of the building at various places, so that some means of safe access from the interior

CONSTRUCTION D'UN HÔPITAL CONTOURNANT UN HÔPITAL

Ce papier demontre la preparation et l'execution pour la construction d'une addition de 90,000 pieds carrés de la présente existante de 294,000 pieds carrés des soins speciales qui consiste de 434 lits.

Ces methodes démontrent la necessité de modifications aux services techniques des hôpitaux qui sant necessaire durant la construction.

Sa concerne de la resolution des problemes concernant le feu, les interruptions d'urgences durant la construction de la présente et la nouvelle structure. En plus une sortie d'urgence pour les patients et le personnel et des malades extérieur et du malade. Inclu sont des communications pour les soins speciaux et l'entrainment aux nouvelles méthodes et au nouveau équipment.

Les points principaux de cette présentation sont de assurer. Toute consideration des services speciales durant cette construction.

of the existing building would be available to the construction crew as the building was being built. This of course assisted construction workers in their efforts to connect the two buildings, but also provided fire fighters and those who wished to inspect the construction from within the safety of the existing building a method of getting into the construction area in a reasonably safe manner. A great many services for the new addition had to pass through the existing areas of the hospital, a notable area was the basement of our Laboratory where many pipes for chilled water, steam, and domestic water services had to pass through an existing ceiling. In order to facilitate the smooth installation of this pipework, an evening shift was arranged with the contractor. Our Lab personnel worked on a 6.30 am to 3.30 pm period during the day; the contractor started at 3.30 pm and installed piping until around midnight — 1 am when Housekeeping staff went through and mopped up to prepare for Lab operations of the next day. By arranging to do this work in this manner, we managed to get this piping through the Lab area in a two-week period, a temporary fire separation was made at the end of the Lab and the construction continued on the other side of this separation, with welding, etc being done and the piping extended on through the new construction.

At the beginning of the project, the contractor was given the locations of air intakes into the various parts of the building, especially Laboaratory, OR's, the Labour and Delivery. Every effort of course was made by the contractor to keep machinery away from these air intakes and not to allow diesel equipment to idle in these areas, however, even small amounts of fumes from such things as form oils and this type of thing, and even the adhesives used to glue down roofing membrances do cause problems in areas of this type, especially in the OR, and it was found necessary on many occasions to check out complaints of odours in cirtical care areas. I found that by writing to these people and explaining what was going on that often times we could make the staff more tolerant of these intrusions into their work areas.

The Hospital is served by an Air Ambulance and the Heliport is immediately east of the existing emergency wing. As you can see in this picture, we had to excavate to a depth of approximately 20 ft up the roadway between the hospital and the heliport in order to install new sewer services, while at the same time keeping the air ambulance operating. As this work was progressing, we made regular contact with helicopter air service management to advise them of changing conditions at the hospital. In this manner, we managed to get through some very difficult times without any unexpected events when a helicopter arrived on site. The erection of the tower crane also proved to be an interesting one from the point of view of the air ambulance, however, after checking with our Ministry of Transportation and the Air Ambulance management people again, we found that this particular piece of equipment posed no treat to the Helicopter and things proceeded quite smoothly again by making sure that everybody was aware of just exactly what was happening on the site. In spite of all of our efforts, sometimes the best planning can still be thwarted in some way by people who are not familiar with the dangers involved. This picture shows a breach in a temporary fire separation between the basement of the construction area and a very small mechanical room in which there is a reciprocating compressor. Someone in the mechanical crew in searching for a route to run their new chilled water piping took this separation apart and of course left the door into the compressor room wide open and this makes an excellent path for a fire directly into an area where we have exposed medical record film stored. This type of accidental penetration of fire separations really is an ongoing situation. There is always someone who has not heard why the separation was put in or something of that nature and so a constant effort needs to be made to tour the building, and tour the site so that both sides of the walls are surveyed to ensure that no-one has thwarted the intent of the fire safety separations which are put in place.

At the beginning of the project, a construction newsletter was developed. We used our Hospital Foundation and Community Relation staff to create this newsletter. It was a valuable tool in the beginning of the project to keep the hospital staff involved in what was going on with the project. Most people within the hospital really don't understand the workings of a major construction project and it is good to keep them advised of what is going on. They see things out there that they don't understand and this is one method of explaining the process to them. One unexpected advantage of the newsletter was that the construction workers took great interest in seeing that their work was being described to hospital staff. We then began to use the newsletter to interview people on the site and this created quite a bit of interest on both sides of the construction fence.

Nursing division of the hospital assigned our Director of Critical Care Nursing to be the contact for the entire hospital. This was a very fortunate move as this woman had been the unit supervisor in charge of Emergency Department during the planning and design stage of the project. She and I held regular meetings throughout the entire project so that any concerns of nursing staff could be addressed by myself in conjunction with the architects and/or the construction company. She also acted as a liaison for me to relay the needs of the project to the hospital staff in general. Major areas such as womens' lockers rooms, office occupancies were involved in some way with the project and all of these people had to be moved, or put out in some way and the communication line between project management and the hospital staff in general was a very important one.

After the major construction was well into the stage where the building was out of the ground, we formed a Hospital Equipment Acquisition Committee, which consisted of our Purchasing people and again the Director of Critical Care Nursing, myself, and our Executive Director. We detailed a program for purchasing all of the hospital equipment which was to be installed by the Contractor. We arranged for suppliers to provide shop drawings of the equipment which I reviewed and had the hospital's consultants review. These drawings were then passed along to the contractor so that long before the equipment arrived on site, he had accurate drawings by which to make his rough-in and fabrication of support details. This ensured a smooth method to provide for the installation of equipment for which the contractor was not responsible at the purchasing stage. An area was set aside in the new construction for the storage of this hospital equipment and hospital staff were trained the policies put in place to receive, store, and catalogue this equipment so that when it was time to have it installed, it could be turned over to the contractor in an orderly and reasonable manner. This procedure also gave us the opportunity to examine all incoming equipment to make sure that it was (1) as ordered (2) in good shape and (3) complete so that at the time of installation we would get no surprises. Training sessions for hospital staff on equipment supplied by the contractor for the project were arranged. One of the most notable was demonstrated by the supplier of the diesel engine for maintenance staff. Previously the hospital had two rather old small diesel stand-by generators and these were largely replaced by a new 600 kW 900 hp V 16 Detroit engine with ultramodern control.

After the installation was completed by the electrical contractor, the supplier of the engine and generator came up to the site to give the engine a load test under field conditions. At this time, selected members of the electrical contractor's staff and key members of the hospital staff were trained in the operation of the diesel. This was done on this particularly small scale because this engine was to be used to supply a major portion of the hospital's power requirements while the cables which would supply power from the new utility connections were connected during the month of January. Also at this time a new 44,000/4160 volt transformer had to be installed and so for a short period of time the entire hospital was forced to operate on less than optimum power requirements. Some time after this power changeover had been completed and when the diesel generator set was commissioned to stand-by power use, the entire operating and repair staff who would need to be familiar with its operation and its characteristics, were trained by the contractor and by the supplier of the unit. At the same time, while mechanical and electrical services were being installed in the newly constructed areas, hospital maintenance staff were taken on regular tours so that they might inspect the locations of the various valving and controls for the equipment as they were installed. Hospital electricians were given tours and instruction in the new major electrical distribution centres as they were being insalled, and were encouraged to review plans so they might ask appropirate questions of the construction electricians on site. The same process of course applied to the mechanics who were also asked to review mechanical drawings so that any questions they might have could be addressed to contractor personnel while they were actually installing the mechanical equipment. This type of training was given as a backup to the usual maintenance manuals which are turned over to the hospital at the end of the project in the hopes that maintenance staff would be able to visualise rather than read about the methods which were used to install the equipment. Due to the fact that this project increased the size of our hospital by approximately one-third, quite early in the project I felt that a great amount of familiarisation would be necessary for all staff. The Hardhat Herald, previously mentioned in this address, was one method which was used to familiarise staff with what was happening to the hospital. Also, early in the project, as soon as there were areas of the building closed in, I set aside Friday afternoons when normally construction workers were not at work, so that I could take tours of various interested people in the hospital to familiarise them with what was going on in the construction project, and as the project progressed familiarised them with what their departments would look like. This type of procedure was especially helpful for the nursing staff in the Emergency Department. Most hospital staff I believe find it rather difficult to visualise the finished project from plans and specifications, descriptions etc and it is much easier for them to visualise what their new surroundings will look like, even when the project is at the stage of erecting partitions. Our Unit Director in charge of emergency had been making attempts to train her staff in some of the new types of administrative duties which would be necessary in the expanded department and the tours of the actual location enhanced their understanding of what it was that they needed to address before moving in to the new quarters. Similar training and visual inspections were carried out with members of each department that would be moving into the newly constructed areas.

This is one small phase of the Project Manager's work, but I suggest to you that it might be one of the most important in that this is the way that hospital staff are included in the construction process. In this way, the entire staff feel a part of what is happening in their hospital.

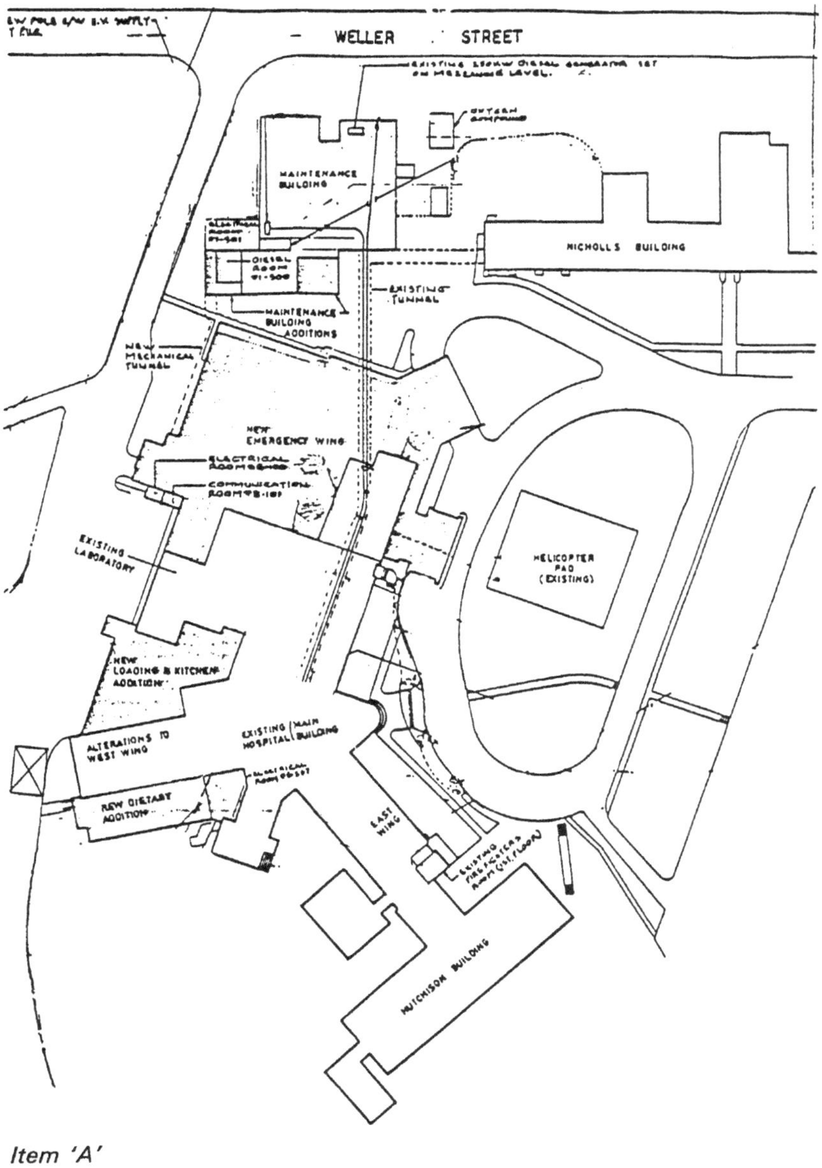

Item 'A'

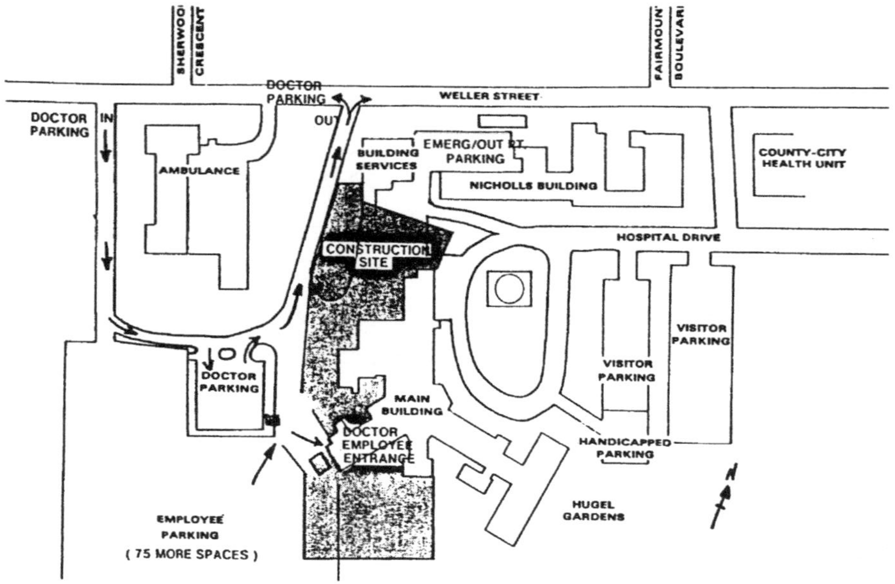

Item 'B'

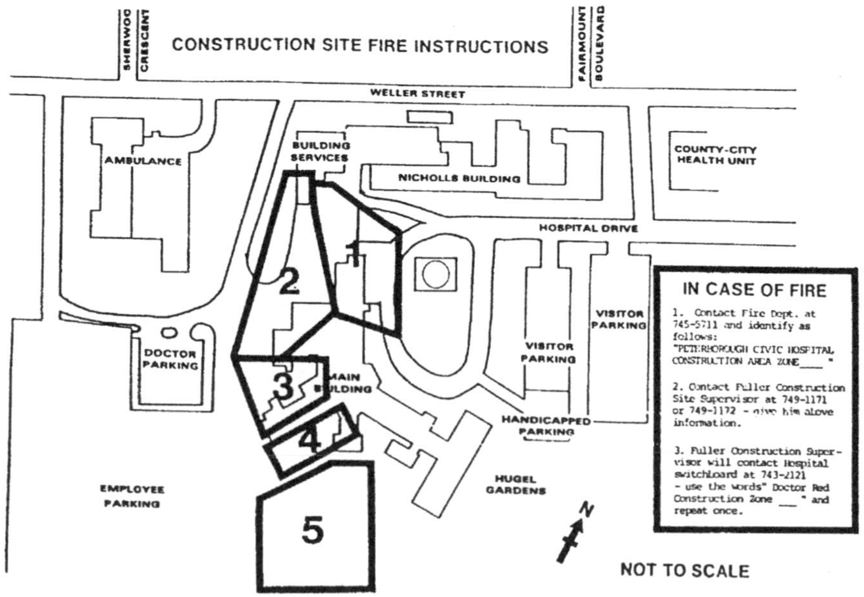

Item 'C'

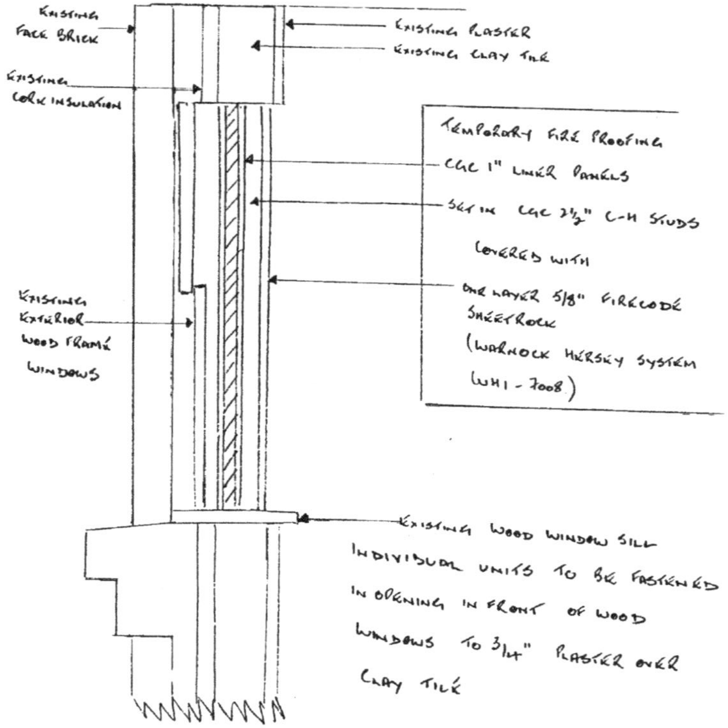

Item 'D'

An Updated Communication System at the New Pietralata Hospital in Rome

by

Arch Paola M. Falconi
Regione Lazio
Assessorate Lavori Pubblici
Roma, Italy

1. Health Care Organisation in Latium, The Rome Region

In 1978 Italy started its National Health Care Service: a country wide organisation to assist every citizen, regardless of his income.

This organisation, which is similar to the British, splits the Regions into Local Health Care Units (LHCU), to program and take care of all HC activity, including hospitals.

Latium, which we discuss in this paper is one of the 20 Italian Regions, having Rome as its centre. Our Region is split into 51 LHCU's; these are co-ordinated by the regional government. Latium has 5,000,114 residents (1981), of whom 57% live in Rome.

Latium has 96 hospitals with 30,773 beds, of which 12,719 are managed by the LHCU's and 9,054 by Teaching Hospitals, by various scientific Institutes and by semi-public hospitals (the so-called classified hospitals).

Rome has, as a whole, 18,643 public bedplaces, housed in 24 public and 17 classified hospitals.

2. Health Care Building Programmes in Rome

In 1983, Region Latium started an updating programme for its Rome Hospital network, by creating HC points in the densely inhabited outskirts and preventing overcrowding in the town.

This was the reason for building two new hospitals, at Ostia Lido (West of Rome, 360 beds) and Pietralata (East, 384 beds); North of Rome, the Sant'Andrea Hospital (650 beds) is being built.

This rationalisation also includes a functional modernisation of the old downtown hospitals involving reducing the bed numbers and increasing facilities.

The plans for completely revamping six major hospitals have been released. The regional infectious disease hospital, 'L. Spallanzani', (South) is being altered in order to provide for the increase of AIDS patients. This programme for hospitals building involves an investment of 430 milliards liras for Rome between 1990 and 1992.

3. The Introduction of the Oxford Method

Until the early eighties, the average time for building a 300 bed HC structure in our Region was about 10 years, due to budgetary constraints and to the tender system, where tenders accepted were split between many Contractors making on site co-ordination very difficult.

In order to reach European standard construction times, Latium tried out new techniques when constructing the Rome Ostia Lido Hospital. The salient features of the new policies, aimed at optimising hospital construction times, were:-

- immediate availability of 80% of the total construction sum;
- the use of a modular industrialised construction system so as to allow integration of prefabricated construction with standardised work practices.
- assigning all works responsibilities to one firm.

This experiment gave real benefits. Osta Lido Hospital (360 beds; 89,800 cu m; 24,270 sq m) was erected, ready to start-up, in 24 months, on a turnkey basis.

The Rome Pietralata Hospital was erected (384 beds, 105,500 cu m, 31,200 sq m) by adopting the same policies. Work started on 3rd September 1987 and ended on 4th December 1989 — 27 months, and the Hospital is now ready to function.

For constructing these two hospitals, Region Latium used the British 'Oxford Construction System', which is industrialised in Italy by an ENI Group (State Participated) Company. Such system is based on the following items:-

- Design base module 30 cm and multiples.
- Steel holding structure both vertical and horizontal.
- Technical interfloor over the ceiling of any floor, to allow for horizontal distribution of water, technical, conditioning facilities etc.
- Carton gypsum prefabricated partitions internally hollow, for the vertical passage of facility distribution lines.
- Peripheral closures with prefabricated elements.
- False ceiling for every technical floor, making services completely accessible.

4. Modifications and Integrations to the System

It is not my intention to illustrate such a system, as it is well known and also replaced in the UK by the 'Best Buy' system; but rather briefly to expose those modifications and

REORGANISATION DU SYSTEME DE COMMUNICATIONS AU NOUVEL HOPITAL DE PIETRALATA A ROME

Dans son introduction (lere section), le Dr S. Giovannetti, ingénieur en chef, décrit la situation actuelle du système de santé, et les programmes de construction de ce domaine dans la ville de Rome.

A Rome, l'Hôpital du district de Pietralata vient d'être construit. Le système de communications illustré dans la deuxième section y a été installé selon une méthode de construction d'Oxford, adaptée aux données culturelles italiennes.

Dans cette deuxième section, ie Dr P. M. Falconi, architecte, présente le système de communications prévu pour cet hôpital. Il s'agit d'un système de communications duplex, avec indications lumineuses et acoustiques, qui comprend une salle de terminaux micros. Le système peut fonctionner soit à partir d'une station centrale contrôlant tout l'hôpital, soit à partir d'un certain nombre de sous-stations, dirigées chacune par une infirmière en chef (système décentralisé), ou encore les deux (système mixte). Il permet d'appeller soit le personnel soignant, l'infirmière en chef, ou un médecin, selon les besoins. Mais il permet aussi l'intercommunication avec d'autres domaines des soins de santé, la sécurité, la prévention des accidents, EDP, les équipements administratifs etc.

integrations we have introduced in the system, featuring what is called the Italian Style. Variations introduced in the construction of Pietralata Hospital have allowed us to achieve the following goals:-

- A mixture of the functionality of the Oxford method and the Italian architectural taste and culture.
- The construction system provides for the different habits of patients and personnel.
- Adaption of the system to the different construction criteria, different materials, different climate, different anti-fire rules and regulations, etc.

Concerning the first item, the architectural style in most Oxford method buildings was modified by changing the internal layout and introducing facade decoration elements of architectural structure.

These changes were achieved by redesigning safety staircase element by using a different construction technology. Views from inside are improved by the increased glassed surfaces, and by wall surface treatment combining aesthetics with conservation requirements. The external wall colour scheme was chosen to match the prevailing ones in Rome town.

Covering the air conditioning system by a steel — polycarbonate structure has directly influenced the architecture.

Concerning the second item, the 6-8 bed ward, quite common in the hospitals built according to the Oxford system, was replaced by 2-4 bed wards for increased privacy.

The centralised rest rooms of the Oxford method have been transformed into a private WC in every ward.

The windows have been widened to allow the patient to enjoy the scenery. We also took into consideration the behaviour difference between British (more quiet) and Italian (more aggressive) hospital personnel: for example, to limit maintenance expenses we decided for a Klinder lining in the bathrooms, and a shock absorber layer along the corridors and the bedhead.

This latter device, to prevent beds and trolleys damaging the walls, resulted in a decrease in the internal partition's metal support reference line from 60cm (Oxford) to 40cm, so as to account, for a higher rigidity of the shock absorber section;

Additional modifications were:-

- Double gypsum panels were used (two for each side, ie 24mm per side instead of 12) for the partitions, resulting in more rigid walls and a better acoustic isolation.
- A subterranean floor was built, at foundation level, to facilitate maintenance of the sewage system and to allow expansion, if required: this level also contains connecting stations (substations) for gas and liquid, as well as power, and also a corridor for transporting dirty linen to the laundry and corpses to the morgue.

Concerning materials, especially for finishing, research was used to improve the interior decorations by the wide use of colours (on doors, walls, floors etc), in order to enhance the psychological effect on the patient.

As for the windows, the blinds for living areas have been replaced by external aluminium shutters, wound on coils, in the typical Italian style.

The difference in climate requires summer ventilation in the wards (2-3 volumes per hour), with air-temperature cooled at 3°C less than outside, while using double glazed windows for better thermal insulation.

I hope this Italian adaptation of the Oxford method in the Rome area has proved of interest to you.

Section Section

1. Foreword

By communication system we mean the equipment used to transmit and remotely receive, messages and signals, as well as information; it minimises staff personnel movement between areas of the hospitals which are sometimes very far apart.

Sometimes these movements repeat themselves quite regularly and greatly reduce the effective use of health care staff. The internal communication system is, therefore, of fundamental importance for the efficiency of the hospital, in reducing the running costs and contributing to an efficient patient service.

We believe an efficient communication system can reduce staffing levels by increasing their productivity, while cutting down management costs, particularly as personnel costs are 70% of hospital expenses.

2. The Updating of Communication System — Today's Trends

In the past few years we have seen several generations of communication systems even though their characteristics seemed up to date at the time they appeared on the market. At the same time the need for integration of the various internal communication systems grew, with the tendency to limit some of them to particular uses, such as the intercom in the outpatients area, radio paging to medical or technical personnel, telephone for outer communication, etc.

For example the 'light trace nurse call' is now just as archaic as 'bell ringing'.

Some 20 years ago the first 'simplex' system communication systems appeared; followed by the 'bus line technique', 'microprocessor systems' and 'duplex' systems. At the same time, there was discussion about the best use of such systems, hence the need for centralisation, or decentralisation of information and therefore, of the communications etc.

After years of research, discussions, requests, all complicated by the fact that all manufacturers introduce a new electronic generation every 3-4 years, some key aspects were spotted:-

- The system must be universal, therefore anybody must be able to contact anybody.
- The possibility of operating locally, ie ward by ward, must be available depending on the time of day.
- Continuous operation must be possible even in case of absence of a main operator, or when the matron is not in her office.

3. How to Inform — To Communicate — To Be Present on the Spot — The System Philosophy

3.1 The Triangle: Information Communication Presence

Certainly, in the hospital, internal communications provide the basis for security if we consider this to be presence in the right place at the right time with the right tools.

Basically, it can be stated that security *is* bound to the triangle 'information — communication — presence'; but, additionally, quantity, quality and the need for precise information are essential to ensure that staff have correctly understood the call.

3.2 The Philosophy of the System

The philosophy on which our communication system is based is that information must be full and precise; communication easy and targeted; response must be quick and efficient.

The ability to talk with missing staff within a few seconds of pushing the button makes possible the long awaited 'humanisation in the hospital'. In fact, the 'human voice' acts as a re-assurance for the individual and, if this is valid for any person in general, it is particularly valid for a sick person.

This system, at the same time, is very much accepted by the staff, and not only because walking is reduced, but also because the nursing staff are given, in every room, information and control which was unthinkable in the past.

They are also likely to increase their own professional attitude and satisfaction because factors such as:-

(1) efficient managing system;
(2) security for the patient; and
(3) humanitarian health care and tranquility for the patient provide the best result. After filtering therefore, those cases which really need personal attention are spotted and dealt with, while simple voice communication solves other cases where the human voice can replace the need for a human presence. Additionally, responding after a verbal communication is more effective, as the nurse can be prepared by the communication beforehand.

3.3 Continuous Information on Personnel Location

The system adopted in the Pietralata Hospital is based on knowing, in real time, the location of nurses, matrons and doctors throughout the various wards and stations.

This data is obtained by presence marking made by such operators whenever entering or leaving the ward, or any other designated important rooms. It is necessary to mention that *presence marking* is mandatory, as effective functioning of the system depends upon it.

4. Type and Functioning of Plant-Component Elements

4.1 How it Operates

The plant can be visualised as a tree, on whose roots stands the main control station, where the main knots are the matrons' stations, and the branches are the wards or departments. The plant can function with most operating versions, with no need for changing any structure when making modifications.

In Pietralata Hospital we wanted to offer the following operating versions:-

(1) Centralised communication over colour videographic monitors, operated by light pen.
(2) Decentralised communication with *or without* substation.
(3) Mixed (centralised plus decentalised) communication.

Undoubtedly, in most conditions, the centralised system is the best option; but the plants must also be able to function efficiently when decentralised; simply because centralisation is often temporarily impossible (when restructuring; when starting up; or when operators are missing).

4.2 Applicable Regulations

The communication system is built up by means of smart microcomputer operated room terminals, according to DIN and VDE regulations (ICE compatible):-

* DIN 41050: Part 1 and 2
* DIN 57833/VDE 0833 Class 2
* DIN 57834/VDE 0834 Part II

4.3 System Basic Components

4.3.1 One consulting colour graphic video, reporting all hospital plan drawings.
4.3.2 One operating colour graphic video, reporting, in detail, the required area (usually 2-3 wards), similar to that fitted in air traffic control rooms for controlling aeroplanes with radar. Notice that functions are highlighted by using the light pen on the video screen.
4.3.3 Ward Station: This communication equipment is located in the matron's room, that is in the heart of the wards. It allows processing of duplex calls, presence markings, answers and general announcements.
4.3.4 Room terminal: Communication equipment located in every important room. It is meant for making duplex calls, cancelling them, answering, marking presences and making various types of announcements.
4.3.5 Patient hand unit: This allows calls, conversations, radio receiving, six channel wire broadcasting, volume control, light and TV control.
4.3.6 Bathroom call: Wire operated, it allows no conversation. It is usually installed in showers, bathrooms, etc.
4.3.7 Corridor lamp: Holding different colours, they indicate calls and personnel presences, as well as memory for them. It is a sort of safety measure for the patient as it gives a clear indication of staff where they must go.

5. The Room Terminals

Room terminals include a smart microcomputer with built-in microphone and loudspeaker. This allows easy two-way communication. Additionally, six buttons are built in the keyboard: the three lower ones — green, yellow and orange, allow marking presences of staff: green for nurse, yellow for matron, orange for doctor. The upper buttons mean: red button: nurse calling; orange button with galenic symbol: nurse calling doctor and white button with question mark: determines the start, end and types of any conversation.

The room terminals are really the greatest asset in the system. They allow the operation in every room of a considerable range of functions, other than just call and presence; and besides qualifying the intervention level, they allow personnel to call the doctor, to memorise where to go next, to answer any 'type of call and to cancel them remotely, to make announcements separately for guests and personnel, to select audio and TV channels, etc. In brief a terminal is today a third-level central station. The proof of this is that two of them constitute the basis for a complete plant.

6. Light Memory in the Corridor Lamps

These light indicators may furnish a large number of indications even without a preceding communication. The steady light gives an indication of who is present in the room (doctor, matron, nurse). When blinking it shows who is required in the room.

The blinking of the red light indicates an emergency call, made either by staff or by a machine.

The white light in the corridor means a call from the toilet: in the toilet itself this corresponds to a red light in the patient call, and a green light in the nurse cancel pushbutton: alarm cancellation can be done by the nurse only when entering the bathroom.

7. Type of Calls — Automatic Priority Device

7.1 Type of Calls

The types of calls are continually increasing. Since the call is the first step of the process and therefore, as explained, the basis for any safety measure, let us see how it must be structured.
7.1.1 Patient call: It must be as simple as possible. The patient must be in a position to push just one button, and the decision whether this should be considered as an emergency or not must be left to personnel or the room computer.

In Pietralata, we have chosen the patient hand unit, which ensures more privacy and is easier to operate than the unit built in the night table, normally used for example in Germany.

7.1.2 Alarm caused by the call unit being pulled out. A typical security feature.

7.1.3 Call and conversation from room terminal. Of the type: nurse speaks with nurse.

7.1.4 Call from bathrooms or WC's. No conversation expected: an immediate presence is necessary.

7.1.5 Emergency Call: It can be operated, both by a patient and by a nurse, but is always expedited by the latter: immediate presence of a nurse is necessary following the communication.

7.1.6 Alarm from a monitoring equipment. Again, it is a matter of security. Typical connected equipments are infusion pumps, ECG's, lung ventilators, microphones. Voice connection is not necessary.

7.1.7 Request for doctor. As stated before, it must be initiated only by the nurse. It brings about a voice connection, and the doctor must be reached outside the called ward.

7.1.8 Alarm from Intensive Care Stations. It is initiated by the nurse from a terminal (sometimes a desk terminal that is directed to the IC team by connection through the paging system. An orange flashing light outside the door indicates the area requiring assistance.

7.1.9 Telephone follow-up call. If a telephone call to the matron's room is not answered then the call is relayed via the communication system.

7.1.10 Automatic priority device. An automatic device allows the most urgent call to be processed first (in the priority order listed below). In case two or more calls are made at the same time, this device allows the top priority call to be processed first. Only when this is cancelled will the next call show up as requiring an answer.

Priority	*Type of Call*
1	Request for doctor
2	From monitoring equipment
3	From bathroom, shower, etc
4	Emergency room terminal
5	Emergency from bed
6	Normal terminal call
7	Normal bed call or for patient unit displacing
8	From telephone

8. Extension and Interfacing

The system is easily interfaced with radio paging, telephone, or TV. The system allows the patient a number of options, such as:-

- reading light switching;
- television switching, including a simple (one button) remote control by cable, thus avoiding interference with electro-medical equipment, if any;
- telephone paying system facilities; and
- radio controls, wire diffusion, in-house voice programmes etc.

All this though, must be easily operated since the patient may for example, only have very limited physical capability; it is also necessary to avoid the necessity for the patient continuously to call the nurse to ask for information.

Additionally, television may be used for therapeutic purposes by making the extra channels available for the doctors only (eg for reading the patients sick notes in the patient room itself).

9. Security Functions — Breakdown Controls

9.1 Data Memory

The system retains the data in memory in case of power failure, for a minimum of 30 minutes and restores it to the original position when power is restored.

9.2 Breakdown Control

The system also allows control of all terminal microcomputers, of the data and communication transmission lines, by distinguishing between 'breakdown' and 'out of service'. This information is given both at the central station in the control room and at the corresponding substation in the matron's office. When a breakdown on the upper level occurs, the plant automatically switches itself down to the immediately lower level, ie from central station to sub-stations, and from these to the terminals. The functions 'light calls', 'acoustic call', and 'communication' are always assured. No system blackout is possible.

9.3 Circuit Test Functions

A lamp test button can control, room by room, function of any lamp, light diodes, buzzers. The plant is thereby self controlling and it shows in real time the presence and location of 'breakdown' and 'out of order', or just burnt lamp.

10. Conclusions

The communications system, produces efficiency and speed in patient care, allowing the nurse a direct and continuous access to the patient. This presence gives confidence and peace of mind to the patient and is of fundamental importance psychologically in recovery from illness. The communication system integrated with TV and telephone allows the patient not to feel a prisoner in the hospital, but to keep his contact with the outside world unchanged. The system, therefore, contributes significantly, not only to the behaviour of the nursing personnel, but also to the humanisation of the hospital, that is, making hospital life closer to the patient's way of life.

Staff and Patient Communications – Trends and Technologies

by

Paul Warminger BSc(Eng), MBA
International Product Manager
Communications Systems
Ohmeda, a Division of BOC Health Care

1. Introduction

The 1990's is a decade where resource constraints and increasing activity focuses even more attention on the drive towards efficiency.

Demographic effects of a greying population together with the advancement of medicine and methods of treatment are increasing patient numbers. Yet shortages in the labour market are limiting the supply of trained nurses.

Greater patient throughout is increasing the volume of inter staff/patient communications — so much so, that some hospitals are discovering that their traditional communication systems no longer have the capability to cope with these increasing demands.

Communications in hospitals are particularly complex because of the whole interaction of various groups such as nursing staff, doctors, administration, specialist departments, engineering support, and the interaction of this organisation with patients, visitors and outside agencies.

A large part of this communication is characterised by short messages which have high urgency but are only valid for a limited time. Therefore, if their requirements are to be fulfilled, these must be spontaneously formulated, safely transferred and quickly received.

In response, most hospitals in West Germany and the US have adopted integrated hospital wide communications systems incorporating speech and available to all patients and staff.

This trend is now global, with hospitals in the UK and an increasing proportion of hospitals in Holland, Italy, France and other parts of Europe as well as the Far East following their lead.

A variety of hospital speech systems exist but their configuration can be broadly characterised as being either decentralised or centralised.

With both approaches, patients can call a nurse or other ward staff and request assistance. Staff also have the facility to pass messages to each other.

Decentralised systems consist of independant group systems, each with its own master console usually located at the nurse station. In this mode, staff to staff communication via the system is within the department. The main system features at the console are:-

- speech communication;
- call answer/hold/cancel;
- identification of call source and call category;
- display of nurse presence positions by category;
- selective room, area and staff announcements; and
- interface capability to other systems.

Centralised systems integrate these separate system groups at a hospital central console which is manned by an operator. Various other departments are added in, such as Theatres, X-Ray, Accident and Emergency etc so the benefits to all staff increase as messages and the co-ordination of activities becomes inter-departmental. Experience has shown that communications traffic approximately doubles in this mode as the benefits for organisational efficiency are optimised.

The central operator (who often has previous nursing experience) answers all calls and relays messages, undertaking the organising of tasks such as the transfer and movements of patients etc as requested by calling staff. Other responsibilities might include the instigation of emergency procedures, monitoring of other central systems such as gas alarms, fire alarms, security screens and carrying out some central administrative duties. The exact scope of the role is determined by the hospital and its operational policies.

So what of the origin and development of these systems, and the technology that support them? And what challenges lie ahead for their future development so that they may meet the needs of hospitals in decades to come?

2. Development of Voice Communication Systems

Todays advanced hospital speech systems originate from the development of nurse call. In early times, this activity was not systemised; patients in large open wards waving and calling to attract the attention of a nurse. Nurses had to maintain high visability of patients to prevent calls going unanswered.

The introduction of formal systems which followed using lights and buzzers is still in use in many hospitals today and, over the years, its development has led to better design and more features. Special mention should be given to the development of patient handset design in the UK where attention to ergonomics, hygeine and minimum maintenance has led to the incorporation of surface mount technology, membrane switching and more sophisticated interfacing with entertainment and lighting controls.

The first speech system was installed in the US, in 1935, but their general introduction was in the 1960's at a time where new large hospitals were being built. The objective of speech systems have been to overcome the inherent limitations of traditional nurse call and to tackle the difficulties of staff organisation.

The principles limitations of lights/buzzers nurse call are:-

- a patient can call but cannot communicate a request;
- the patient's call is only answered when a nurse arrives

LA COMMUNICATION ENTRE MALADE ET SOIGNANTS

Le système traditionel d'appel se fait peu a peu remplacer par la communication à vive voix. Ceci tend à une efficacité accrue ou de plus en plus de malades sont soignés par de moins au moins de soignants. Le malade peut aussi demander une aide spécifique a l'infirmière, celle ci peut si nécessaire demander l'assistance d'une collégue ou passer un message.

Ce mémoire rappelle la développement de ces systèmes à vive voix, et expose les techniques employés pour leur construction: on y trouve une discussion des avantages des systèmes multiplex pour le transport des informations et le contrôle continu des circuits primaires ainsi que de la bonne marche du système dans son integrité.

L'auteur commente aussi des éxigences des evolutions courantes des systèmes de provision des soins et de l'effet de celles-ci pour les hôpitaux dans l'avenir.

on the scene which leaves the patient in doubt of when the call will be answered;

- many patients will not call if they feel their need is trivial and will interrupt the nurse's tasks;
- all the ward staff are alerted, often resulting in more than one nurse attending. Staff have to attend every call even if the caller only requires information;
- there is no facility to call the nearest or most available nurse and the result is excessive walking distances;
- nurses cannot give a call a priority and so may have to leave a current task unfinished to attend the patient;
- usually, an additional journey is required to fetch what is needed;
- the locating of particular or additional staff is hampered by poor staff/staff visability; and
- system faults can often go undetected.

Such limitations led to a total re-think of system solutions for a modern hospital. Speech systems have come a long way since the 1960's, and todays solutions employ advanced data transmission techniques which has improved systems capability and has enabled such solutions to be more easily afforded.

Todays systems overcome the limitations or traditional nurse call as:-

- partients can communicate their request to a nurse who answers the call from a remote location. The system advises staff of the call type (patient, WC, staff/staff, Emergency) and, after speaking to the patient, the nurse can prioritise calls and collect anything required en-route;
- nurses can locate and communicate with various other staff from the nurse's station master console by utilising nurse presence indication and speech facility;
- centralised systems enable messages to be passed between staff all over the hospital quickly and efficently;
- systems are *active* and so include self monitoring and self diagnostics; and
- such systems help to fulfill higher patient expectations of care.

3. Serial Data Transmission

The exact techniques of transmitting and receiving signals around the system varies slightly between manufacturers, and there are advantages and disadvantages between each. However, to provide a technical perspective, further explanation is given here to the techniques as employed by Ohmeda.

A modular distributed system concept is adopted which uses intelligent terminals installed in each room and which interact with others within a total system group. Groups are installed so that their boundaries normally reflect the natural departmental boundaries within the hospital.

Each group is controlled by an intelligent micro processor control unit which is installed anywhere along the systems wiring. This control unit incorporates a data transmission interface to transfer various signals and conditions around a common bus line linking each room.

The intelligent room terminals transmit and receive information appropriate to the corresponding rooms's condition and, on receiving this information, the group control unit decides on what response to initiate. For example:-

- commanding visual and audible prompts at the master console;
- opening of speech lines;
- cancellation of calls; and
- automatic forwarding of calls to nurse locations if the master console is unattended.

4. System Wiring

As Figure 1 shows the communication bus line cable links all rooms by the most efficient and practical route.

The bus line consists of six cores — two for speech plus a screen, and three for signal multiplexing which includes a OV reference, a data and a clock line.

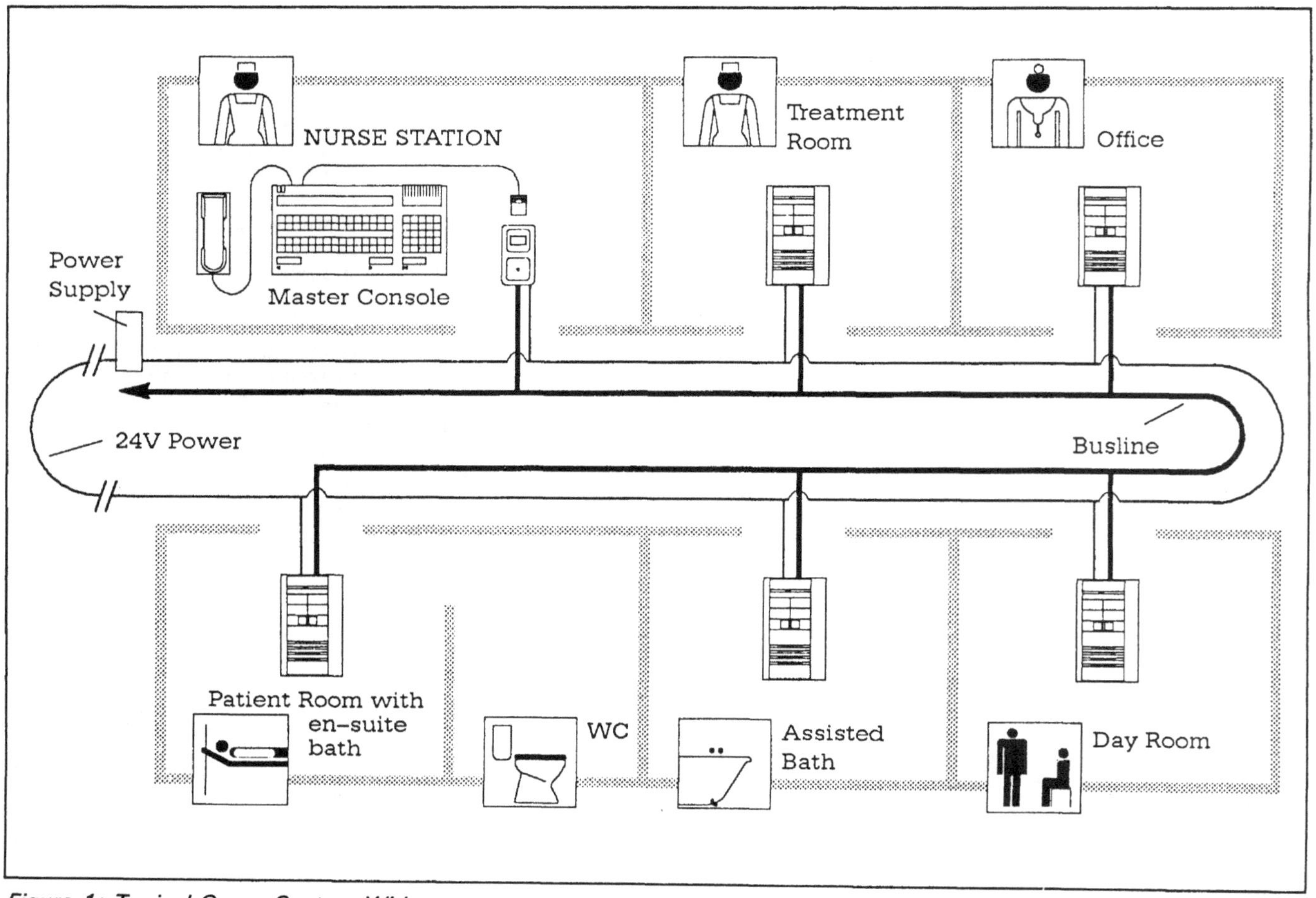

Figure 1: Typical Group System Wiring

Within rooms, the room communication terminal interfaces the bus line with various room components such as patient call/speech devices, call and cancel switches, staff presence switches and corridor lamps. The room terminal incorporates speaker and microphone modules and this is used for open staff communication and announcements, and various function switches on this unit provide additional features for staff such as call, call answer/cancel (when the nurse station is not attended) etc. Figure 2 shows the typical configuration of a three bedded room with en-suite bathroom.

A two core power cable accompanies the bus line by connecting each room (Figure 1) and is wired in a loop at the power supply unit to minimise voltage drop.

The power supply is rated at 24V, 10A and features fold back compensation in case of high loading, and capacitance protection in case of input peaks from the supply. Figure 3 illustrates the performance characteristics of the fold back compensation.

Significant advantages in installation are provided by this simple wiring scheme, when compared to wiring the installation of various separate alternatives such as traditional star wired nurse call, an emergency system, intercom and public address. System connections are also solderless and most 2nd fix items are simple plug in modules, thereby simplifying connections and commissioning and any requirements for maintenance.

5. Time-Division Multiplexing

Time-Division Multiplexing (TDM) is used and this is driven by the group control processor which provides a bit time of 0.65 ms and therefore an operating frequency of 1.5KHz. The system references 30 bits of information from each room which takes 30 × 0.65 ms = 19.5 ms. Various software can be used depending on the installation size and requirements. With one particular version of software, up

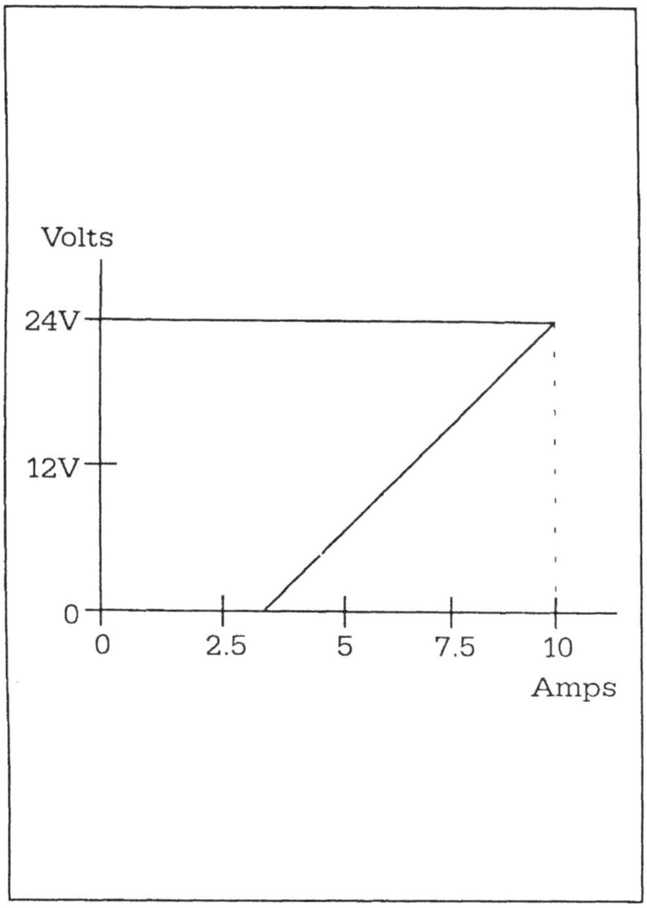

Figure 3: Current limited Power Supply (Fold-back-characteristics)

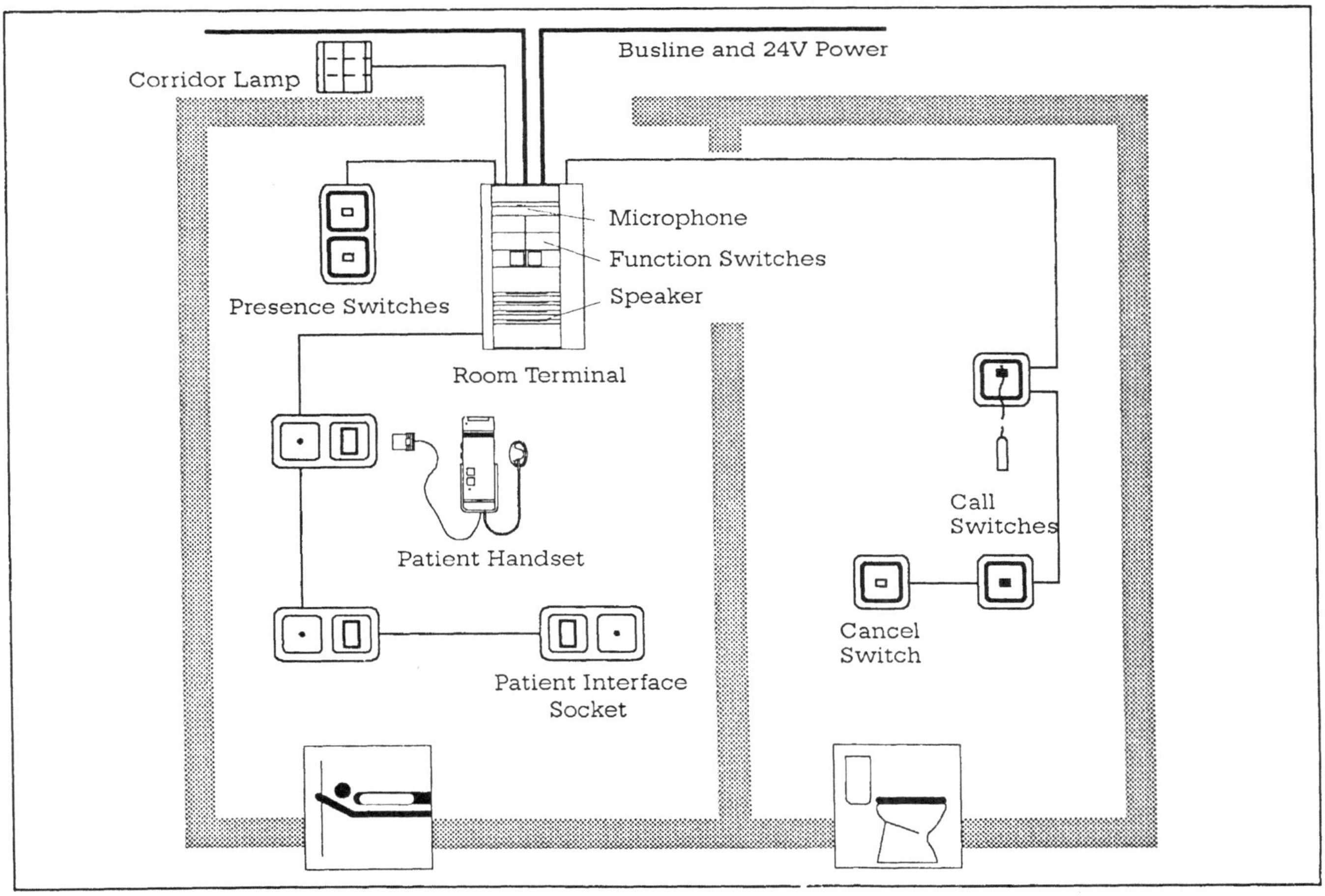

Figure 2: Typical Room Configuration

to 64 room addresses can be connected and this provides a total scan cycle for the system of 1.25 seconds (see Figure 4). This continuous scanning process is *'Active'*, and so even if no action is taking place in a room, the room terminal nevertheless responds to the control processor command. This provides high system integrity since the system is always self monitoring.

Data line signal bits are measures against the OV reference line and are determined as either logic 'O' or '1' Figure 5 represents a logic 1 pulse.

The shape of the signal pulse is sampled to determine whether it is being transmitted accurately, ie whether the bus line has any short circuits or is affected by any voltage transients. The operating frequency and waveform shape are co-ordinated to ensure a high degree of data transmission integrity.

Information about a room's status can be made available to the user anywhere on the bus line via an appropriate user interface such as the master console or room terminals located in other rooms. Flexibility is provided by this approach as the master console can be unplugged from the nurse base and relocated in say, the sisters office perhaps to suit day and nightime operation, without affecting the system's performance.

Looking specifically at the information transmitted and received during the scanning of a single room, Figure 6 shows how bits 1 to 9 are used for address signalling so that each room is considered separately. Binary encoding determines the room's address ie, Room 1 registers a pulse on bit 9, Room 2 on bit 8 and Room 3 on the 8th and 9th bit, and so on.

The following 20 bits of information relate to the condition of the room's status; transmitting information onto the bus line for reading elsewhere as well as receiving commands from the group control processor to alter a rooms status.

For example, bit 10 and 21 are signals transmitted to the room terminal. A pulse on bit 10 cancels the current patient call in that room, having previously received a user instruction from elsewhere in the system.

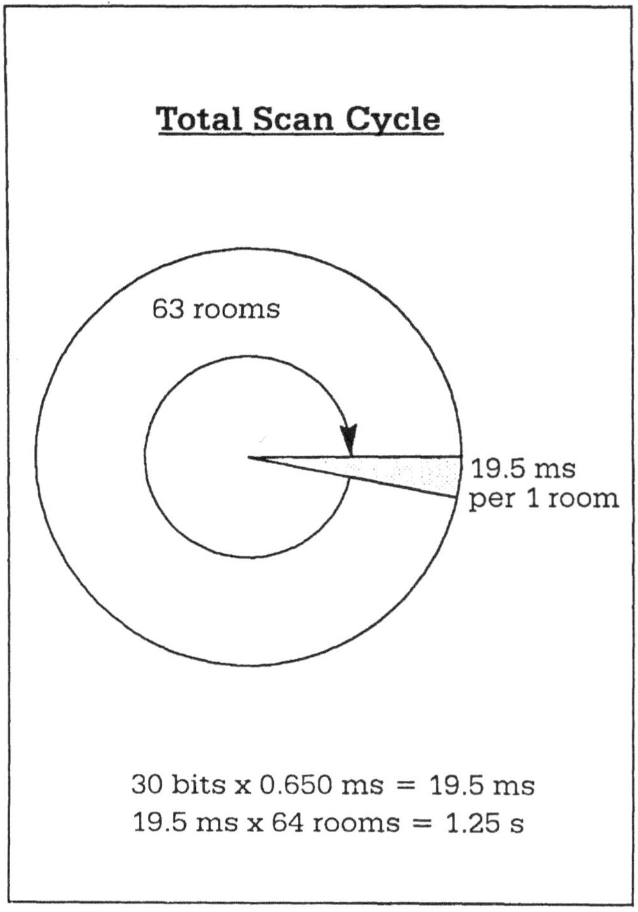

Figure 4: Principle of time multiplexing

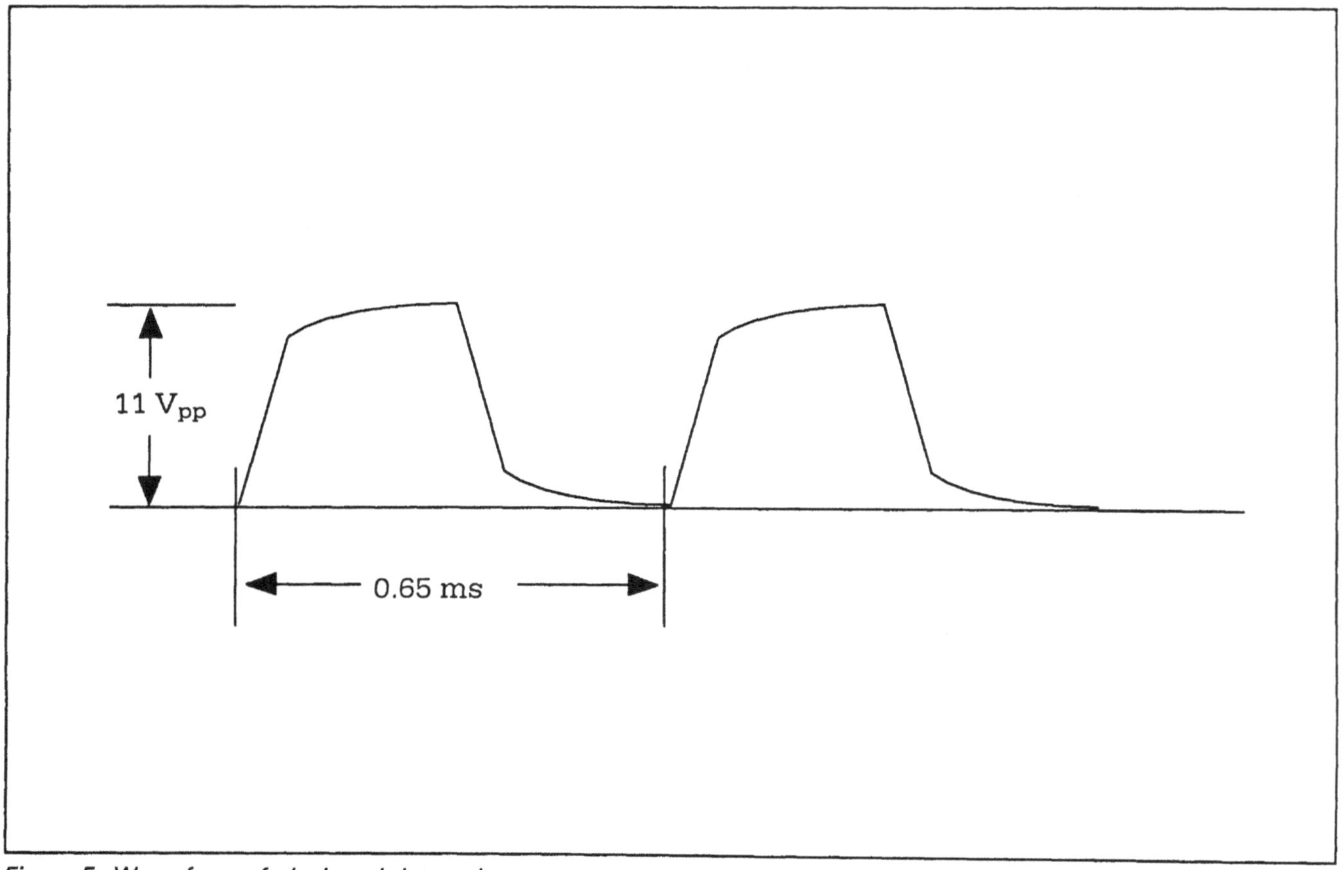

Figure 5: Wave form of clock and data pulses

A pulse on bit 21 commands the room terminal to open the speech communication chennel to a particular patient, the system having identified that a nurse has chosen to answer this patient's call.

Other signal bits represent various room conditions which are transmitted onto the bus line:-

- new call
- held call
- WC call
- emergency/monitor call
- staff presence indication for one or more categories of staff
- bed identification of caller; and
- call forwarded from/to another room.

The system also interprets a combination of signal bits as separate conditions. For example, another call category available on the system is staff assistance (or staff/staff) call, which is initiated by a member of staff to provide open communication into the room, rather than communication via a patient handset. In this situation, system operation is simple since subsequent to activating a presence switch on entry into the room (or automatically via an ultrasonic transmitter), the nurse may activate *any call switch* in the room. This eliminates the need for dedicated staff call switches. The diagram at the bottom of Figure 6 shows the transmitted signals for this case. The room which is addressed number 3 has a pulse at bit 17 which indicates staff presence II (ward sister or manager), and a pulse at bit 12 which indicates new call (bit 13 accompanies bit 12 in preparation for putting the call on hold). The system interpretes this combination as a separate condition, giving the call a higher priority through different signalling to other users in the group.

After the 29th signal bit, the system moves on and, after resetting with a synchronisation pulse at bit zero, the system scans the room with the next address reading. And so the process continues at the rate of one room every 19. 5 ms.

6. System Technology and Construction

The quality of advanced speech systems relies on component choice and design. Performance, reliability, cost, size and appearance are all factors which have to be optimised. Hospital communication systems represent a unique application for combining various specialist technologies, and so certain features deserve a special mention.

The design of microphone and speaker sets together with their mechanical package and amplifier circuits considers:-

- free communication across normal size rooms;
- communication with patient via handset, bedside console or other device;
- announcements; and
- call forwarding.

These components need to cater for varying distance to the caller as well as patients who may not have particularly strong speech. High quality acoustic properties, high sensitivity microphones, automatic gain control and a frequency response curve which eliminates unnecessary high and low frequencies, are key criteria for good design. Mechanical positioning is also important so that the possibility of any feedback and interference is minimised. Figure 7 illustrates the frequency response curve for an essential part of the speech circuits.

The modular items in the system produced in high volume, such as room terminals, require minaturisation and low cost. In the system manufactured by Ohmeda, this is achieved using sophisticated custom large scale integration (LSI) micro chips, one for digital processing and a second for analogue amplification and speech processing.

Miniaturisation and cost advantage is assisted through the advantages of better shape and intricacy available with high quality modern injection moulded plastics. The opportunity of improving aethetic design through shape,

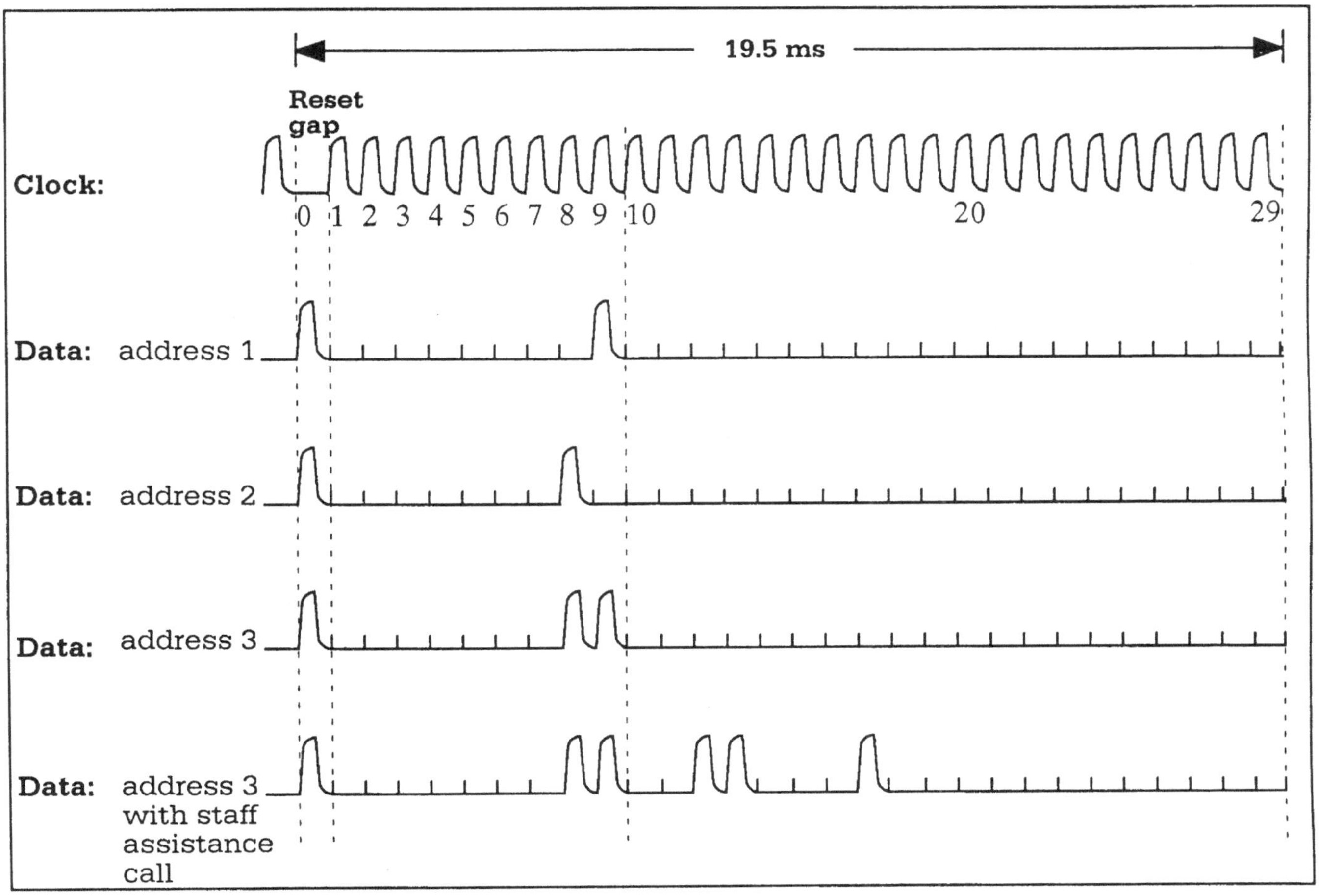

Figure 6: Application of the time multiplex principle

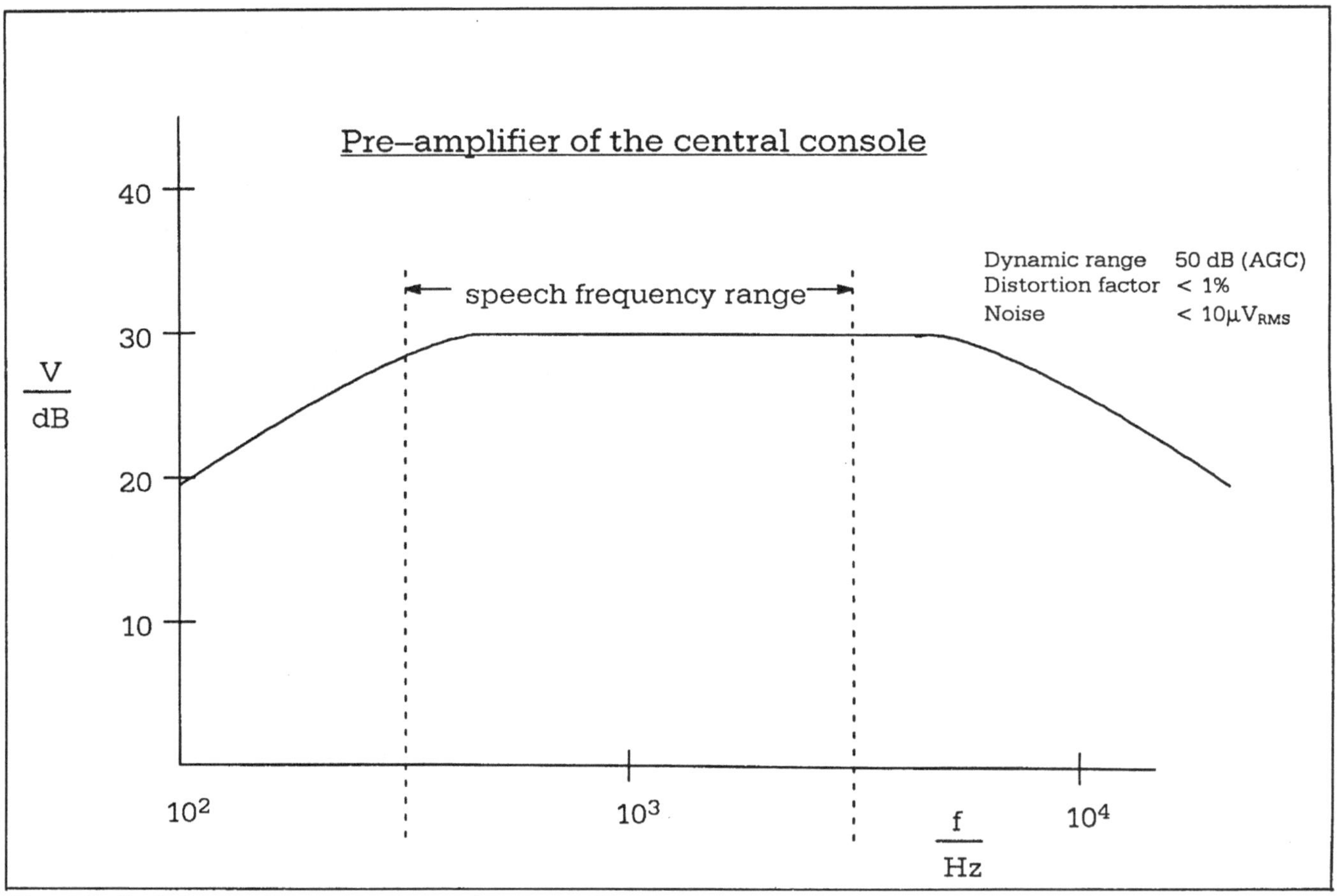

Figure 7: Technical performance of speech transmission

colour and ergonomics provides additional benefits here.

The group controller does not have the same tight constraints of mechanical size and so conventional state of the art 8 bit micro procressor technology is employed.

7. System Integrity

The modular distributed system design concept means that the hospital's system is made up of independant groups, each group's operation is spread across independant rooms. The functions of room terminals and the group controller represent separate building blocks to the system's overall performance. Each is capable of driving some aspect of the system and, if failure occurs, the rest of the group's (and other groups) functions are not affected and/or standby facilities take over.

To explain this further, let's consider the failure of:-

— a single call switch;
— a room terminal;
— the group controller;
— the master console; or
— the hospital power.

End of line resistors on call lines cause any faults to be reported when they occur. This is displayed at the master console with indication of whereabouts on the system the fault can be traced. All other room functions including other call switches operate as normal.

The failure of a room terminal is also reported on the master console display and, depending on the nature of this fault, some of the room's other functions may be unaffected. The remainder of the group is also unaffected.

Failure of the group control processor causes a stand-by processor located in the master console to automatically take over. No information is lost.

Failure of the master console causes the system to trip into call forwarding mode as if the master console was unattended. All calls are forwarded to staff presence positions where they can then be answered at room terminal locations.

Failure of both the group control processor and the master console would cause the system to operate at a lower level and perform as a light call system.

Should the hospital's power supply fail, data retention for 60 seconds allows uninterrupted continuity after change over to standby power.

Such distributed system design maximises system integrity — its continuous monitoring provides the engineer with information regarding the condition of primary circuits and its modularity simplifies fault finding and repair.

Modularity has other advantages:-

— it increases familiarity and user confidence;
— it reduces component and installation cost and spares holding; and
— it enables flexibility through configuration to meet the different requirements of various rooms.

Should any repairs be necessary, then replacement of faulty modules can be carried out without shutting the system down whilst short circuit and cross polarity protection assures system integrity and safety.

8. System Extensions

Data transmission technology, along with the system's modular construction, enables today's advanced speech systems to be extended and upgraded with minimal disruption.

For example, additional functional units and additional rooms may be wired and connected into the bus line at any point.

New rooms are addressed to a particular room response key on the console using a binary coder. The configuration of a groups functions and responses is programmed using EPROM and EEPROM components to maximise flexibility and any later reconfiguration.

System groups may be interfaced to provide the transfer of calls between wards to meet flexible modes of nursing.

Furthermore, system groups may be integrated at one central location and connected to a hospital central console. Many hundreds of hospitals operate in this way — a central operator answering calls immediately, redirecting messages and co-ordinating activities.

Interface with pocket paging, activity recording, patient database and building management systems extends the system's automatic responses — for example, by alerting the cardiac team via pagers with call source data displayed, as soon as a cardiac arrest switch is activated.

Whatever the end configuration, systems available today take account of refurbishment and extension programmes which necessitate an incremental approach to total system installation.

Wards act as independent groups and, as more are added, group coupling interfaces and the possibility of centralisation provides synergistic benefits to the hospital.

9. Future Developments

There are three main considerations:-

- shortage of nurses;
- hospital design; and
- technology.

Nursing shorages are already influencing changes in nursing practices. In some areas, zone nursing is becoming more popular. In others, staff are being given narrower definitions of responsibilities as relate to their training and status. Combined with this, more categories of staff are being introduced. The consequence of these trends is that message communication will become more fragmented. Therefore, the ability to register the presence and locate *all* staff will become more important.

Future systems will continue to be designed with ease of use in mind as they will need to cater for an increase in part time and agency staff as well as staff with greater skill differentials.

Systems will become even more flexible, especially through software, to cater for more flexible (and greater differences in) approaches to nursing. Users will have greater scope to alter parameters of the system functions during use.

Hospital design will move to more single and double rooms to reflect changes in patient expectations, to further minimise cross infection and to facilitate higher bed occupation through better distribution of male and female patients and patients across ward boundaries.

Greater system capability in rooms will lessen the importance of the nurse station, also reflecting trends on wards today, whilst the justifications for hospital centralisation will grow.

System construction will minimise installation costs and diagnostic facilities will benefit fault finding and repair.

Advances in applied technology are revolutionising equipment and systems in hospitals and greater use is being made of information technology. System integration will therefore become an important issue in the future. Information and features of one system will extend the capabilities of others whilst economising on effort and installation by eliminating duplication.

Patient interface units already link into TV, radio and lighting controls, and this trend will continue, with patients being given greater control over their environment and service.

Further miniaturisation of system construction and the development of features will be facilitated by further advances in data transmission techniques, new components, materials and methods of manufacture.

10. Conclusion

From a technical and operational perspective, advanced speech communications systems are appropriate for the drive towards greater efficiency in todays hospitals.

Such systems:-

- optimise the efficiency of inter-staff/patient communications, thereby improving hospital organisation;
- are safe, reliable and have high system integrity; and
- simplify fault finding and repair.

Speech systems are patient orientated as they meet growing patient expectations and provide easy communication which helps the patient feel safe and reasurred.

The changes taking place internationally in the provision of health care will affect the way hospitals are organised. Further developments in hospital communication systems will further optimise efficiency in an ever increasing complex environment.

ISDN — Telecommunication in Hospital

by

Volker Sporleder Dipl Ing
St Josefs-Hospital Wiesbaden
Solmsstrasse 15
6200 Wiesbaden

St Josefs-Hospital at Wiesbaden

The St Josefs-Hospital at Wiesbaden was founded 112 years ago in 1876 by the 'Armem Dienstmägde Jesu Christi' from Dernbach/Westerwald. The oldest building still in operation was erected in 1892. In 1961 until 1965 it was extended and became a hospital with 477 projected beds. In 1973 the nursing school including 100 training places, founded in 1964, could move into the new building and in 1980 a new pharmacy as well as a ward for radiologic therapy could be installed. In 1986 and 1987 the first construction lot of the new medical treatment building was finished and the restoration of the boiler house and transformer central executed. Today the affilate institute of the 'Armen Dienstmägde Jesu Christi' is the manager of these general catholic welfare hospitals for acute cases, with a central medical care ward including 460 beds as well as the wards: Medical Clinics, Surgery, Vessel Surgery, Intensive and Anaesthetic Treatment, Radiology, TNE and the training hospital of the Johann-Wolfgang-Goethe-University at Frankfurt am Main.

Telephone Technics in the St Josefs-Hospital

We regret for not having been able to be informed when and which technics have been employed for the first telephones in hospitals.

However we can prove that until 1959 there was a phone system including two exchange lines and four extensions for the chief surgeon, the administration and the gate keeper.

When starting the construction work for the new building in 1959, a new phone unit with five exchange lines and fifty extensions could be installed.

During the implementation of the new hospital complex, the installation of a lift-off rotary dialling unit with globally 20 exchange lines and 300 extensions could be realised in 1961 and was extended to 600 in 1965, however, without direct in-board dialling. From these 600 extension lines, the patients could only use approximately 100. In each three-beds' room only one phone was installed. Therefore the multiple demands of the patients for a phone could very often not be respected. Moreover the exchange of all incoming and outgoing calls via the central exchange resulted in an enormous work load during the last years and provoked long waiting times for callers. Not only the demand for shorter distances to the patients, but also the required installation of a direct dialling system have been a strong argument for the execution of a restructure of the old unit. Until this transformation of the new unit only 12 exchange phones could treat phone calls independantly. However, this fact again formed an extreme load for the exchange lines and consequently to frequent blocking of the global system.

Technical Planning

The technical planned with regard to the change-over of the telecommunication unit was performed by the technical department of the hospital. The decision to engage the technical department in this project was taken as it became evident that only collaborators excellently aware of the local and organisatory problems within the hospital were able to perform this task independantly. Considerable problems arose due to the fact that the enlargement of the phone system up to 1,200 extensions could only take place in the compass of the complete restructure of the extension line numbers to four-digit-numbers and the additional displacement of lines until the implementation.

For assistance and communication purposes a 'Communication Committee' was founded, including the following departments:-

- Administration
- Technics
- Nursing
- Data Treatment
- Information

This committee worked regularly from the beginning of the planning phase until the implementation and will exist furthermore in view of extensions, improvements and the required adaptions, especially within the application of digital services as there are telex, teletex, btx, telefax, data transfer and the use of personal computers.

The execution of technical planning included:-

As-Is Anaylsis of the existing phone connections on the basis of the existing documents and in the compass of an inspection walk. The determined data could be treated in view of a later application.

Determination of requirements concerning the number, situation, technics and the optimum remedies required for organisation of the telecommunication on the basis of an intense inquiry, analysis and consulting work for each individual work place, as well as the discussion of the data in the 'Communication Committee' and the entry into EDT-units for later use.

Tender of the global unit on the basis of the data on the requirement determination under consideration of the technical and financial decision finding.

Installation of the telecommunication unit within a timely limited frame, including placing of the new lines for the patients' phone and the installation of the phone on the wall

LES RESEAUX ISDN — DEUX ANNEES D'EXPERIENCE DANS UN HOPITAL

Quand la morbidité naturel du malade est restreint, les moyens de télécommunication prennent une importance accrue. Le téléphone est souvent le seul moyen de liaison avec parents et amis. Le télécommunication elle — meme devient part des système de thérapie, qui ne doit pas être sousestimée.

Un téléphone pour le malade entraine des consquences nombreuses, quelles soient techniques, financières ou administratives toutes à prendre en considèration. Pour le malade l'emploi du téléphone doit être aussi facile qu'à la maison.

Les techniques digitales (ISDN) offrent de nombreuse avantages autant pour le malade que pour le personnel de l'hôpital.

Les systèmes duplex (BBD) avec une vitesse de transmission de 64 K bit est la base de communication des ordinateurs, du téléfax, du téléx, du télétext et du videotext.

L'auteur fait la revue historique de l'installation, la mise en route, et la pratique de l'operation d'un réseau digital avec 1.200 branchements dans un hôpital à 460 lits.

and on the moveable supports near the bedside tables.

Training of all collaborators before and after the implementation in order to realise an increased acceptance and the optimum utilisation of all performance characteristics.

Implementation of the unit on the day X without interruption of the global communication system, including the particular problems of the new phone numbers to be dialled-in from outside and the new extension line numbers within the hospital.

Cost control and anaylsis of the given financial corner values including the as-is data to secure the financial base.

Installation at the Bedside

With regard to the installation of phones at the bed side, there is a multiplicity of various possibilities, depending frequently on the scope of apparatus manufactured. These are the following basic requirements for the patients' phones to be respected from our point of view:-

- packed mounting near the patient;
- simple and one-hand operation;
- operation like 'at home';
- invoicing on the day of leaving; and
- all-time detectability of the patient by the central operator by means of the electronic phone directory.

The picture shows the swivelling-type installation of the phones as near to the patient as possible with no place required on the bedside table. The apparatus can be operated equally with one hand by the patient in bed. Even during the night time a small glow indication lamp facilitates dialling. From the actual experiences and inquiries among the patients with regard to this type of unit, there are only positive results underlining the correctness of this decision for this type of apparatus and its mounting. Invoicing is also accepted. After the handing-over of the application for a phone, the connection will be executed immediately. The patient gets his invoice only on the day of leaving. Only the permanent phone occupiers are asked to pay after a certain period in case of a prolonged stay in hospital. This quality to move is certainly another reason for the increased load of the system.

Another advantage not to be underestimated should be discussed also. The exchange personnel can recognise on their data terminals on which bedside and/or under which phone number a patient can be called up. As a multiplicity of calls to patients must be exchanged by the central operator, even in case of direct dialling-possibility, this is also an important information not yet realised within other actual systems.

From our point of view the ideal solution is the following: When taking-up the patient, a phone chip card is handed-over to him, indicating his phone number, his name and his address. This card can be plugged into any phone. On the data terminals the actual position of the card is shown. Cards that have not been plugged-in are shown with their last location and marked particularly. On the leaving day invoicing takes place on the basis of the chip card, a solution allowing for all imaginable encashment systems. There is also the possibility to use the card for further services. The development of electronics will offer a similar solution.

ISDN — Technics in Service

The Deutsche Bundespost actually places at disposal various line systems for the different communication types:

Telecommunication System for the telephone service, telecopy unit (Telefax), viewdata systems (entry of participants), data communication (couplers, Modem), and teleoperation (Temex).

Datex-L-System for the teletex service, telex service and data transmission.

Datex-P-System for data transmission and viewdata entry into large-scale data processing units.

Direct-In-Dialling System for data communication.

The individual systems show different user system interfaces, digit indications, numbering, transmission speed, tariff structures and tariffs.

ISDN is the attempt to unify and standardise these various sytem types.

ISDN stands for Integrated, Serviced, Digital, Network.

Which are the Advantages of Such an Integrated System?

Some of the most important advantages of this system are:-

- Improvement of the existing telecommunication services including simultaneously an increased service comfort.
- The standard transmission speed of 64 kbit/s as only connection to language, text, picture and data.
- The multiple economical use of existing lines by means of the simultaneous operational possibility for two different services under one uniform dialling number and a similar tariff structure.
- The ISDN socket is a standardised unit and enables the liberalisation within the final unit sector, enhancing therefore the technical innovation up to the multifunctional phone for language, text, picture and data.

What is the Practical Importance of these Advantages for Communication Inside and Outside the Hospital?

Phone

Considerable improvement of phone language quality. Performance data as there are:-

- central and individual abbreviated dialling;
- party line for three subscribers;
- repeating of dialling;
- taking over of calls;
- transfer of calls;
- automatic recall;
- indication of dialling number of calling subscribers;
- knocking and broker's call function;
- digital memory service for language, data, text and picture;
- list of calls;
- partical and global blocking;
- 'call stop';
- fee indication;
- individual connection evidence;

enable a comfortable operation and the facility of daily operation. In this compass let us indicate some practical examples:-

In the mode *Abbreviation Dialling — Central* all important service telephone numbers are stored and may be dialled-in directly from all wards.

Taking-Over of Calls simplifies work. No more jumping between the phones.

The *Automatic Recall* renders superfluous the permanent repeating of phone calls. In case the occupied receiver terminates his call, the desired connection is reinstalled immediately and independently.

The experiences in hospital are all positive. However, we shall not suppress that training as well as an individual repeated information for all collaborators is very important, in order to make the characteristics of the new service effective for the hospital. Of special interest is certainly the implementation of some of this performance data into ISDN, when the effect becomes also evident in telecommunication.

A particular practical element is the *Language Information Server*, usually called call indication or call responder. This digital language information server is placed at the disposal of all authorised callers, who make an individual call and install the indication or responder operation. This language memory will be used in the meantime:-

- by the secretariat of the chief physician for the indication of unoccupied times and as phone responder, as a service for the callers;
- as a technical service for order acceptance;
- to provide information for the indication of patient movements; and
- within the nursing and administration section as a quick means to store information too unimportant to write down or for paging.

Another advantage is the possibility of operating the language information service from any phone connection in the world by means of the multifrequency technics (infotip).

Teletex

Telextex enables the interchange of documents between electronic memories (memory type writer, personal computer) at a speed of 2,4kbit/s via the Datex-L-network and a X.21 interface. A transmission to the telex-system enables the communication with all telex participants in the world.

Within ISDN the telex service was developped and increased by 30 times for a speed of 64 kbit/s.

In our hospital teletex is basically used within the central purchasing department for ordering via telextex and telex. In the medical sector there are actually data settlements only with foreign patients. In the future one may consider the dispatch of medical correspondence between remote clinics. Within the hospital the use of teletex is actually verified for a rapid transport of X-ray treatment results.

Telefax

These units enable the transmission of maximum DIN A4-sized documents and even handwritten documents at a resolution of up to 200 × 200 screen elements/inch. The transmission period via the phone network takes approximately one minute, acc. to the number of details and the transmission speed.

The ISDN the resolution will be increased up to 400 × 400 screen elements/inch. The transmission minutes correspond to those of the teletex service and the period for 1 DIN A4-page takes only approximately five seconds. Here we can see the possible savings for postage and telephone expenses. Information of a DIN A4-page may certainly not be transmitted to a phone partner within 5 and/60 seconds. When analysing the phone calls with regard to their contents one can see that more than 60% of all official calls include a one page information transmission. In this case the telefax gives place to the introduction of rationalisation.

In the St Josefs-Hospital the telefax system is used by the central purchasing department for ordering, by the technical department for the transmission of drawings, orders and quick information and by the medical service for the transmission of urgent results from other clinics.

Viewdata Systems

Viewdata Systems is a dialogue-guided calling system for information and the transmission of information for private and official use. The access takes place actually by a Modem and the postal phone network at a speed of 1,200/75 bit/s.

In ISDN the use of BTX is extended by a multiplicity of performance data and moreover to speeds of 64 kbit/s, ie by 50 times.

This will certainly influence positively the acceptance of the viewdata system.

In the St Josefs-Hospital the BTX is actually used at the information desk as information system, in the pharmacy (pharmaceutical information) and in the administration (keeping of drawing accounts).

Certainly the ISDN will be used for other purposes.

Data Communication

Data Communication is actually a non standardised service without uniform minutes, working at speeds in the system of up to 4,8 kbit/s and up to 9,6 kbit/s in the Datex-L-Network.

In ISDN standardisation takes place under consideration of ISO and CCITT. The increased maximum transmission speed of 64 kbit/s in the ISDN-network will enable a development with regard to a user-friendly and cost-saving use of data transmission.

In the hospital a simultanous data transfer is possible via the same line, via V24 interfaces for switching the data terminals and the PC into operation. However, one should not forget that in case of increased data numbers speeds of 2-10 Mbit/s may be executed during the transport via coaxial cables. In this case a transport via ISDN would hinder the system operation. When projecting the ISDN extension units one should therefore always consider the actual and future planning of the central data processing units.

Transmission of Moving Pictures

Transmission of Moving Pictures will be offered by the postal services as the most important event of ISDN. Besides a comfortable use for private purposes, there is actually a multiplicity of utilisation possibilities in professions. For the hospital we can already find test units in the surgery, transmitting for example surgery treatment to local specialists being able on the other side to contact the surgeon via the phone line. However, these applications seem to be very utopian, but should be discussed and used in practice in the future.

After the installation of the 'luxury services for the patients', phone and television, the future provides the installation of a picture phone at each bed side.

Or could it be a jump to the portable, wireless, worldwide useable picture phone of satellite transmission?

Financial Concept

The reasons for purchasing a new telecommunication system were clear and have been supported by all relevant departments: administration, nursing, technics, data technics and patients. However, a transformation of the demand requires considerable financial input. The financial situation of the public authorities did not allow much hope for a short-term provision of finance. Moreover, they couldn't find a sponsor, so that an exact verification of costs and possible reimbursements by means of installation fees must be performed.

When looking for hospitals of the same size, with a phone connection for each patient at each bed side, many problems could be faced. The best basis for the elaboration of a financial plan would have certainly been a similar experience project. Due to the fact that such a project could not yet be found, a multiplicity of individual data from similar objects could be collected, analysed and taken as a basis for calculation.

How Many Phone Leasing Days?

They have been the basis for the following calculation data of St Josefs-Hospital.

When starting from a projected bed number of 460, one phone unit can be placed at permanent disposal at each bed side. For an average reservation of 83.5%, we get the maximum number of 140,160 phone leasing days. The average value for the load of the phone system resulting from the data established, takes approximately 80%. Due to the fact that these are not values from a full-time phone service, we started from a possible load of 60%. There we get realistic results with 230 connections × 365 days =

SOLL		IST
	PATIENT	
460	Bettenzahl	460
83,5%	Belegung in Jahr	83,5%
60%	Telefonauslastung	61,2%
230	Vermietete Anschlüsse	235
365	Anzahl Miettage	365
83.950	Miettage pro Jahr	85.775
5	Einheiten je Miettag	4,6
419.750	Einheiten pro Jahr	394.565
83.950,–	Einnahmen Grundgebühr	85.775,–
54,567,50	Einnahmen Einheiten (0,40 - 0,27 DM)	51.293,45
138.517,50	Summe Einnahmen	137.068,45
	PERSONAL	
160	Wohneinheiten	160
60%	Belegungsdurchschnitt	78,8%
12	Mietmonate	12
20,-	Monatsgrundgebühr	20,-
52	Einheiten je Mietmonat	112
23.040,–	Einnahmen Grundgebühr	30.240,–
1.797,12	Einnahmen Einheiten (0,30 - 0,27 DM)	5.080,32
24.837,12	Summe Einnahmen	35.320,32

Table 1

83,950 leasing days and/or at a basic daily fee for use of f.ex.DM 1 – per day, resulting in 83.950 DM/year.

How Many Units

Much more difficult than the preliminary calculation of the telephone leasing days was the determination of the average fee units per day, patient or phone connection per year. When summarising the as-is values of other systems, we could see important differences. Those differences had multiple reasons like dialling practices of the patient, age structures, local situation of the hospital, the basic day fees as well as the fees for units and the limit of the eight-minutes' sequence. Certainly a scientific analysis of these reasons would have been very interesting. For our calculation we decided to take the experienced value of five units per leasing day of a comparable hospital with the same number of beds and the same fee for the units. After the multiplication with the calculated 83,950 phone leasing days, we got a global fee amount of 419,750 units per year. For fees of 0.40 DM/unit and after the deduction of approximately 0.27 DM/unit as effective postal expenses, we got proceeds of 54,567.50 DM/year.

Telephone within the Apartments

Not only the patients but also resident staff are asking for a personal telephone extension from the exchange. The facility of an extension from the exchange is advantageous for all involved. In-house official and private calls can be made cost-free. The application for and the countermand of main connection becomes superfluous. There are no application fees for employees. The basic expenses per month and the fees per unit may be settled variably. For the 160 apartments in our house we suggested a load of 60% of the existing phone lines, as well as an average unit consumption of 52 per leasing month. For a basic monthly fee of DM 20 – and unit expenses of 0.30 DM we got proceeds from the basic expenses and the units of DM 24,837.12 per year.

These costs are mainly required for the purchasing, installation and maintenance of the additional extension apparatus.

Financial Frame

The determination of the individual values are executed very carefully, in order to objectively estimate the possibility of making spare acquisitions and the realisation of control of the performed calculations. Therefore the execution of projects could base upon globally 163,354.62 DM.

Financial Control

After the implementation of the global unit a monthly control of the relevant data took place on the fee computer. The result of the control of all values after nearly two year's operation period could confirm basically the theoretical preliminary calculations. Larger differences between the set and the as-is values could only be determined for the apartments of the employees. A comparison of these values is indicated in Table 1. The load of the apartment connections takes on the average 78% as against the estimated value of 60%. The fees exceed the expected 60.000 units by the triple value. This results from an increased load of the leasable connections on the one hand and an increased unit consumption than expected on the other hand. The estimated units of 52 per connection per month are surpassed by the effective 112 unit per connection per month, ie by more than 100%. Globally the effective results surpass the estimated values by approximately 6,5%.

The confirmation of the estimated proceeds and the comparison of the a.m. set and as-is values shows clearly the certainty by which the estimated values for the average load of the phone connections may be determined. The amount of the proceeds obliges, however, to reflect on another point of investment. The investment costs for the patients' phones in the compass of actual technics must be settled at 900. – DM/connection. On the other side we get average proceeds per patient connection from my example of approximately 298. – DM/year. However we should subtract the amount of approximately DM 85. – for current costs in the compass of the yearly maintenance and renovation work.

Rentability

Based on net proceeds of 213. – DM/year per connection, the investment costs of 900. – DM/connection with interest on the invested capital of 7% result in a depreciation period of 4.4 years.

Cost Damping by Communication Technics

A phone system for the patient is absolutely required for communication with the outside and may be considered as a certain type of therapy. However, such a comfort at the bedside is not absolutely necessary for the direct recovery or regeneration process during the patient's stay in the hospital. For this reason we should discuss whether financing of such type of services by the public authorities can be justified. This problem is underlined by the performed rentability calculations, as the auto-financing of these services for a depreciation period under five years can be realised. Shouldn't public means be taken for the urgent financing of new diagnostical, therapeutical and the related constructional equipment as well as for space acquisitions within these sectors? Here we can see a contribution to cost-damping for health care.

Future Aspects

The ISDN-phone on the bedside with language, text, picture and data will certainly no longer be a science fiction in future. However, we shouldn't forget the auto-financing of such luxury services as a basic condition.

ST. JOSEFS - HOSPITAL WIESBADEN
COMMUNICATIONSYSTEM HICOM 3W 3000

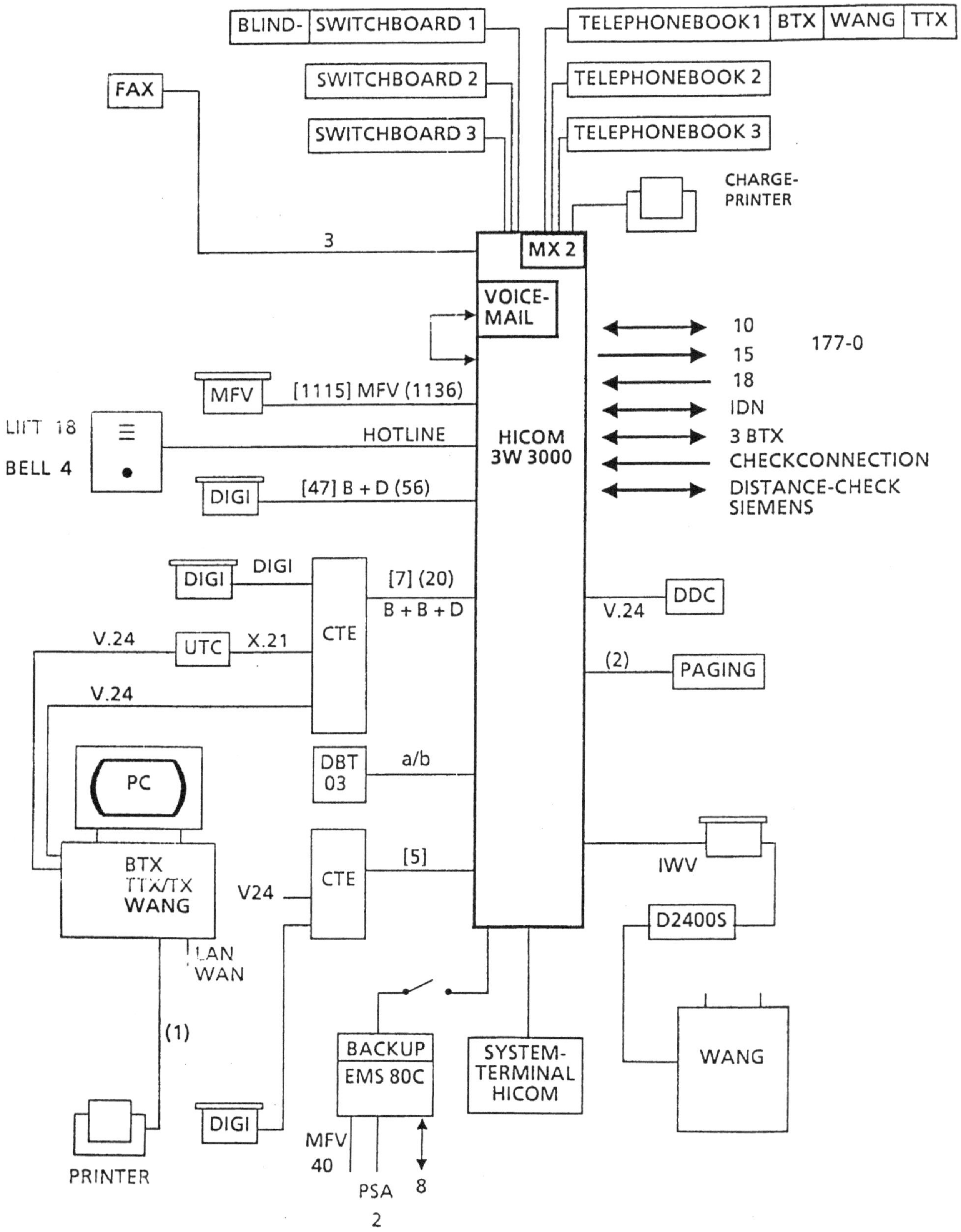

The Use of Communication Systems in Planning Hospitals — The Example of Bologna

by
A. Lena
Chief Engineer of Technical Service
St Orsola University Hospital
Bologna (Italy)

C. Pipoli
Engineer Architect Planner
Bologna (Italy)

The evolution of the individual habits, the change in social needs, the age of the population, the spread of some pathologies or the change in the causes of mortality, and finally the swift, technological process are gradually modifying health needs.

Therefore it's necessary to have continuous planning in order to adapt the old structures to the new needs, while it's necessary for suitable design to realise new flexible structures that can be modified easily.

- Some restrictions and difficulties often exist so that these two requirements can't be realised.
- For instance it isn't always possible to modify the territorial sites of the existing health buildings, or to build new buildings freely because of the restrictions imposed by neighbouring buildings.
- All this happens to a lot of Italian Hospitals especially in the big hospitals in the biggest cities which have ancient origins and famous traditions.
- In spite of this, their restructure is often indispensable in order to adjust them to new health needs. Modern medical equipment to realise these purposes, is often necessary with all the available means of the newest and most advanced technology.
- Where it isn't possible to modify the hospitals, planning and the design can help by using modern means of communication, transport and the exchange of information.
- The use of electronic systems in the communications, the automation of some plant and equipment, and the telecasting of health diagnoses allow a lot of progress and updating.
- We are going to show some examples of what we said above as evidence of the advances achieved in some of the biggest Italian Hospitals.

One example we believe to be one of the most significant is represented by the Bologna Hospitals complex.

Bologna is a city of about 500 thousand inhabitants, capital of Emilia — Romagna Region, with about 10 million people.

She had one of the oldest Universities in Europe for 900 years, in which the Medicine faculty has famous traditions.

For these reasons the Bologna Hospitals group has a large number of specialisations and receives many patients from all Italian regions.

The main three located in different sites in the territory are:-

- in the NW: the 'Ospedale Maggiore' containing about 1,200 beds;
- in the Centre the 'Ospedale St Orsola' containing about 2,500 beds; and
- in the SE: the 'Ospedale Bellaria' of 800 beds.

That represents a total of 4,500 beds.

Most of them are dedicated to specialities dept by the University clinics.

In the next 10 years, they plan to modernise the existing health structures with a budget of 400 to 500 billions Italian lires.

Besides the 'Ospedale Maggiore', which is a monobloc one, the two others are pavilion hospitals and, due to their dimensions, communication and transport aspects assume a great importance.

For this last reason we will concentrate our attention to these systems giving some examples.

1. Centralised Booking of the Medical Services

(That we called CUP —Centro Unificato Prenotazioni)

This system is already operating in Bologna.

Actually 25 centres offer to the habitants the possibility of booking their medical needs such as: laboratory visits, specialities, etc in any place in the city and at least close to their home.

Besides this 100 family doctors will receive the hardware in order for them to book directly from their surgeries.

In the near future every doctor will have that possiblity.

The computerised heart of this system is located in a bunker within the St Orsola Hospital area and gives much useful information for all departments.

2. Optical Fiber Networking

The three hospitals will talk to each other using a complete optical fiber network.

Besides general information, the network will transport diagnostic images and results in real time.

As for CUP, this technology will permit the statistical use of information in order to improve departments.

Their treatment will be realised in the same computer centre connected to other sections.

3. Physical Automatic Transport

This problem is being tackled by using transportation robots permitting the horizontal (underground tunnels) and vertical (lifts) conveyance of most products used daily.

4. Centralised Nurse Call System

Here again centralising a system which to day is used only in small departments, in order to optimise their functions.

We could examine other aspects but we believe that developing the above mentioned is already a challenge.

As a conclusion, besides the facilities given to users, these technologies in communication systems will permit the optimisation and the improvement of managerial and financial performance.

UTILISATION DES SYSTEMES DE COMMUNICATIONS DANS LA PLANIFICATION DES HOPITAUX L'EXEMPLE DE BOLOGNE

L'évolution des habitudes individuelles, les changements de besoins sociaux, le vieillissement de la population, le développement de certaines pathologies, le changement dans les causes de mortalité ont tous une incidence sur les besoins en services de santé, sans oublier les rapides progrès de la technologie.

Il est donc nécessaire d'avoir recours à une planification continue afin d'adapter les anciennes structures aux besoins nouveaux, mais il est aussi nécessaire de prévoir de nouvelles structures flexibles, qui elles aussi, pourront s'adapter.

Cet article présente les facteurs dont il faut tenir compte dans ces processus, et examinent le rôle important des systèmes de communications dans la modernisation des hôpitaux, dont Bologne représente un exemple.

The Application of Modern Nurse Call Systems to Flexible Nursing

by

W. T. Colman
Ms, BSc, CEng, MIEE,
Managing Director, Static Systems Group plc
United Kingdom

Introduction

This paper traces the historic development of nurse call communications from the early direct wired systems through the still widely used low speed multiplexed equipment to the new concept of high speed multiplexing.

Good communications in hospitals undoubtedly increase efficiency and saves money. The rapid progress now being made to offer a much extended service with simplified wiring and at a reduced cost will be explained.

The versatility of this new generation of equipment is illustrated by using the example of flexible nursing. This allows the nurse call and monitoring system of individual beds to be transferred to adjacent wards enabling the size of wards to be adjusted to suit patient demand.

Traditional Systems

In the early days, hospital wards tended to be open plan or Nightingale style with rows of patients all within view of the staff. Electrical nurse call was limited to lights and buzzers. No speech or entertainment facilities were provided. The wiring for such a system was simple.

As wards became smaller communication became more difficult and speech systems were introduced. Most of these also require a nurse presence facility to enable the location of the nurse to be determined. The wiring of the nurse call becomes much more complex with eight to ten cores required as well as screened cables for the speech signals.

Radio entertainment has traditionally been provided by typically six tuners feeding separate power amplifiers. The output of these are distributed round the hospital on 100V lines. A pair of bulky wires are required for each channel. At the entrance to each ward a step down transformer for each channel is needed to reduce the voltage to an acceptable level before on going transmission to every bed. This system is illustrated in Figure 1.

This system suffers from numerous technical problems. It will require 200W of audio power for each channel for a 300 bed hospital. Cross talk between channels is always present. A fault at any bed will cause degradation of performance at every bed in the hospital. If, for example, channel 2 is shorted to channel 4 at one bed anyone in the hospital listening to one of these channels will hear the other signal superimposed.

System Improvements

To reduce the number of wires between bed units slow speed multiplexing was introduced about 15 years ago in Europe and is still considered state of the art by many manufacturers and it is widely used. This technique allows many of the nurse call signals to be carried down a single pair of wires. This reduces the nurse call wiring considerably but it is too slow to handle the bandwidth needed for speech or the entertainment distribution.

The first example of the use of modern computer signalling techniques was introduced in 1984 in the design of hand units inspired by a British Department of Health study group. This is the unit used by the patient to call the nurse, switch the lights and control the entertainment. Traditionally to control all these features the patient either had to stretch to a locker controller, or an overhead cantilever unit or have a hand unit with a thick stiff multicore cable.

By the use of a microprocessor in the hand unit and another one in the wall unit behind the bed the cable can be reduced to a thin, flexible data cable which is terminated by a simple plug which will snatch easily from the wall if it is pulled. Since their introduction these units have been improved considerably. The new models can be dip sterilised and can withstand the very high static electric build up experienced when man-made fibres are used for bed linen in dry conditions.

Figure 2 shows an example of the latest design which is waterproof to IP 67 for sterilisation purposes. It can also withstand a 70,000V static charge.

This was ergonomically designed for ease of use. The purpose of each feature is self explanatory. The nurse call push is back illuminated for location at night.

High Speed Multiplexing

To reduce the bulk of the wiring between each bed unit in the carcass of the building an entirely new approach was required. The existing slow speed multiplexing system could not cope with either the speech or the entertainment distribution.

In 1986 we introduced the first high speed multiplexing digital entertainment distribution system. We called this CODEM standing for 'Compact Digital Entertainment Multiplexer'.

This consists of a small central unit which can be easily accommodated on a shelf in the reception area. It contains up to 15 signal sources such as tuners and microphone amplifiers, the outputs of which are fed into a digital encoder. This combines all the signals and launches them as a digital stream into the hospital down a slim four core data cable. This is illustrated on Figure 3.

By using advanced techniques a single module can include either four FM tuners or two AM tuners.

Extra channels are inexpensive with CODEM, so in a multi bed ward where loudspeakers cannot be used, a convenient

APPLICATIONS DES NOUVEAUX SYSTEMS DE COMMUNICATIONS AVEC LE PERSONNEL INFIRMIER EN SITUATION FLEXIBLE

Cet article rappelle le développement des systèmes de communications avec le personnel infirmier, depuis la liaison délégraphique directe, en passant par le système toujours très répandu des équipements multiplex 'lents', jusqu'à celui des nouveaux multiplex grande vitesse.

Un bon système de communications en milieu hospitalier augmente l'efficacité des services et économise de l'argent. Des progrès rapides viennent de s'acomplir dans ce domaine, permettant d'augmenter le réseau de services ainsi que de simplifier le système et de réaliser des économies.

Afin de démontrer la capacité d'adaptation de cette nouvelle génération de matériel, nous allons utiliser l'exemple des personnels travaillant en situations flexibles. Le système permet aux appels d'infirmière et aux contrôles de malades fonctionnant à partir de lits individuels de se transférer á un service voisin. De ce fait, la taille des services peut s'adapter aux besoins des malades particuliers à un moment donné.

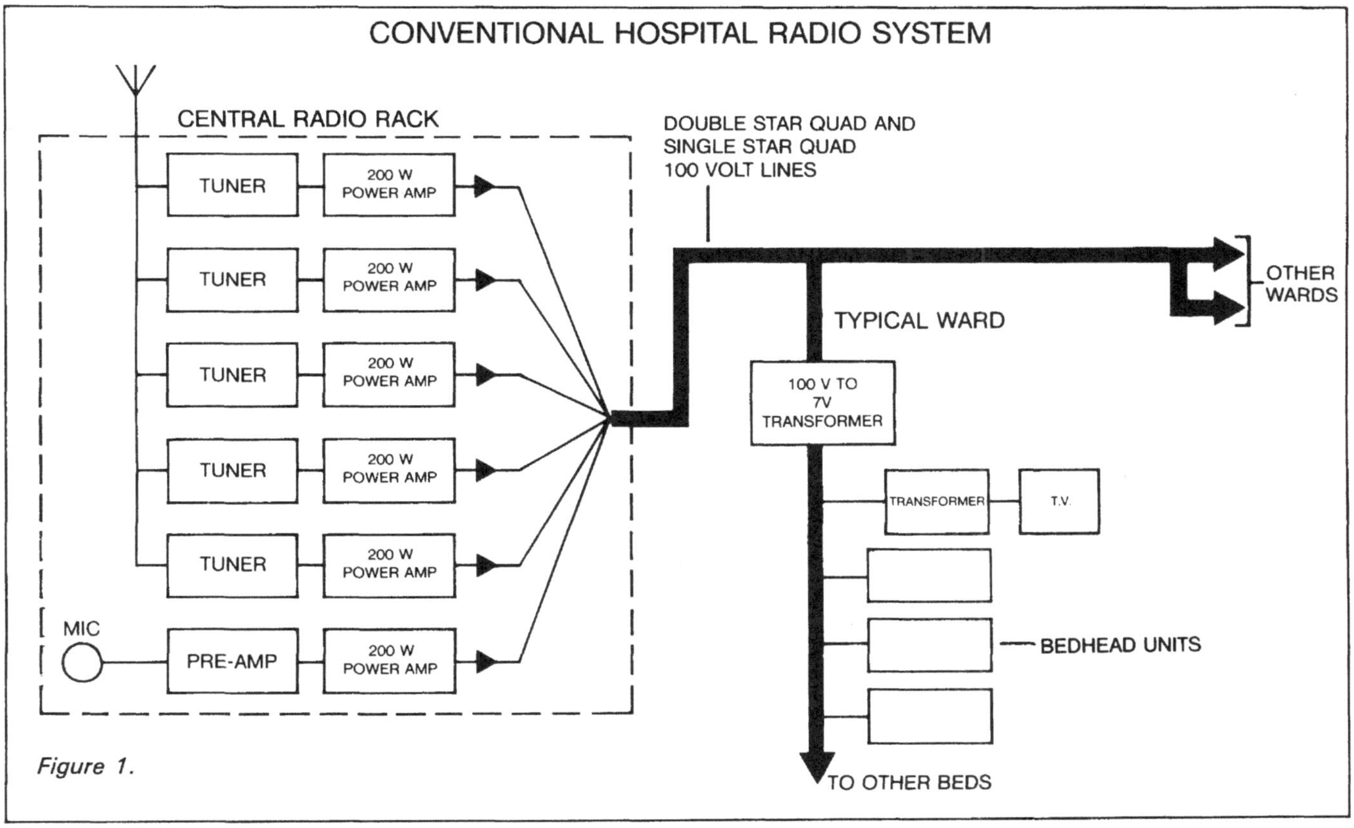

Figure 1.

and economical way of providing television sound is by distributing all the sound channels on the system. This also avoids the need to modify the individual television sets to feed their sound signal to the correct head sets within each ward.

At the entry to each ward area an isolator is fitted which ensures that any wiring faults within that ward area do not reflect back and cause degradation in other parts of the hospital. The digital signals have to be decoded back to analogue signals at each bed unit, where the channel selection and the volume control is via the patients handset.

A loudspeaker unit can be fitted for use in single bed rooms and day rooms.

If a run of data cable exceeds more than 300m a simple repeater is installed to maintain the integrity of the signal.

This system has many advantages:-

(1) The central unit is compact and uses little power.
(2) The data cable is thin and cheap so small conduits can be used.
(3) The sound quality is enhanced with no degradation from partial wiring faults.
(4) Up to 15 channels can be distributed on a single data cable.
(5) There is no limit to the number of beds that can be fed from one central unit.

The CODEM equipment described so far is limited to the distribution of entertainment and public address only. It can only communicate in one direction radially out from the central unit to every bed.

Full Communication Integration

Having installed at fast data link to every bed it is a relatively small step to make the system bi-directional, so that it can also communicate back from the bed to a ward station or a central console. This opens up a whole new set of opportunities.

The design specification for CODEM was carefully drawn up to reserve several spare channels. These can now be used to carry signals back from the bed.

The industry is now starting to refer to this development as CODEM II.

To do this using high speed multiplexing involves the use of more complex bed head unit electronics. A compact solution is only possible by employing the latest surface mount technology where minute circuit components are placed on the top surface of a printed circuit board by robotic machines.

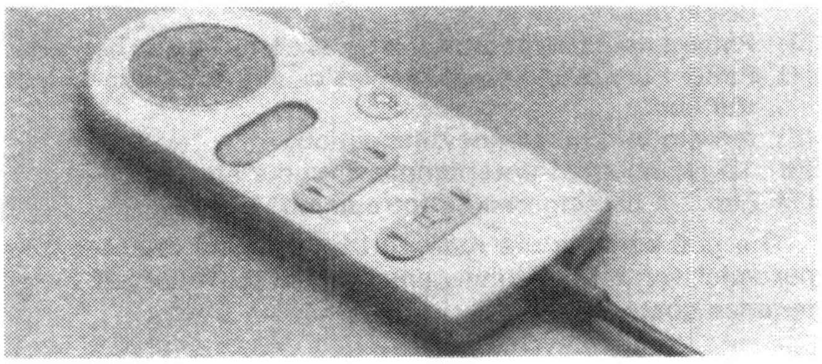

Figure 2.

The enormous advantage is that all nurse call, speech and all entertainment channels are carried on a slim four core data cable.

The only wires now required to feed each bed unit are the four core data cable and a 24V supply. This compares with a typical direct wired system of:-

2	Power supply lines
10	Nurse call control wires
2	Core screened cable for duplex speech
12	Core twisted pairs for 6 channel entertainment
26	

In practice each cable is looped in and out of each bed unit making the total number of connections to be made 52.

It is difficult to compare the cost of CODEM II with the traditional approach because it depends on the facilities required and the hospital layout but in general the extra bed electronics cost is more than offset by the saving of cable and conduit.

Control wiring is one of the greatest maintenance costs the hospital engineer faces. It is now proven that it is well worth increasing circuit complexity to reduce interconnecting wiring. Professionally designed modern circuits are now so reliable little trouble is experienced and as they are all

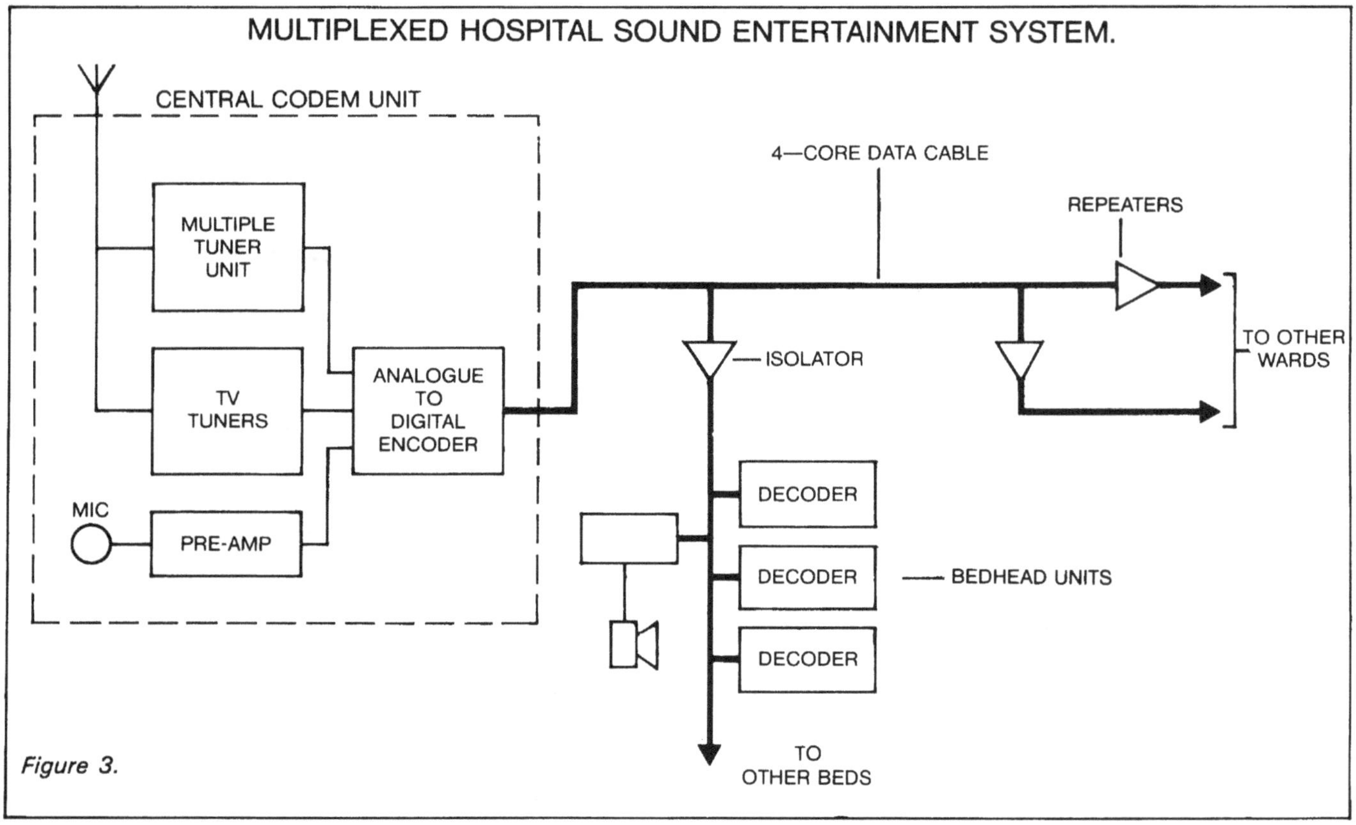

Figure 3.

plug in, they can be changed easily.

Having once installed a high speed data cable to each bed position in a hospital numerous new opportunities arise. For example:-

(1) Several medical alarm signals can be scanned.
(2) continuous patient monitoring can be remotely displayed.
(3) Patient medical records can be available at the bed side.
(4) Patient drugs and consumables can be accounted for at the bed.
(5) remote bed occupancy indication.
(6) 15 channels of entertainment, some stereo.
(7) Flexible nursing can be introduced.

The real benefits are realised in the added features, the potential for future enhancement and the reduced maintenance costs.

Flexible Nursing

Traditionally hospital wards have been of fixed size and the nurse call system has been hard wired to operate in this situation. However the number of patients in a hospital at any one time will vary by sex and category. To make full use of the installed beds a means of flexing the ward boundaries is essential. At the design stage of a hospital this is relatively easy to accommodate physically.

Until this new generation of nurse call equipment became available it has only been possible to transfer the control of whole wards to another station to facilitate night nursing, for example. There was no simple way of engineering a system that would give sufficient flexibility to enable individual bed rooms to be transferred. This limitation is now removed.

Figure 4 shows the plan view of a tower block with four wards on each floor forming a hollow square. Under traditional management each ward has its own nurse station where all the calls from the ward are received.

A flexible nurse call system will allow authorised staff to transfer individual bedrooms within a ward to either of the two adjacent wards. This is achieved by selection in the local ward. When this happens a 'transferred out' light is illuminated at the local nurse station and a 'transferred in' light is illuminated at the adjacent ward nurse station. Any

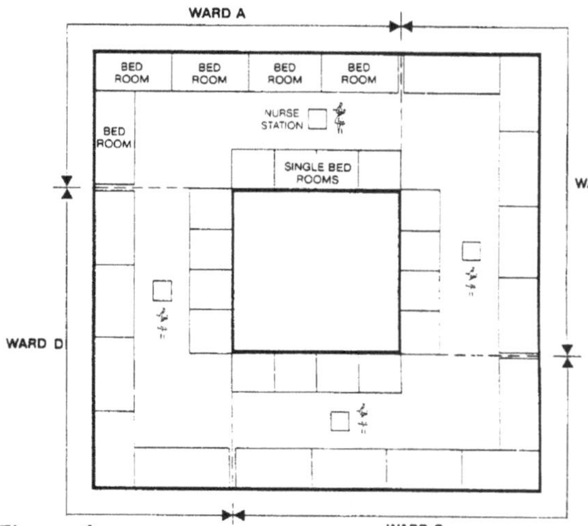

Figure 4.

calls now made from that bedroom will be received at the adjacent nurse station.

Referring to the diagram it is therefore possible, for example, to transfer one or up to all the bedrooms in ward 'A' to ward 'B' or 'D'.

Thus, an adjustable boundary between each ward is achieved.

Future Trends

Numerous new applications will be found to exploit this technology. We think that it is unlikely that even faster data rates will be employed economically in the near future because of the constraints on cabling imposed by very quick signalling.

Summary

This paper has shown how modern digital technology is being applied to nurse call systems and how integrated bed head services can be provided using the minimum number of cables and offering the maximum facilities within a very modest cost increase.

Computerisation of Hospital Engineering

by

Donald L. Britton
Memorial Medical Centre
Springfield, Ill 62781-0001

1. Introduction of Memorial Medical Centre

Memorial Medical Centre is a not-for-profit 600 bed teaching institution. It is accredited by the Joint Commission on Accreditation of Healthcare Organisations, and a member of the Amercian Hospital Association. Memorial offers a complete range of services to the people of central and southern Illinois.

1.1 Affiliations of Memorial Medical Centre

To provide quality patient care, and an atmosphere for clinical education and research, Memorial is affiliated with:-

- Southern Illinois University School of Medicine;
- Voluntary Hospitals of America (VHA);
- Visiting Nurse Association;
- Sangamon State University;
- Lincoln Lane Community College; and
- School District 186.

1.2 Memorial's Centres of Excellence

Over 2,400 Memorial employees direct their efforts, to providing personalised patient care and to supporting the following 'Centres of Excellence':-

- Regional Oncology Centre;
- Regional Kidney Centre;
- Regional Perinatal Centre;
- Regional Burn Centre;
- Neuromuscular Science Centre;
- Heart Care Service;
- Radiology Service;
- Radiation Therapy Service;
- Emergency/Trauma Centre;
- Level 1 Rehabilitation Centre; and
- Healthline Programs.

Memorial also provides support, through Shared Service Programs, to approximately 100 surrounding hospitals and clinics.

1.3 Memorial's Engineering Department

Memorial's Engineering Department consists of 66 employees. We are responsible for:-

- Preventive and Corrective Maintenance;
- Clinical Engineering;
- Planning/Designing of In-house Remodelling;
- Construction/Redecoration of In-house Remodelling;
- Co-ordination of Exterior Construction;
- Management of Utilities;
- Grounds; and
- Installation of New Technical Equipment.

1.4 Engineering's Computer System

In 1985, with the support of senior management and Information Systems, our Engineering Department began to computerise its activities. Our current computer system consists of stand-alone and network of personal computers. Using various software packages, we developed a system that is flexible and expandable.

In this presentation, we will discuss three of our software packages:-

- Asset Information Management System (AIMS);
- Computer Aided Design and Drafting (CADD); and
- Project Construction Cost Control.

2. Asset Information Management System

AIMS software enables us to track all important information on our equipment such as:-

- original cost;
- life expectancy;
- maintenance history information such as:-
  - PM and CM hours/cost;
  - employee name/number; and
  - material/parts used;
- inventory information.

2.1 What is AIMS?

AIMS is an exclusive series of computer programs, designed and developed by a group of hospital engineers and software experts. It is a tool designed to manage all of a hospital's physical assets, as well as the labor required to maintain them.

2.2 Our Engineering Department Uses the Following Aims Software

- Equipment Information;
- Preventive Maintenance (PM)/Corrective Maintenance Work Order Control;
- Materials Control; and
- Employee Accountability.

2.3 Equipment Information Software

Equipment information is added to our History file and is used to provide a complete inventory of our hospital's equipment.

LE ROLE DE L'ORDINATEUR DANS L'INGENIERIE HOSPITALIERE

L'auteur decrit un systeme de contrôle par ordinateur des functions des Services Techniques du Memorial Medical Centre, Springfield, Illinois, USA, flexible et capable d'expansion. Le système consiste en un nombre de programmes independents et liés permettant une suite d'operations liés.

Le programme de contrôle des équipments et des constructions, leur entietien preventif et correctif, fiches d'execution, les matières premières de l'activités du personnel. Ces programmes ont aidé le maintien par les Services Techniques d'un haut niveau de rendement, d'un contrôle effectif des équipment et des constructions de prévoir le renouveau de l'equipment, de justifier le niveau courant et dans l'avenir du personnel, de contrôle des inventaires. On espère dans l'avenir, cessurer une haute qualité de l'inspection et de l'entietien des équipments.

Les programmes de dessin et de préparation de devis servent à la prèparation de dessins exacts, proffessionels, ainsi que des graphiques et autres présentations techniques, ils ont permis le temps de préparation d'un plan d'implantion de cinq à un jour et aussi une gestion plus efficace du travail. Nous avons l'intention d'incorporer d'employer ce système pour tous les plans de nos batiments.

En ce qui concerne nôtre propres personnel technique, un programme de contrôle des dépenses sert à fournir au service des comptes le détail des dépenses sert a fournir au service des comptes le détail des dépenses pour chaque project.

C'est l'avis de l'auteur que l'emploi de ces systèmes a permis aux service Techniques d'accomplir leur tâches j'une facon exemplaire, à bon prix.

In 1988, using our equipment software we tracked 5,500 pieces of equipment.

2.4 PM and CM Software

We use our PM and CM software to automatically schedule and track our maintenance as required by regulatory agencies. It provides:-

- automatic printed work orders;
- procedure to be performed; and
- predetermined time to complete procedure.

Once our maintenance is completed, the PM or CM information is added to our system. This will provide a permanent record for our Clinical Engineering Department, Regulatory Agencies, and for the respective departments.

In 1988, this software tracked 11,900 PM work orders and 30,700 CM work orders.

2.5 Work Order Control Software

Our Work Order software provides a totally automated work order printing and tracking system. It also provides the following information:-

- Open Work Order Report;
- PM/CM Hours Report; and
- Charge Back Capabilities.

After a work order request is entered into the system, it will be listed on an open work order report until it is closed. A work order is closed when the completion date, material, and labor hours are entered into the system. The system now has the capability to calculate and charge back the labor and material costs to other departments.

In 1988, our work order software tracked a total of 42,600 work orders.

2.6 Materials Control Software

We use our Materials Control software to track and control materials, supplies, parts, minimum reorder level, and maximum restocking level.

This software has reduced the time and cost of counting our annual inventory by 70%.

In 1988, this software tracked and controlled an inventory of $304,000 for maintenance and construction.

2.7 Employee Accountability Software

We use our Employee Accountability software to track our productive and our non-productive hours and costs. This information is provided in the following reports:-

- Monthly Accountability Analysis; and
- Monthly Accountability Graph.

2.8 Monthly Accountability Analysis Report

(See Figure 2.8)

The Monthly Accountability Analysis Report provides detail and summary totals of productive and non-productive hours per employee and division:-

Productive Hours

(1) Preventive Maintenance;
(2) Corrective Maintenance;

MEMORIAL MEDICAL CENTER
AIMS - ACCOUNTIBILITY ANALYSIS
FOR PERIOD: 06/01/89 - 06/30/89
FOR SERVICE RANGE: 40 - 40
FOR SERVICE CENTER: 40 - PLUMBING DIVISION
FTE HOURS AVAILABLE: 874

PAGE 1
PROGRAM A10510
RUN DATE 07/07/89

EMPLOYEE CODE & NAME	PRODUCTIVE HOURS PM	CM	OTH	OVT	PROJ	TOT PROD	NON-PRODUCTIVE HOURS VAC	HOL	SICK	TN	TOT NON	TOT HRS
401	0.50	54.00	51.70	3.25	30.00	139.45	8.00	8.00	16.00	0.00	32.00	171.45
402	24.00	59.20	2.80	4.50	69.75	160.25	0.00	8.00	8.00	0.00	16.00	176.25
403	3.80	35.50	0.50	0.00	50.25	90.05	80.00	0.00	0.00	0.00	80.00	170.05
404	16.80	61.30	1.50	15.00	63.00	157.60	16.00	4.00	8.00	0.00	28.00	185.60
405	11.50	23.00	3.80	8.25	78.75	125.30	48.00	0.00	0.00	0.00	48.00	173.30
PLUMBING DIV.	56.60	233.10	60.30	31.00	291.75	672.65	152.00	20.00	32.00	0.00	204.00	876.65
	①	②	③	④	⑤	⑥	⑧	⑨	⑩	⑪	⑫	⑭
ACCOUNTIBILITY						77% ⑦					23% ⑬	100%

Figure 2.8.

(3) Other (travel, phone etc);
(4) Overtime;
(5) Project Construction;
(6) Total Productive;
(7) Percentage of Productive;

Non-Productive Hours

(8) Vacation;
(9) Holiday;
(10) Sicktime;
(11) Training;
(12) Total Non-productive;
(13) Percentage of Non-productive; and
(14) Total Productive and Non-productive.

Our managers use this report to determine where the productive and non-productive hours were used. It is also used to justify our current and future staffing needs.

2.9 Monthly Accountability Graph

(See Figure 2.9).

The Monthly Accountability Graph is used to identify the percentage of productive and non-productive hours for each division. It also provides us with a department average.

A manager may use this graph as a quick and easy reference to spot any changes that affected a division.

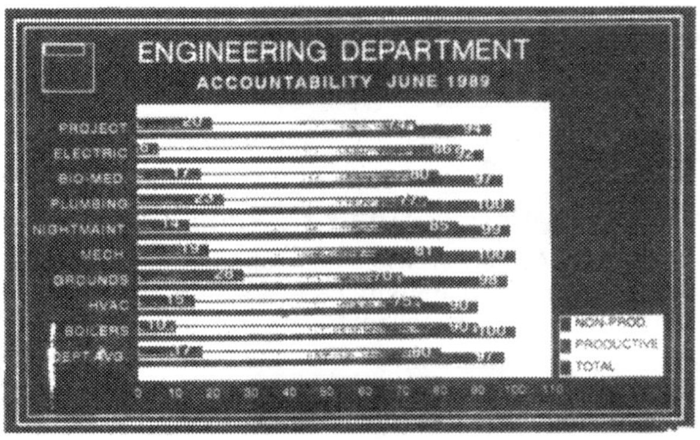

Figure 2.9.

This concludes the presentation on our AIMS Software. Now, let's discuss the CADD System.

3. Computer Aided Design and Drafting (CADD)

We use the CADD system as a high speed, high quality, drafting tool to provide architectural drawings, organisational charts, and graphic presentations. In this presentation we will discuss three different types of drawings:-

- Architectural Drawing;
- Capital Budget Workflow; and
- Scope of Projects.

Lets look at an actual architectural drawing from our CADD System.

3.1 Architectural Drawing

(See Figure 3.1).

An architectural drawing will allow the Requesting and the Engineering Departments to plan, develop and organise a project, to ensure that all necessary elements are included such as:-

- architectural changes;
- mechanical requirements;
- electrical requirements;
- type of finished materials (wallpaper, paint, carpet tile, etc);
- cabinetry; and
- any special communication systems.

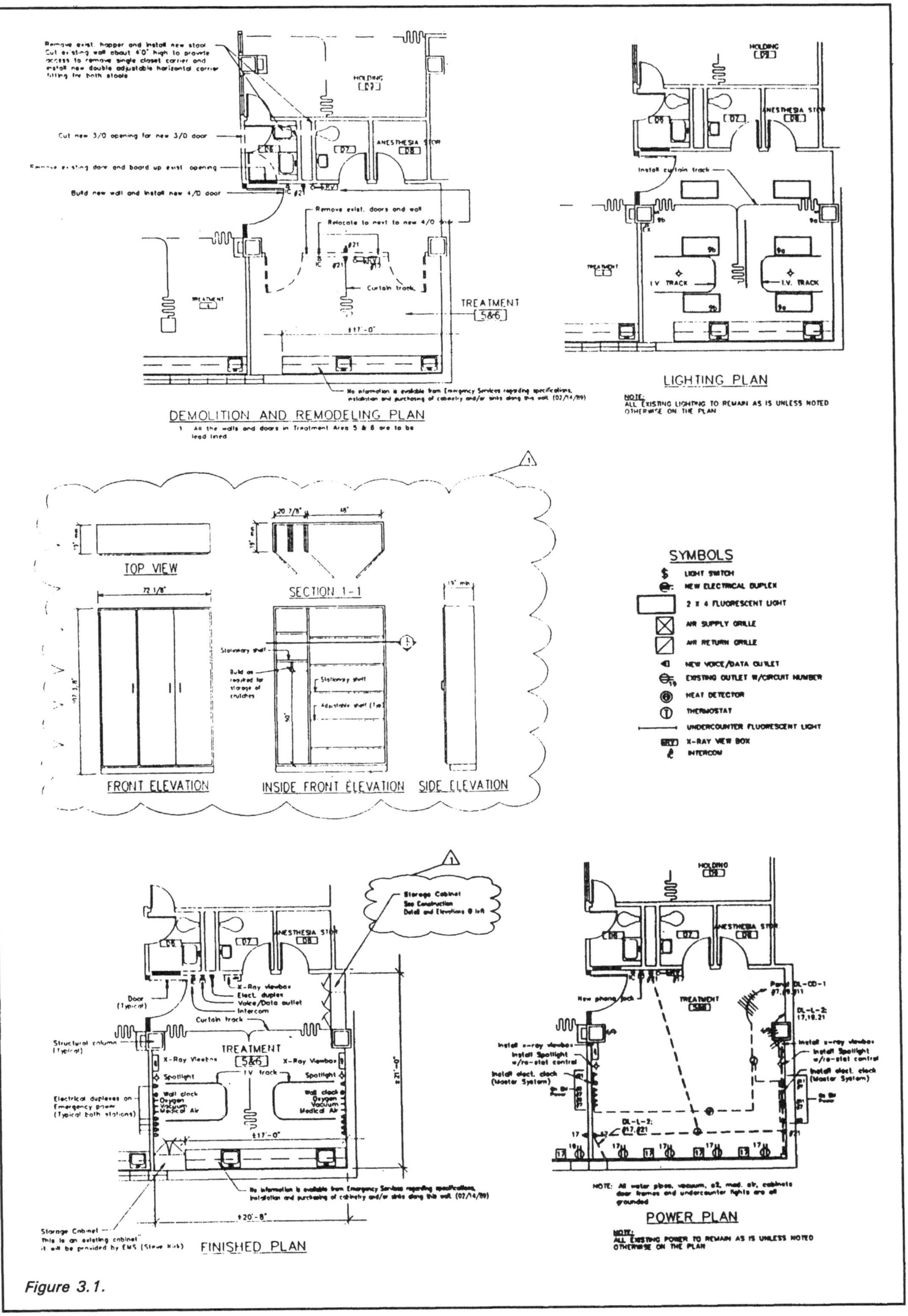
DEMOLITION AND REMODELING PLAN
LIGHTING PLAN
TOP VIEW
SECTION 1-1
FRONT ELEVATION
INSIDE FRONT ELEVATION
SIDE ELEVATION
SYMBOLS
LIGHT SWITCH
NEW ELECTRICAL DUPLEX
2 X 4 FLUORESCENT LIGHT
AIR SUPPLY GRILLE
AIR RETURN GRILLE
NEW VOICE/DATA OUTLET
EXISTING OUTLET W/CIRCUIT NUMBER
HEAT DETECTOR
THERMOSTAT
UNDERCOUNTER FLUORESCENT LIGHT
X-RAY VIEW BOX
INTERCOM
FINISHED PLAN
POWER PLAN
TREATMENT
HOLDING
ANESTHESIA STOR

Figure 3.1.

3.2 Capital Budget Workflow

(See Figure 3.2).

By the use of the CADD system, our Engineering staff developed a Capital Budget Workflow chart. This chart depicts 11 procedural steps used for budgeting new or renovation construction and installation of equipment. These steps are:-

(1) proposed construction/installation;
(2) preliminary costing;
(3) budget committee review;
(4) preliminary operations approval;
(5) feasibility study;
(6) final operations approval;
(7) planning;
(8) budget approval;
(9) preparation;
(10) implementation; and
(11) final inspection/acceptance.

Our hospital uses this procedural workflow to:-

- control financial responsibilities;
- control communications;
- ensure all code requirements are met (building, licensing, etc);
- ensure all activities are consistent with Memorial corporate objectives and goals; and
- plan, control and implement projects for least disruption of normal daily hospital activities.

The CADD system also works as a scheduling tool for our construction projects.

3.3 Scope of Projects Schedule

(See Figure 3.3).

As stated in a procedural step of the Capital Budget Workflow, the Engineering Department is required to develop a Scope of Projects Schedule for the next budget year. This schedule will include:-

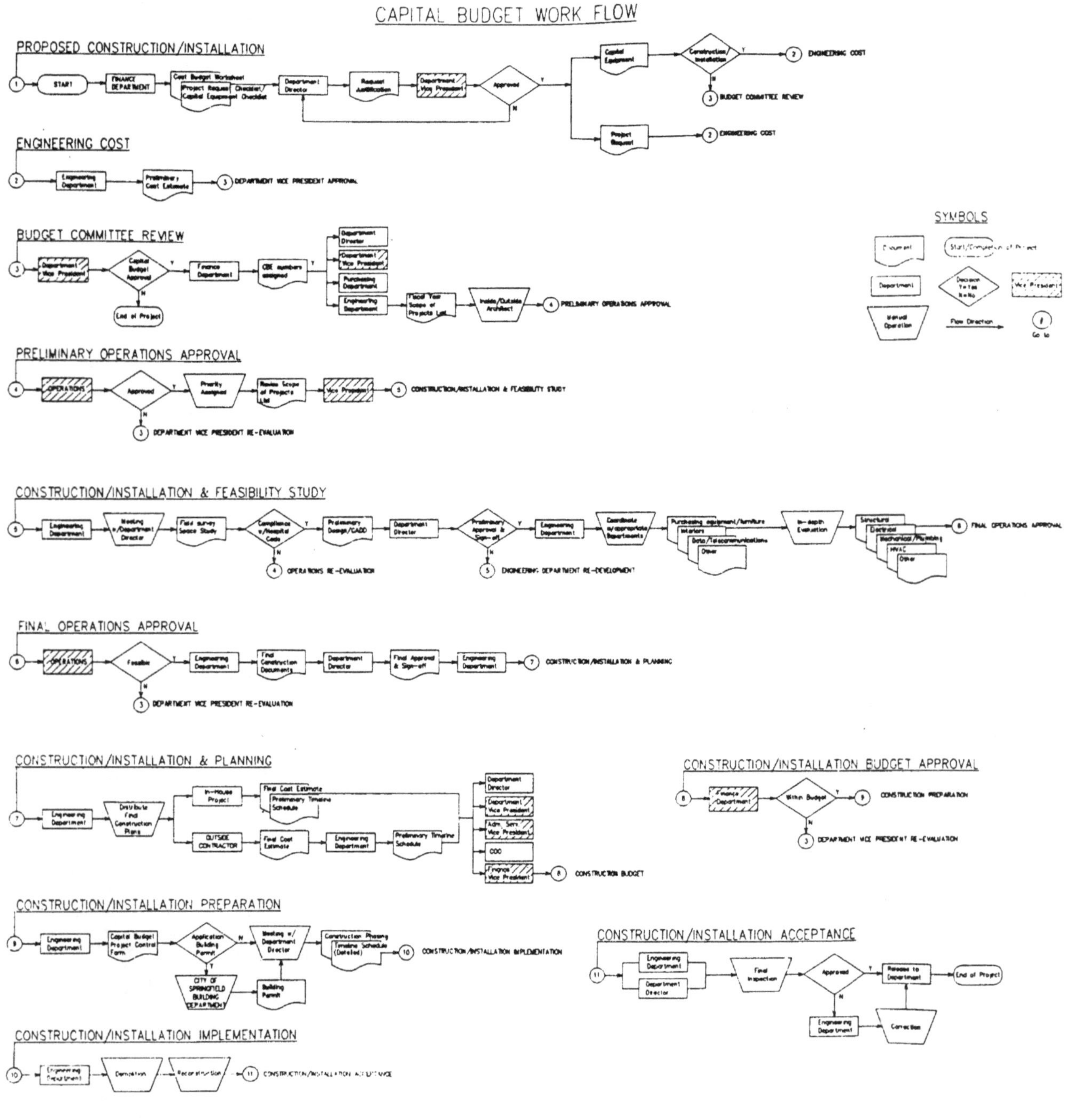

Figure 3.2.

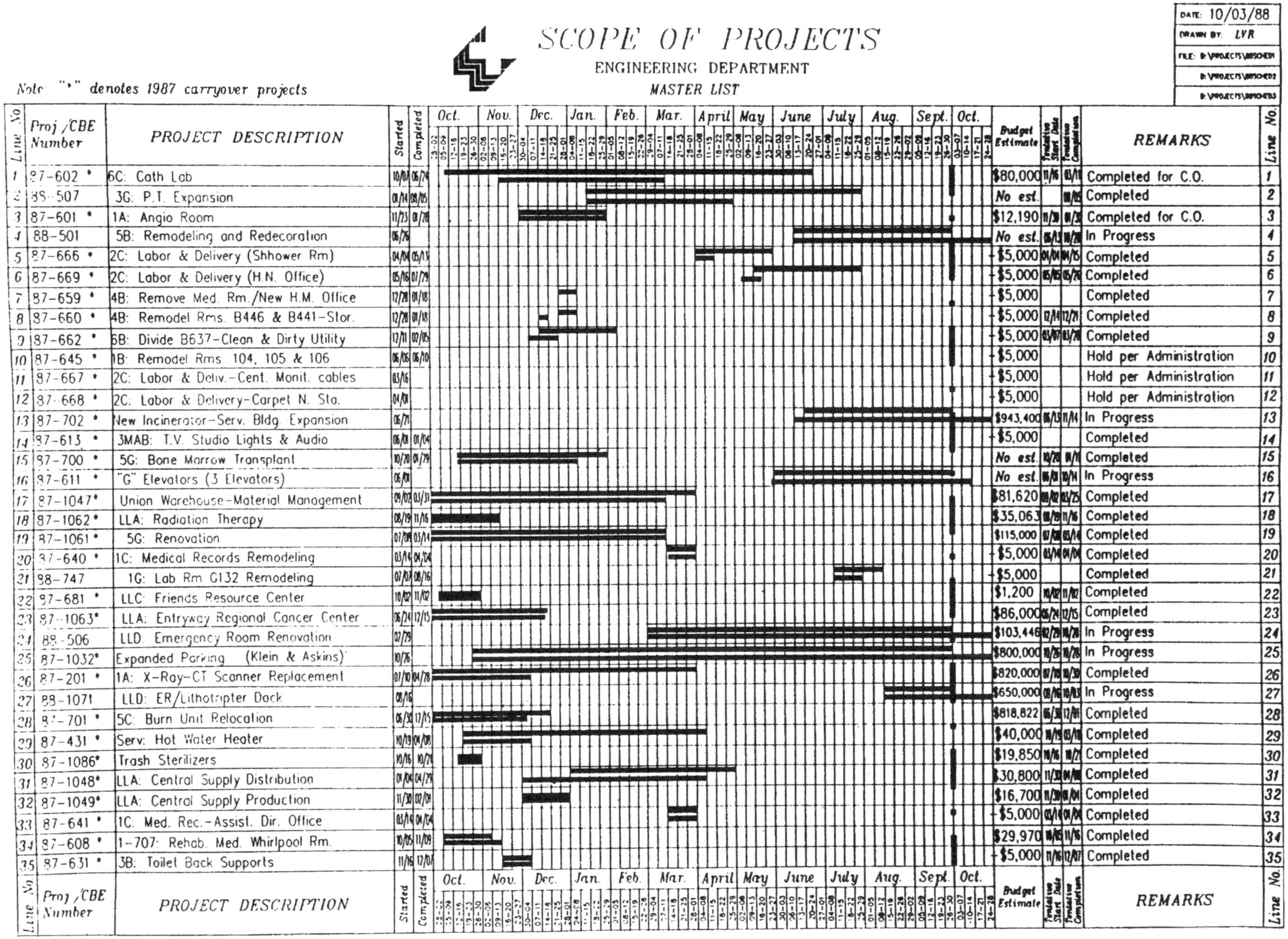
SCOPE OF PROJECTS
ENGINEERING DEPARTMENT
MASTER LIST
DATE: 10/03/88
DRAWN BY: LVR
Note "•" denotes 1987 carryover projects
Line No. | Proj/CBE Number | PROJECT DESCRIPTION | Started | Completed | Budget Estimate | REMARKS
Oct. Nov. Dec. Jan. Feb. Mar. April May June July Aug. Sept. Oct.
1 87-602 • 6C: Cath Lab $80,000 Completed for C.O.
2 88-507 3G: P.T. Expansion No est. Completed
3 87-601 • 1A: Angio Room $12,190 Completed for C.O.
4 88-501 5B: Remodeling and Redecoration No est. In Progress
5 87-666 • 2C: Labor & Delivery (Shhower Rm) $5,000 Completed
6 87-669 • 2C: Labor & Delivery (H.N. Office) $5,000 Completed
7 87-659 • 4B: Remove Med. Rm./New H.M. Office $5,000 Completed
8 87-660 • 4B: Remodel Rms. B446 & B441-Stor. $5,000 Completed
9 87-662 • 6B: Divide B637-Clean & Dirty Utility $5,000 Completed
10 87-645 • 1B: Remodel Rms. 104, 105 & 106 $5,000 Hold per Administration
11 87-667 • 2C: Labor & Deliv.-Cent. Monit. cables $5,000 Hold per Administration
12 87-668 • 2C: Labor & Delivery-Carpet N. Sta. $5,000 Hold per Administration
13 87-702 • New Incinerator-Serv. Bldg. Expansion $943,400 In Progress
14 87-613 • 3MAB: T.V. Studio Lights & Audio $5,000 Completed
15 87-700 • 5G: Bone Marrow Transplant No est. Completed
16 87-611 • "G" Elevators (3 Elevators) No est. In Progress
17 87-1047• Union Warehouse-Material Management $81,620 Completed
18 87-1062• LLA: Radiation Therapy $35,063 Completed
19 87-1061• 5G: Renovation $115,000 Completed
20 87-640 • 1C: Medical Records Remodeling $5,000 Completed
21 88-747 1G: Lab Rm G132 Remodeling $5,000 Completed
22 87-681 • LLC: Friends Resource Center $1,200 Completed
23 87-1063• LLA: Entryway Regional Cancer Center $86,000 Completed
24 88-506 LLD: Emergency Room Renovation $103,446 In Progress
25 87-1032• Expanded Parking (Klein & Askins) $800,000 In Progress
26 87-201 • 1A: X-Ray-CT Scanner Replacement $820,000 Completed
27 88-1071 LLD: ER/Lithotripter Dock $650,000 In Progress
28 87-701 • 5C: Burn Unit Relocation $818,822 Completed
29 87-431 • Serv: Hot Water Heater $40,000 Completed
30 87-1086• Trash Sterilizers $19,850 Completed
31 87-1048• LLA: Central Supply Distribution $30,800 Completed
32 87-1049• LLA: Central Supply Production $16,700 Completed
33 87-641 • 1C: Med. Rec.-Assist. Dir. Office $5,000 Completed
34 87-608 • 1-707: Rehab. Med. Whirlpool Rm. $29,970 Completed
35 87-631 • 3B: Toilet Back Supports $5,000 Completed

Figure 3.3.

- Capital Budget Equipment (CBE) Number;
- Description (name of project);
- Actual Date Started;
- Actual Date Completed;
- Graphic Bar Chart for Next Budget Year;
- Budget Estimate;
- Tentative Start Date;
- Tentative Completion Date; and
- Remarks (completed, in progress, etc).

On a monthly basis, the Engineering Department will update this schedule, as directed by Administration. This schedule will serve as communication tool between the Engineering Department, Administration, and other departments (such as when renovation or construction will begin).

In 1988, we used our CADD system to produce 700 drawings.

This concludes our presentation of our CADD' System. Now let's discuss our Project Construction Cost Control.

4. Project Construction Cost Control

We use our Lotus Software and information from our daily work orders to prepare a Project Construction Cost Report.

This is a two page report used to list a project's labour and material costs.

Project Construction Cost Report

(See Figure 4.1).

Page 1 of the Project Construction Cost Report provides the previous and monthly detail costs by division for:-

(1) Labour;
(2) Overhead;
(3) Hours;
(4) Materials;
(5) Supervision;
(6) Outside Contractors;

Page 2 provides the following cost-to-date summary information by division:-

Cost-to-Date Totals

(8) Labour;
(9) Overhead;
(10) Materials;
(11) Supervision;
(12) Change Orders;
(13) All Contractors;

MONTH END PROJECT CONSTRUCTION COST REPORT - DETAIL PAGE 1 OF 2
FOR ENDING MONTH OF AUGUST 1989

4B ORTHOPEDIC RENOVATION & DECORATION

89-400 LABOR EMP#	PREVIOUS HOURS	RUNNING LABOR CST	COST TOTAL	JUNE HOURS	JUNE LABOR CST	JUNE TOTAL	JULY HOURS	JULY LABOR CST	JULY TOTAL	AUG HOURS	AUG LABOR CST	AUG * TOTAL
PAINTER, 104	0	0.00			0.00		8.50	81.60		22.50	216.00	
PAINTER 101,06	24	294.00		19.25	235.81		13.50	165.38		9.25	113.31	
ELECT 202, 210	158.5	1,521.60		4.00	38.40		111.25	1,068.00		76.75	736.80	
ELECT 201,03,06	6.5	79.63		5.50	67.38			0.00		0.00	0.00	
PLUMB 402,03,04,05	91	1,114.75		66.75	817.69		88.50	1,084.13		104.00	1,274.00	
PLUMB 401	8	120.00		10.50	157.50		2.50	37.50		5.00	75.00	
DRAFTSPERSON 102	0	0.00		2.00	19.20			0.00			0.00	
HVAC 802,03,05,06	17.75	170.40		1.50	14.40		11.00	105.60			0.00	
HVAC 801	0	0.00			0.00			0.00			0.00	
CLIN ENG 302,03,08	5.5	52.80			0.00		4.50	43.20			0.00	
CLIN ENG 301,06,07	15.75	192.94		6.00	73.50			0.00		4.00	49.00	
PLASTERER 107	46	563.50		30.00	367.50		64.00	784.00		32.00	392.00	
LABORERS 806,123	0	0.00		5.50	35.75		15.50	100.75		7.50	48.75	
CARPT 120,607	24.75	237.60		28.00	268.80		78.75	756.00		22.75	218.40	
CARPT 112,130	239.75	2,936.94		124.50	1,525.13		71.50	875.88		75.00	918.75	
CARPT 110,11,13	227	3,405.00		114.50	1,717.50		101.50	1,522.50		82.50	1,237.50	
CAB CARPT 114	206.5	2,529.63		91.75	1,123.94		36.00	441.00		32.25	395.06	
CAB CARPT 109	5.5	82.50		28.75	431.25		18.50	277.50		20.50	307.50	
MILL/MECH 603,04,06	9	110.25		2.75	33.69			0.00			0.00	
TOTAL LABOR COST		13,411.53	(1)		6,927.43			7,343.03			5,982.08	
OVERHEAD 20%		2,882.31	(2)		1,385.49			1,468.61			1,196.42	
HOURS	1,085.5 (3)			541.25			625.50			494.00		
MATERIAL												
PAINT		62.58			33.75			73.22			116.12	
ELECTRICAL		3,105.22			2,552.00			1,084.43			1,448.65	
PLUMBING		1,063.06			406.83			1,761.84			1,581.00	
HVAC		189.21						42.33			277.51	
CLINICAL ENG												
PLASTERING		115.90			75.99			115.89			30.48	
CARPENTRY		1,284.48			619.90			626.55			285.58	
CABINETRY		858.33			558.97			136.71			645.37	
MILL/MECH		57.32									0.00	
KEY SHOP		43.71			107.64			30.80				
MATERIAL TOTAL		6,779.81	(4)		4,355.08			3,871.77			4,384.71	
SUB TOTAL			22,873.64			12,677.99			12,683.40			11,563.20
SUPERVISION 10%			2,287.36 (5)			1,266.80			1,268.34			1,156.32
TOTAL			25,161.00			13,934.79			13,951.74			12,719.52
OUTSIDE CONTRACTORS												
ILLINI PELLA		540.96									0.00	
ANDERSON ELECTRIC		2,000.00			2,000.00			1,500.00			0.00	
CHRIS ULN		652.00									0.00	
LIFE SAFETY DESIGN		17,278.00			6,692.00			6,692.00				
J & E DISTRIBUTING		1,800.00			4,035.84							
H.F. FRITSCH & SONS		11,000.00			12,000.00						80.00	
SIM'S CABINET CO					7,410.00							
#8												
#9												
#10												
OUTSIDE CONT TOTAL		33,270.96	(6)		32,137.84			8,192.00			80.00	

Figure 4.1.

MONTH END PROJECT CONSTRUCTION COST REPORT - DETAIL PAGE 2 OF 2
FOR ENDING MONTH OF AUGUST 1989

PAINTER 1	297.60		
PAINTER 2	908.50	ALL PAINTERS	1,106.10
ELECT 1	3,364.80		
ELECT 2	147.00	ALL ELECTRICIAN	3,511.80
PLUMBER 2	4,290.56		
PLUMBER 2	390.00	ALL PLUMBERS	4,680.56
DRAFTING	19.20	DRAFTING	19.20
HVAC 1	290.40		
HVAC 2	0.00	ALL HVAC	290.40
CLIN ENG 1	96.00		
CLIN ENG 2	315.44	ALL CLIN ENG	411.44
PLASTERER	2,107.00	PLASTERER	2,107.00
LABORERS	185.25	LABORERS	185.25
CARPT 1	1,480.80		
CARPT 2	6,256.69		
CARPT 3	7,882.50	ALL CARPENTERS	15,619.99
CAB CARPT 2	4,489.63		
CAB CARPT 3	1,098.75	ALL CAB CARPTS	5,588.38
MILL/MECH 2	143.94	MILL/MECH	143.94
		CTD LABOR	33,664.05 (8)
		CTD OVHD 20%	6,732.81 (9)
TOTAL HOURS	2,746.25 (7)		

CTD MATERIALS

TOTAL PAINT	285.67
TOTAL ELECT	8,190.30
TOTAL PLUMB	4,812.73
TOTAL HVAC	509.05
TOTAL CLIN ENG	0.00
TOTAL PLASTER	338.26
TOTAL CARPT	2,816.51
TOTAL CABCARPT	2,199.38
TOTAL MECH	57.32
TOTAL KEY SHOP	182.15
CTD MATERIAL	19,391.37 (10)
CTD SUBTOTAL	59,788.23
CTD SUPERVISION	5,978.82 (11)
CTD TOTAL COST	65,767.05

(12) CHANGE ORDERS

#1 CHANGE 4 DOORS TO 20 MIN. FIRERATED DOOR. AND INSTALL 4 DOOR CLOSURES $2,733.00

#2 REMOVE BATHTUB IN RM 433 AREA TO BE USED FOR STORAGE $561.00

#3 PROVIDE TWO ADDITIONAL 3 DRAWER BASE UNITS AT N. STATION AND SHELF IN NURSE OFFICE $723.00

#4 ADD 3 OUTLETS IN ORTHO TECHS ROOM B451 $232.25

#5 ADD OUTLET IN LOCKER RM 448R $212.24

#6 FABRICATE, STAIN AND INSTALL X-RAY FILM HOLDER $93.37

#7 INSTALL WOLF GORDON JACKSON" MATERIAL TO CORRIDOR WALLS $69r

TOTAL CHANGE ORDERS TO DATE $244.87

CONTRACTORS

CONTRACTOR	PAID TODATE	BID	% PAID
ILLINI PELLA	540.96	540.96	100% (15)
ANDERSON	5,500.00	5,500.00	100%
CHRIS ULM	652.00	T & M	0%
LIFE S.D.	30,662.00	39,901.00	76.85%
J & E	5,835.84	5,138.84	113.56%
FRITSCH	23,080.00	32,890.00	70.17%
SIM'S	7,410.00	7,410.00	100%
*8	0.00	0.00	0%
*9	0.00	0.00	0%
*10	0.00	0.00	0%
CTD	73,680.80 (13)	91,380.80 (14)	

SUMMARY	EST COST	COST TO DATE	% OF EST	SQ. FEET	COST/SQ.FT.
OVERALL CONST.	207,313.00 (16)	139,447.85 (17)	67.26% (18)	13,500.00 (19)	10.33 (20)

Figure 4.1a.

(14) Contractors Bid;
(15) Percent of Bid Paid Per Contractor;
(17) Overall Construction;
(18) Percent of Estimate Paid;

Other Totals

(7) Hours;
(16) Overall Construction Estimated Cost;
(19) Number of Square Feet Per Project; and
(20) Cost Per Square Foot.

Our Engineering and Finance Departments will use this information to track all labour and material costs for construction projects It is used to ensure that costs are controlled within the budget constraints and for future planning.

In 1988, we used our Lotus Software to track and control 189 construction projects.

5. Summary

In 1985, with the support of senior management and Information Systems, Memorial's Engineering Department computerised its activities to provide a system that is both flexible and expandable.

Our system provides us with a complete automated tracking system by utilising various software packages.

We use our Asset Information Management System to track and control equipment, preventive and corrective maintenance, work orders, materials, and employee accountability information. This system has helped the department maintain high productivity levels, control assets, forecast equipment replacement, justify current and future staffing needs, and control inventory. Our future goal is to ensure the quality of inspection and maintenance of equipment.

We use our Computer Aided Design and Drafting software to provide professional, accurate architectural drawings, charts, and graphic presentations. This software has reduced the time to manually draft a floor plan for five days to one day, and to more efficiently and effectively schedule our workload. Our goal is to enter all of our existing building design into this system.

Because we have our own in-house construction staff, we use our Project Construction Cost Control System to provide our Finance Department with the actual costs-to-date that have occurred for each project. This ensures that all costs are controlled within budget constraints.

Our computer system has helped our Engineering Department provide the highest level of service in all areas of responsibility in a cost effective manner.

Engineering Aspects of Aeromedical Transport

by

A. D. Blackler
NZCE, REA, LAME, NZIM Man Dipl
Electronics Engineer
Canterbury Area Health Board
Christchurch, New Zealand

History

The first recorded Air Ambulance flight was in 1870 when balloons were used to airlift 160 soldiers out of Paris, while under seige from the Prussian forces. Aeromedical Transport has developed considerably since that first flight. Today a wide variety of aircraft are used, internationally, for transport, of a diverse range of patient categories, internationally. Aircraft typically available to undertake the aeromedical transport role include:-

(i) commercial jets with pressurised cabins;
(ii) turboprop — commercial aircraft with pressurised cabin;
(iii) light aircraft — private or commercially owned; and
(iv) helicopters.

New Zealand by comparison with many international countries could be considered small. Total land mass of the two islands is 103,736sq m with a total population of 3.3 million. The geography of the two islands is such that the population is concentrated in about four principal cities and as such these cities become the locations where sophisticated medical care is available. Between many of the regional towns and the major cities there is often terrain which is not conducive to transport of critically ill patients by road ambulance. The requirements for an air ambulance will vary from centre to centre, and the frequency of air ambulance flights may well be such that there is no dedicated air ambulance facility. Those aircraft which are specifically designated for air ambulance work are usually rotary aircraft whose principla role is trauma work.

All aircraft are required to work within the operational and airworthiness requirements of the regulatory authority of the country in which that aircraft is operated.

New Zealand Air Ambulance Categories

The current categories of air ambulance as specified by the New Zealand Civil Aviation Authority are:-

Category A

An aircraft capable of flight under Instrument Flight Rules (IFR) and hence multi-engined. The aircraft is suitable for flight both day and night anywhere within New Zealand. Treatment of the patient may be continued during the flight.

Category B

Aircraft able to operate under Visual Flight Rules (VFR) and configured in such a way that treatment may continue during the flight.

Only Fixed Wing Aircraft may be certified in Category A and B.

Category C

VRF Helicopters which are suitable for short distance flights by day. Treatment of the patient must be able to be continued during the flight.

Category D

VFR Fixed Wing Aircraft with similar capabilities to Category C.

Category E

Covers VFR Helicopters fitted with an external stretcher with facilities for carriage of a medical attendant. Suitable for carriage by day from inaccessible areas to a point where a surface ambulance or air ambulance of higher category take over.

As previously indicated aircraft must be operated within the airworthiness requirements for the country of operation. Part of that requirement is that all modifications are carried out in accordance with airworthiness standards.

With any aeromedical transport there is the need to know the specific capabilities of the aircraft being used and the medical equipment required. This equipment may be a mixture of that provided by the aircraft operator and the referring hospital. It has been our experience that the aircraft operator has a good understanding of the aircraft capabilities and the medical team similarly are aware of the capabilities of the medical equipment. However there have been many instances demonstrated when the understanding of the combined medical/aircraft requirements have been deplorably absent.

Engineering Requirements

To meet the airworthiness requirements any equipment carried on the aircraft or modifications to the aircraft must be assessed against the following criteria.

1. Gravitational Forces

All items must be able to withstand the following gravitational forces:-

Down — 4.5G
Forward — 9.0G
Up — 2.0G
Sideways — 1.5G

The importance of adequate restraint can not be stressed too much. If an aircraft flies into turbulence, items of

ASPECTS DES MÉCANIQUES DU TRANSPORT AÉROMÉDICAL

Le transport aéromédical s'est developpé sensiblement depuis le premier vol enregistré en ballon, en 1870. N'importe quel transport d'un patient doit satisfaire les exigences de navigabilité du pays en question. Il est nécessaire d'avoir conscience de l'aviation et des exigences médicales pour assurer que tous les besoins sont satisfaits. La co-opération entre Canterbury Area Health Board et Air New Zealand a permis la modification d'un Vickers 77 Transport — Couveuse qui permit le transport (à bord d'un avion commercial passagers) des enfants du premier âge, qui ont besoin de soins intensifs.

L'emploi d'Air New Zealand et Royal New Zealand Air Force s'est démontré d'être bien efficace pour transporter des adultes et des enfants ensemble. Air New Zealand les transporte à bord des services reguliers des passagers. On utilise RNZAF pour transporter un patient des hôpitaux plus petits et des hôpitaux d'urgence aux hôpitaux principaux, quand un patient peut avoir besoin d'une specialité particulière comme la chirurgie cardiaque.

equipment used for patient care must not become projectiles around the aircraft cabin. An inappropriately restrained oxygen cylinder may become a lethal projectile if the regulator assembly was snapped off in severe turbulence.

2. Power Supply

Small aircraft typically have a 12VDC power supply available similar to a road ambulance. Other power supplies available on larger aircraft are not initially compatible with medical equipment.

Available Supplies

12VDC	— Small aircraft
28VDC	— Fokker F27, Hercules C130
24VDC	— Iroquois Helicopter
115V AC 400 Hz	— DC10, Boeing 737, 747, 757, 767

3. Oxygen

FAA Regulations must be followed for all matters relating to oxygen use. Concerns raised in the formulation of the regulations include contamination of dispensing equipment and the requirement for cylinders to be certified by a testing authority.

In a pressurised aircraft a sudden decompression would cause freezing of regulator equipment if water vapour content was excessive.

4. Interference

Any equipment must be free of electrical interference both electromagnetic and transmitted via the incoming power supply. Sensitive aircraft avionic equipment must not be disrupted by equipment radiating unnecessary interference.

5. Documentation

It is most essential that any modifications or equipment additions are fully documented. The documentation should include the aircraft maintenance and procedures manuals and the hospital manuals.

6. Approval

Any equipment carried on an aircraft becomes an integral part of the aircrafts systems and as such must have passed all the usual airline certification processes.

Medical Equipment Difficulties

Documented cases of particular problems or incompatibilities have only been forthcoming in recent years. The items listed below highlight the need for trial of equipment prior to actual use.

1. Drop Pumps

Obvious difficulties will be experienced with pumps which count each drop by way of an Infra-Red Sensor. Problems experienced with interference from propellors and random alarms, as the result of movement, make this type of pump totally unsuitable.

2. Stethoscropes

Internal cabin noise in the majority of aircraft types will make the use of stethoscopes difficult.

3. Pacemakers

A patient with an implanted pacemaker had a noteable increase in firing rate when in the aircraft. On arrival at the destination the rate returned to normal. The rate responsive pacemaker was responding to the aircraft vibration with a resultant change in firing rate.

Unsuitable Equipment

Mercury — Shygs
— Thermometers
Unsealed batteries
Materials without flame resistant capabilities

Neo Natal Transport Experience

Problems experienced with transporting premature twins from the Chatham Islands some years ago to a suitable Neo Natal Intensive Care Unit, highlighted the fact that equipment designed for conventional road transport was not, in its basic form, suitable for use in an aircraft. In an attempt to overcome this problem discussions between Air New Zealand and Hospital Staff were held, to look into the possibility of making the Vickers 77 incubator suitable for aircraft use.

Vickers 77 Transport Incubator System

1. Description

The Vickers 77 incubator in its most basic form provides a safe warm environment for infants requiring transport from hospital to hospital or within a facility. The addition of the air-compressor module and ventilator along with monitoring equipment provides a compact integrated system capable of ventilating a neonate while maintaining a safe environment (Figure 1).

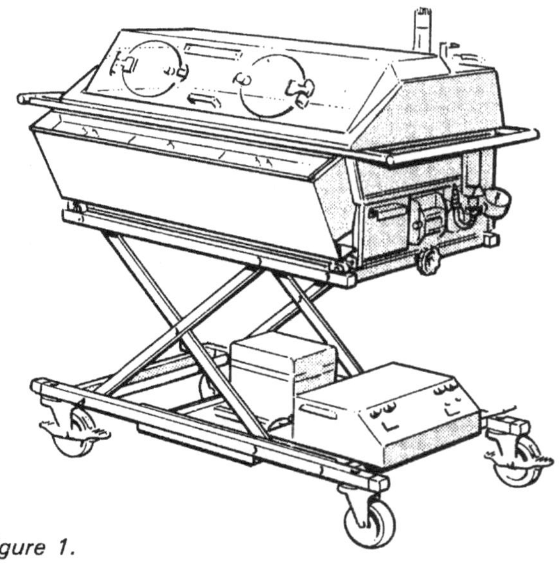

Figure 1.

2. Modifications Required

(a) Power Supply — The standard unit had both 12V DC and 230/115 VAC capability. However the supply from 230/115 VAC was split with one supply for incubator and ventilator and one for the air compressor. The power supply was redesigned to permit a single point of entry for the AC Supply and provide adequate protection for each supply by way of fuses.

Various options were investigated for the 28V DC Supply including DC voltage regulation and commercial inverters. After much research a 700 VA 115V 400 Hz aircraft static inverter was purchased. Thus ensuring that clean power was provided with no disruption to aircraft avionics.

(i) Battery Charger Modifications — Provision of a visual indication of battery life was considered necessary. Rather than a voltage indication a bar graph display of available battery time has been incorporated into the battery charger.

(b) Restraint — An important aspect of the modifications for aircraft use was consideration of all aspects pertaining to restraint of the infant and the incubator system.

(i) Infant — A restraint system for the infant and the internal bassinet was designed to permit free access to the baby and permitting flexibility to accommodate varying infant size and treatment requirements.

(ii) Canopy — Catches were installed on the lid of the

incubator to avoid unscheduled lifting of the lid in turbulence.
(iii) Body — Close inspection of the incubator body to frame restraint indicated screws threaded into a fibre glass body which may well have pulled out in extreme conditions. Additional restraining straps were thus added to each end of the incubator.
(iv) Incubator/Trolley — Overall restraint was investigated for aircraft use.
(v) Incubator
Commercial A/C — The incubator sits in two conventional aircraft seats and is restrained by specially modified seat belts which are wrapped around the handles and clipped to the anchor points of the conventional aircraft seat belts.
Air Force F27 — A full restraint system has been designed by Air NZ to ensure the incubator system, complete with trolley, is adequately secured. The sideways method of restraint is preferred to fore and aft to avoid clinical difficulties with the infant during the climb and descent phases of the flight.
(c) Oxygen — To fulfill the Air New Zealand requirements for use of oxygen on their aircraft we were required to use standard aircraft oxygen cylinders. A Scotts oxygen cylinder is slid into the incubator adjacent to the existing cylinder and connected into the oxygen system via a non-return valve (Figure 2).

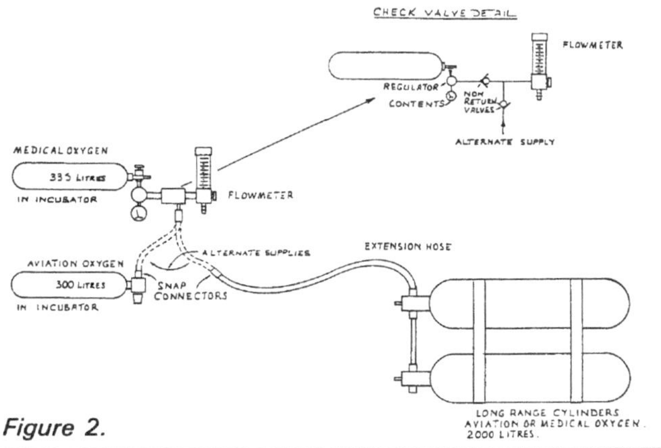

Figure 2.

(d) Suction — The existing compressor for provision of air/oxygen mixtures had the capability to provide adequate suction with minor change to the gas reticulation (Figure 3).

Air New Zealand

Air New Zealand is the national airline carrier for New Zealand and operates both domestic and international services. Their fleet includes Fokker F27, Boeing 737, 747, 767 aircraft.

Air New Zealand have been active in the aeromedical transport field for some years. A wide range of both adult and infants with varying medical conditions are routinely carried. In 1973 as the result of discussion between the airline and hospital staff Air New Zealand purchased a locally produced incubator for carriage of infants requiring basic care on their aircraft. More recently they have purchased a Vickers 77 incubator to fulfill this role.

Modification of the hospitals own incubator had proceeded to the stage of obtaining airworthiness approval in 1982 when it was urgently required to carry a baby requiring full intensive care to Auckland for cardiac surgery. The transport was undertaken on a DC10 travelling on a normal internal sector. This we believe was the first time worldwide that intensive care carriage of a baby was undertaken on a normal commercial passenger jet service.

Since that first flight the system has been refined and other hospitals throughout the country have purchased Vickers incubators and are having them modified and approved for carriage by Air New Zealand.

An essential part of the approval process for the incubator system was the full documentation of the incubator fit in the aircraft maintenance manual. Other sections of Air New Zealand also have their own departmental manuals related to incubator carriage. To assist with co-ordination of the many people involved, the Canterbury Area Health Board and Air New Zealand have compiled a manual for incubator carriage which provides a wider understanding for all who may be involved with the safe carriage of the infant.

To assist with carriage on longer flights, Air New Zealand have developed a long range oxygen kit which consists of a number of oxygen bottles mounted in a frame and anchored to the seat rails.

Adult patients are regularly transported from Christchurch to Dunedin and Auckland for cardiac surgery with an infusion pump and portable defibrillator being routinely carried. Patients requiring carriage on a stretcher needing basic care can be carried on the standard stretcher fit (Figure 4).

Carriage of patients with Air New Zealand has proved a most economic and efficient operation.

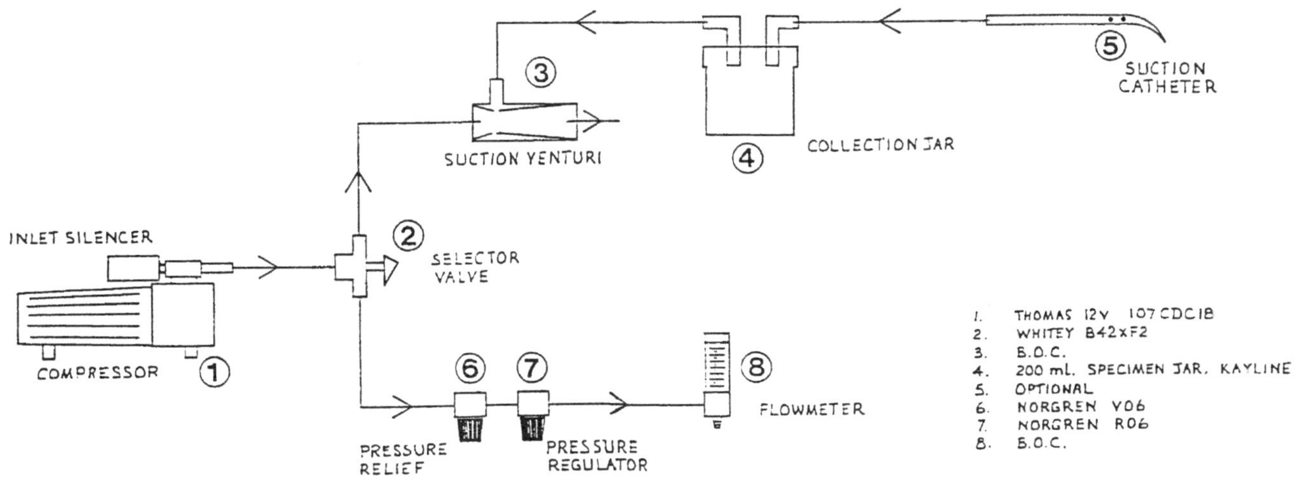

Figure 3.

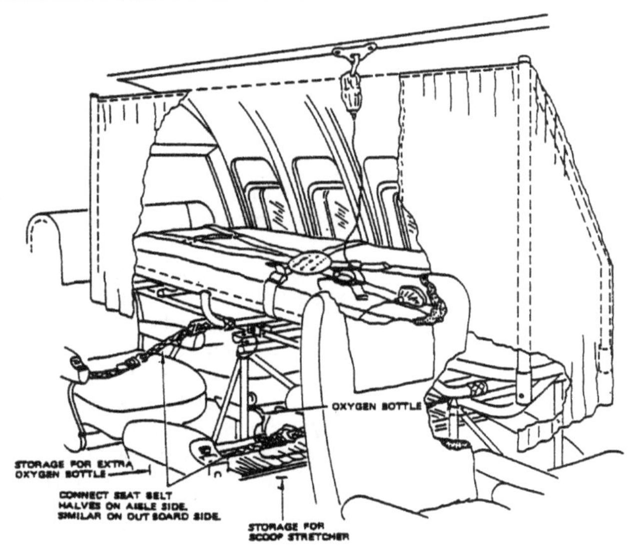

Figure 4.

The Royal New Zealand Air Force

The Royal New Zealand Air Force have a training base at Christchurch with three Fokker F27 aircraft being used as Navigational Training Aircraft. A helicopter detachment of Iroquois aircraft is used often for search and rescue and trauma work and occasionally for hospital to hospital transport.

The F27 aircraft have proved invaluable for patient retrievals, both adult and infant, from smaller outlying hospitals when time has been important, with the medical team from the base hospital stabilising the patient before transport. The skill of the Air Force crews has proved vital when retrieving patients from the West Coast of the South Island and the Chatham Islands where both difficult terrain and airports without night operation facilities make the use of smaller commercial aircraft impractical.

The passenger portion of the F27 may be completely reconfigured thus permitting the carriage of a twin incubator fit and an adult stretcher. Supplementary equipment required for carriage of adult patients such as ventilators, defibrillators and infusion pumps may be optimally located to provide ease of use.

Smaller Commercial Operators

For many years there have been minimal numbers of aircraft available to undertake any aeromedical work. In the last 12 months a small number of operators have shown some interest in this work. It is necessary with each case to assess the requirements for that transport. In all cases we have found that Aeromedical work is secondary to the primary revenue earning role of that operator.

Acknowledgement

The achievements outlined have been possible because of the willing participation of a number of people and organisations. Air New Zealand, The Royal New Zealand Air Force, Ministry of Transport, Canterbury Area Health Board, Air-Shields Vickers and other equipment suppliers have all willingly contributed their time and skills to ensure our goals could be achieved.

References

'Aeromedical Transport: Its Hidden Problems': C. J. Parsons, W. P. Bobechko, CMA; Journal; 1st February 1982, Vol 126.

'Mechancial Vibration and Sound Levels Experienced in Neo Natal Transport': A. N. Campbell, A. D. Lightstone, J. M. Smith, H. Kirpalari, M. Perlman; AJDC; 19th October 1984, Vol 138.

'Mechanical Ventilation of Critically Ill Newborn on Scheduled Flights of Commercial Passenger Aircraft': R. A. Johnson, A. D. Blackler, B. R. Lill, G. B. Evans; Aviation Space and Environmental Medicine; March 1985.

'Accuracy of Blood Pressure Measurements Made Aboard Helicopters': R. B. Low, D. Martin, Annals of Emergency Medicine; 17; 6th June 1988.

'High Altitude Testing of Pulse Oximeter': M. Glenfield British Medical Journal: 10th December 1988, Vol 297.

'Impact of Helicopters on Trauma Care and Clinical Results': Annals of Surgery; December 1988, Vol 208, No 6.

'Defibrillation Safety in Emergency Helicopter Transport': D. K. Dedrick, A. Darga, D. Landis, R. E. Burney, A. Arbor; Annals of Emergency Medicine; 18; 1st January 1989.

'Pacemaker Function During Helicopter Transport': R. S. French, J. G. Tillman: Annals of Emergency Medicine; 18: 3rd March 1989.

Air New Zealand Maintenance and Operating Manuals.

Vickers 77 Service and Operators Manual.

NZ Ministry of Transport — Civil Aviation — 'Air Ambulance Regulations'.

Logistics: The Key to Good Management and Design

by

Howard Goodman and
Prof Raymond Moss
MPA Health Planners,
London NW1 2EW

'The right thing, at the right price, in the right place, at the right time'. Few would disagree with that phrase as a definition of efficiency. And nowhere is that definition more relevant than in the field of hospital planning, indeed it has often been said that management and design are the same process and hence the idea of the operational policy as a design determinent.

In terms of hospitals, 'thing' might be defined as People, Materials, Information and Energy and 'design' as facilitating their arrival at the right place at the right time.

Hence in our modus operandi, we see planning as the process which facilitates the operation of operational policies and we regard it as important because time and effort spent moving things about is expensive — appropriating money which would otherwise be spent on patient care. In an ideal world the patient would be a few metres from the front door, a few metres from the operating theatre and equally close to radiology, laboratories, kitchens and a lot else. But we know this is unrealistic and unachievable.

So, to give the problem some order we need to identify those things in their relative importance. And then, and perhaps even more importantly, we need to quantify them. And last of all we need to know 'when' and how often.

'What goes in, must come out' — in hospital vocabulary: Supply and Disposal, although the form that it comes out in may differ very considerably from the form in which it goes in.

With processes identified and numbers allocated the beginnings of a model emerge: Quantities of People, Materials, Information and Energy; In and Out; continually, frequently, intermittently and rarely.

Looking first at numbers or quantities, we can identify two classes; those over which we have little control and those which as designers or managers we can control. Let us take some examples. The population that the hospital serves is largely fixed, but the number of beds that we provide and how intensively they are used is up to us or, the number of surgical procedures that this population needs is predictable but the number of theatres and their utilisation is up to us. Hence, scale of provision and utilisation are the variables and are related to the levels of efficiency we wish to pay for.

And this is why we link designers and managers. Designers can provide numbers of operating theatres to eliminate queues. But unless the managers ensure that they are fully utilised the investment will be wasted.

To understand and control the problem of management and design we need to classify, in a broad set of groups, the people, materials, information and energy that we are concerned with.

Taking *people* first, as we always must, they fall into four categories; patients, staff, patients visitors and official visitors. I know that we could subdivide these but remember that we are looking for broad groupings.

Similarly *materials* can be almost infinitely sub-divided. We suggest that under 'supplies' come general supplies, sterile supplies, linen, food, pharmaceuticals, equipment, and engineering supplies (including fuel, medical gases etc).

And under 'disposal' come domestic waste, clinical waste, sterile reprocessing, items for return (cylinders etc), food waste, hazardous wastes, and engineering waste.

We hesitate to classify cadavers under 'waste' but clearly they form part of our logistical system.

Information as a category could again be almost infinitely divided but we suggest simply; paper and non-paper (ie ADP, telephone, TV etc). Remember that information includes 'ideas', that intangible asset without which the entire system would fail to meet change and thus ossify.

Energy depends on the fuel source and the methods used to transmit energy around the site, but we would suggest classifying under; fuel, steam, hot water, gas, electricity and recoverable energy.

We are not suggesting that this classificiation is either comprehensive or definitive but it seems to decompose the problem into manageable parts and has relevance to the conventional design process, certainly in the context of our work in the UK.

From the assembled data one has next to predict the amount of traffic under all these heads. This is achieved by combining local surveys in existing situations with national norms. This needs skill in weighting and interpretation as some local patterns depend on the demography and morbidity of the district and some on traditional practice, not all of which may be good! National figures, say for consumption of linen or waste generated, are the basis for most predictions but cannot always be guaranteed to reflect modern medicine. Interpretive skills are much needed at this stage and this usually means experience.

What results are we looking for and how do we use them? Demand for supplies or numbers of visitors gives us a figure for site traffic, car parking, waiting spaces, catering provision and so on. Waste quantities give a picture of volumetric collection requirements, incinerator load or refuse vehicles needed to cart the refuse away. And so on, the scope is almost endless.

Studies such as these have an infinite number of uses; for instance we have been able to predict how much parking would be needed for a hospital being built in a very busy part of London and how much extra traffic would be generated

PROBLEMES DE LOGISTIQUE EN MILIEU HOSPITALIER — POUR UNE GESTION EFFICACE

Les mots d'ordre pour assurer une bonne gestion en milieu hospitalier concernent le contrôle des mouvements des individus, des marchandises, de l'information, avec un maximum d'efficacité, de rendement, et d'économie. La difficulté tient à pouvoir tout d'abord être en mesure d'identifier ces groupes, et ensuite prédire les quantités et les moments appropriés. L'exercice se divise en deux parties: les opérations d'entrée et les opérations de sortie, pouvoir quantifier les besoins et donc exercer un contrôle sur le corollaire: l'évacuation. Par exemple, l'entrée de linge propre correspond à une sortie de linge souillé ou infecté, l'arrivée d'eau propre se traduit par une sortie de quantité correspondante à l'égout. Il faut savoir dans quelle quantité, avec quelle fréquence et dans quelles conditions toutes ces opérations se déroulent. Cet article s'inspire de l'exemple donné par le nouvel hôpital de Westminster et Chelsea (un CHU de Londres). Après l'identification et la quantification des matériels, l'étude presente un système efficace, flexible et rentable.

Il fallait, bien sûr, prendre en compte les dispositions en vigueur concernant la sécurité, la prévention des accidents, et le contrôle des infections dans ces milieux. De plus, il fallait accepter les principes du contexte économique. Il en ressort qu'un système global, prenant en compte toutes les opérations logistiques d'un établissement hospitalier, y compris les impondérables, mais qui soit en même temps fiable, est possible.

L'article établit les critères d'évaluation pour ces systèmes, dans des contextes économiques et sociaux variables et tire les conclusions qui s'imposent.

on local streets. We have been able to design waste disposal systems that are economic, safe and aesthetically acceptable.

There remains the question of when. Whether we are looking at outpatients departments or car parks the same techniques can apply. Space can be used for more than one function if these functions do not occur at the same time, and particularly if no-one 'owns' the space concerned. What was the medical clinic in the morning becomes the childrens clinic in the afternoon. Staff car parking during the day becomes available for visitors in the evening. Indeed, the design of a model timetable for the hospital's activities is as essential as the design of the spaces which contain them.

Perhaps what we are saying is that hospitals need to be designed not only in spatial terms but in chronological terms also. The 'space-time continueum' as someone once said.

Hospital Lift Refurbishment

by

Eur Ing M. B. Clark
DFH, CEng, FIEE, FCIBSE, MConsE
and
P. S. Mantey AMIElecIE

Mr Clark is a Partner and Mr Mantey is an Associate and Chief Lift Engineer with R. W. Gregory & Partners, Consulting Engineers.

1. Introduction

Many hospital lift installations are refurbished without regard to the alternative equipment and technology that is available and they often include dated technology which is inefficient and verges on obsolescence due to on-going developments within the lift industry.

This paper examines two hospital lift refurbishment schemes and concentrates in particular upon the selection of two different replacement drive systems to optimise the use of available technology and achieve high operating efficiencies.

The authors have been involved in the refurbishment of many hospital lift installations taking into consideration all of these problems. They would like to share their experiences of the two separate hospital lift refurbishment projects which both required totally different drive solutions.

The hospitals in question are the Hull Royal Infirmary in Humberside and the Huddersfield Royal Infirmary in West Yorkshire which are approximately 80 miles from each other.

2. Hull Royal Infirmary

Hull Royal Infirmary is a typical high rise hospital built in the 1960's. The main tower block core is served by a group of four bed/passenger lifts comprising 2 lifts at 23 persons at 2.5m/s and two lifts at 30 persons at 2.5m/s.

Due to changes in ward and outpatient arrangements since the original design concept was established (by the same lift department as the authors practice) the traffic intensity of the lifts had increased beyond that which the original relay based controller with mechanical floor selector could cope with.

The DC hauling machines were controlled by a Ward Leonard Drive System utilising large motor generator sets which ran almost constantly for up to 18 hours per day.

The problems with the lifts could be summarised as:-

(1) The control system could not handle the demands upon the lifts.
(2) Slow door operation.
(3) Misuse of controls (stop switches, bed service, key switches etc).
(4) Unreliability due to age and deficiencies of maintenance.
(5) The control of the motors was inadequate causing overlong travel times and poor levelling accuracy.

The specification of a suitable lift control system using microprocessor based adaptive control, the installation of a suitable door operator and a properly specified refurbishment plan resolved problems 1 to 4. Many papers have been written by control and computer experts on the subject of lift controls so this paper is confined to problem number 5 the drive system.

As stated earlier the existing system was by Ward Leonard Control of a gearless DC hauling machine.

Ward Leonard System

A DC traction motor has been the most versatile of hoist motors and has always been relatively easy to control by the use of Ward Leonard method of speed control (Figure 1).

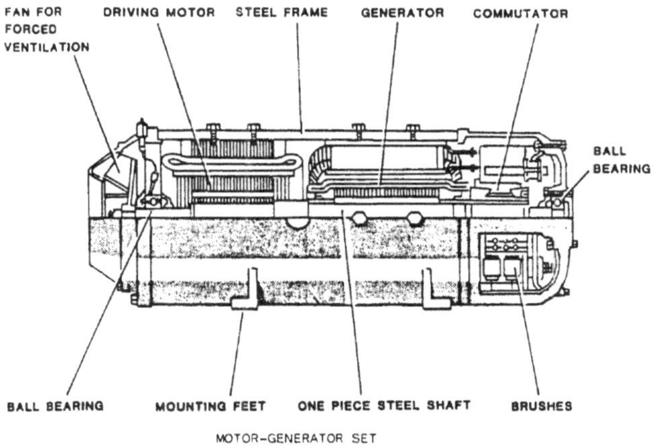

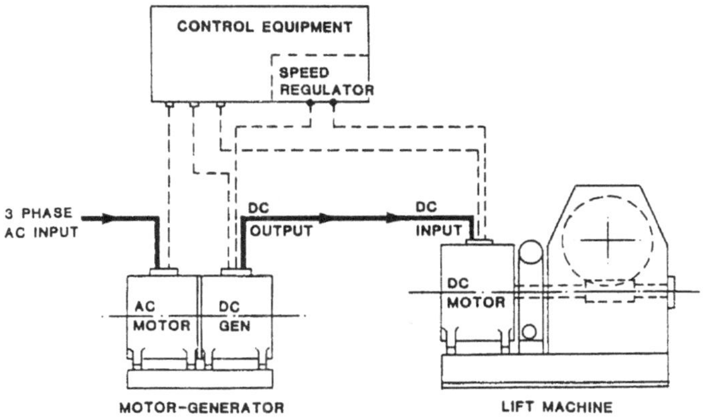

Figure 1: Ward Leonard Drive System.

The Ward Leonard set and open loop control (ie no feedback of the motor speed to the control device) allows tolerable performance over a 30:1 speed range. The Ward Leonard machinery consists of an AC motor on a common shaft with a DC generator, whose armature is in turn connected to the hauling motor armature.

The control of the speed is achieved by switching resistances in series with the generator field. Careful adjustment of the series fields in the machines 'to compound' the machine to equalise the up and down direction speeds is necessary. The characteristics of this type of control are not stable with temperature and time.

LA REMISE A NEUF DES ASCENSEURS D'HOPITAUX

Il se trouve souvent que les ascenseurs d'hôpitaux sont remis à neuf, sans tenir compte des derniers perfectionnements d'équipment et de techniques de contrôle, continuant ainsi l'emploi d'une technologie vétuste, et coûteuse.

Les auteurs, qui ont du prendre la responsibilité de nombreux projets de ce genre font la description de deux mises à neuf récents, dans deux hôpitaux du Yorkshire ou deux techniques alternative d'operation du train moteur ont été employés — le coût des modifications étant rattrapé en moins de deux années — chaque cas individuel requiert sa solution propre.

During surveys the Authors have frequently found that many installed generators are under-rated for the lift size and speed. Consequently the lifts run at less than their designed contract speed theredby adversely effecting the lifts passenger handling capabilities.

The main problems with the Ward Leonard system were related to maintenance and reliability, thus:-

- the generator requires regular attention to maintain it in good condition and requires frequent attention to the field circuit;
- the accumulation of carbon dust from the brushes can cause earth leakage currents to the generator frame;
- incorrect brushes or brush springs and thus incorrect brush pressure can cause scoring of the commutator with consequent sparking and accelerated wear; and
- incorrect adjustment of generators or the application of underrated generators can lead to overheating which in turn reduces the life of the winding insulation.

The inefficiencies of a Ward Leonard set include electrical losses in the AC motor, mechanical friction losses of the combined motor generator set, electrical losses in the generator and mechanical and electrical losses in the hauling motor. Neglecting the hauling machine gears a Ward Leonard drive is typically only 45-48% efficient.

Coming Back to the Hull Royal Infirmary Scheme

The original large gearless DC hauling machines were in a condition whereby they could be readily refurbished. Replacement of the hauling machines of the 30 person lifts was not therefore considered viable.

The inefficiencies of the Ward Leonard system made a like for like replacement of the generator sets undesirable and taking into consideration the condition and significant replacement costs of the large gearless hauling machines an alternative DC drive solution was investigated.

At the time of the proposed Hull Royal Infirmary Lift Refurbishment Project in 1984, Static DC drives were starting to be used for a small number of passenger lift applications in the UK although many of the systems had experienced problems of both audible noise and distortion of the electrical supply. Static DC drives had not been used on large gearless lifts in the UK at that time.

Statically Controlled DC Drives

The Static Converter Drive is an electronically controlled DC power to drive the motor and inverts the regenerated DC power back into AC supply.

There are two basic types:-

(1) single bridge with motor field control; and
(2) two bridge with fixed motor field.

Armature control was utilised at Hull Royal Infirmary, and will be used as an example. (Figure 2).

The power conversion in armature controlled drives is achieved with the use of two thyristor controlled, three phase bridges each utilising six thyristors. Using phase control the DC output power to the motor can be controlled from zero to full output of the drive motor.

In the overhauling situation, light car up or full car down, the motor acts as a generator and the excess kinetic energy can be returned to the mains supply.

The waveform of the current drawn from the supply to a static converter is basically a square wave. This has the effect of producing harmonic currents in the supply which interact with the supply impedance to in turn cause harmonic voltage distortion.

In the UK the only present standard relating to harmonic limits is the Electricity Council's Document G5/3, which is not as stringent as the European VDE equivalent standard, level 'K' requirements, but it does approximate to level 'N' requirements of the VDE standard.

The harmonic orders produced by a static converter are related to the pulse number of the converter by the simple formula:-

$$KP \pm 1$$

where K is any integer and P the pulse number of the converter.

The harmonic orders produced by a 6 pulse converter are therefore 5, 7, 11, 13th etc.

The harmonic current levels and orders produced in a three phase bridge converter (6 pulse) can be reduced by the use of two bridges in parallel with the supply to the bridges phase displaced by the use of double wound transformers (12 pulse) however, no Lift Maker was utilising any such arrangement at the time of the Hull Royal Infirmary Project because the additional bridges and transformer resulted in a

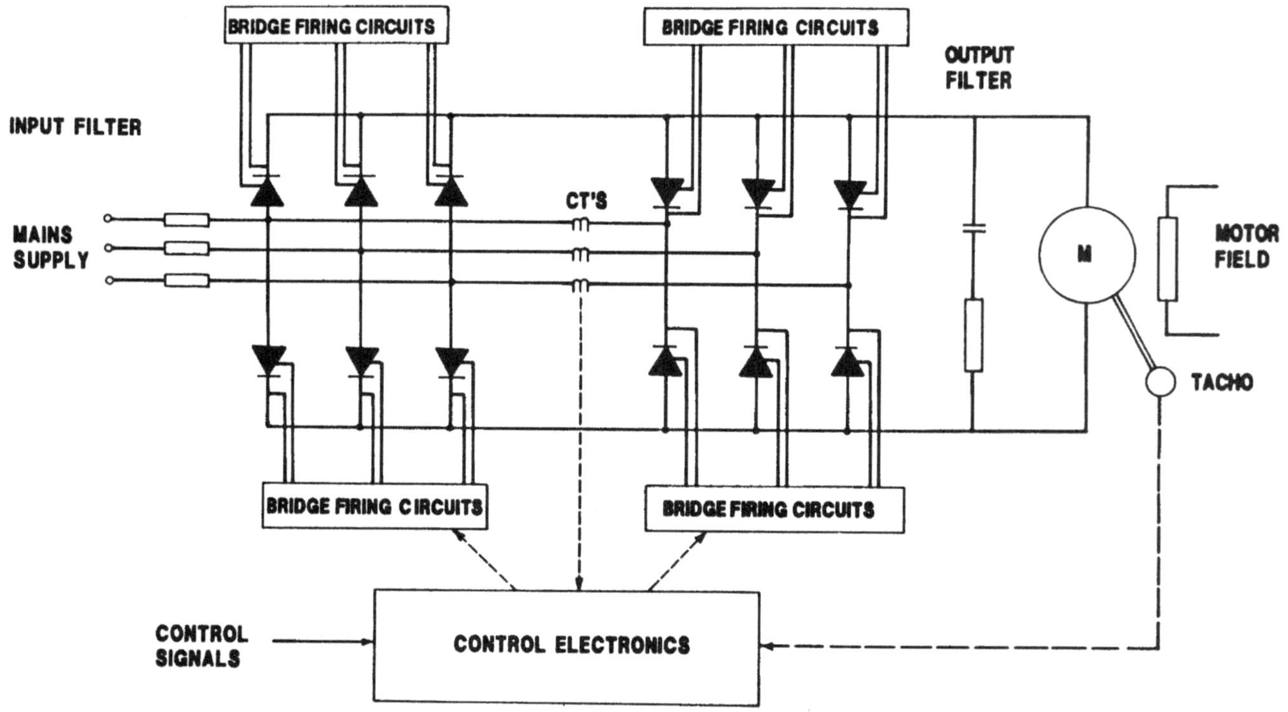

Figure 2: Armature Control Static Control DC Drive.

drive which was not then commercially viable for the lift market.

The potential problems of harmonics have now caused one Lift Maker to offer a 12 pulse system.

The 6 pulse bridge static converter was therefore investigated but the problems of harmonics and audible noise in a hospital environment were of particular concern.

Following investigations and harmonic measurements of other static DC drives, albeit on supply systems of different impedance to that of Hull Royal Infirmary, the proposed solution included input filters consisting of inductor and RC networks of values selected to minimise the distortion on the supply. Such filters both protect the thyristors from damage during switching and act as voltage disturbance and harmonic attenuators.

The output of the 3 phase bridge produces a ripple on the DC output to the motor. On a 50 Hz supply the ripple frequency is 300 Hz. This would have resulted in an obtrusive audible noise in the hauling machine which may have been transmitted to the building structure and down the lift shaft via the traction ropes.

Tuned RC filtering circuits in the DC armature loop were utilised to attenuate the ripple frequency to an unobtrusive 'hum' restricted to the immediate area of the machine room. Without this filtering in the DC loop it was anticipated that the ripple amplitude would have been up to 4% of the DC output.

Following competitive tender the Static DC drive system selected was a 6 pulse, armature controlled drive incorporating the foregoing specified requirements.

The resulting drive system provided an electrical efficiency of approximately 95%, providing a power saving over the Ward Leonard system of in excess of 30% and produced full spectrum harmonic currents and voltages on the supply of less than 3%.

The Hull Royal Infirmary project attracted the interest of several hospital authorities and Hull Health Authority provided considerable publicity to the success of the project.

The power supplies and lift operation were monitored before and after the refurbishment programme and revealed astonishing results.

The combination of the microprocessor group control system and the Static DC drive system provided an annual power saving of 50.4% compared to the system prior to refurbishment. This produced a payback period of just over two years for the small additional cost of the static drive system compared to a like for like Ward Leonard replacement.

The combination of the improved drive system with direct floor approach and the microprocessor group control system incorporating the specified operating characteristics provided an improvement in lift service. The average Waiting Interval was reduced by 33% to 25.4 secs.

3. Hospital No 2 — Huddersfield Royal Infirmary

Huddersfield Royal Infirmary was also constructed, in phases, during the 1960's and is a medium rise hospital constructed on a sloping hillside. It has two primary ward blocks of eight storeys in total. Each ward block is served by four main lifts for public use opening onto a common lobby area. In addition, several other Passenger Goods Lifts are provided at locations along the hospital street for specific functions restricted to staff only.

The ward allocation and hospital management policies at Huddersfield Royal Infirmary had altered over the years since the lifts were installed. The lifts were providing poor passenger service, poor reliability with an increasing intensity of breakdowns.

The original lift installations were geared Ward Leonard Drives running well below their stated contract speed of 200 ft per minute (1.0m/s) controlled by electro mechanical relay panels with mechanical floor selection. The door operators included a gearbox and hydraulic damping. The door closing was protected by retractable mechanical safety edges which were the most frequent cause of the lift failure.

In each of the groups of lifts the four lifts each had independent controls. This arrangement resulted in intending passengers calling all four lifts by pressing all four landing push buttons in turn.

The lift control arrangement had imposed an unrealistically high usage on the lifts resulting in their poor reliability and extreme inefficiencies.

The Client brief was to refurbish the lift installations whilst providing the minimum disruption to the hospital. Improved passenger handling and reliability was the aim.

The correct specification of a microprocessor controlled group control system, specified special controls for rear entrances, replacement door operators, improved indicators and replacement drive systems were all necessary and included in the refurbishment scheme but it is again the selection of the drive system that this paper addresses.

The motor generator sets were in a poor condition and several motors had already been refurbished however, the original gearing appeared to be in good condition.

The hospital's original electrical power distribution system had been subjected to numerous additional loads over the years and the lift supply switchboards for two groups of lifts were some considerable distance from the supply source. The problem of poor voltage regulation on the supply due to the starting of the lifts became an important consideration in the selection of a replacement drive system.

The virtually constant running of the Ward Leonard motor generator sets of the original system meant that the existing supply was *not* subjected to regular surges of current during starting of the lifts.

Variable voltage AC drive systems were initially considered, being the predominant alternative to geared Ward Leonard lift applications up to 1.6m/s. However, even the most sophisticated variable voltage lift drives that were available had starting currents of 2.5 times the motor running currents and had significant electrical losses as they were not able to compensate for motor 'slip'.

With the consideration of the possible voltage regulation problem and the requirement that the lift ride should be improved other drive system solutions were investigated.

The eventually selected system was a variable voltage variable frequency control system driving a squirrel cage AC motor.

4. Variable Voltage Variable Frequency Drives (VVVF Drives)

A simplified circuit diagram of a VVVF drive is shown in Figure 3.

The drive comprises a line filter and diode bridge converter, which produces an intermediate Direct Current. This Direct Current is smoothed and fed to a controlled inverter bridge which by means of a pulse width modulation technique converts the intermediate Direct Current into a three phase alternating current of variable voltage and variable frequency, fed in turn to the induction motor.

To understand the benefits of Variable Voltage Variable Frequency (VVVF) control the effect of controlling the stator frequency must be understood. (Figure 4).

The figure shows that with VVVF the drive may be utilised as a four quadrant drive ie driving and braking in both directions of lift travel. Only the linear part of each individual torque curve is utilised therefore the rotating speed can be easily altered by altering the frequency of the supply to the stator.

As with a 50 Hz non frequency controlled AC induction motor, changes in the motor load will reduce the actual rotating speed of the motor. To compensate for the speed reduction the stator frequency must be increased, this is

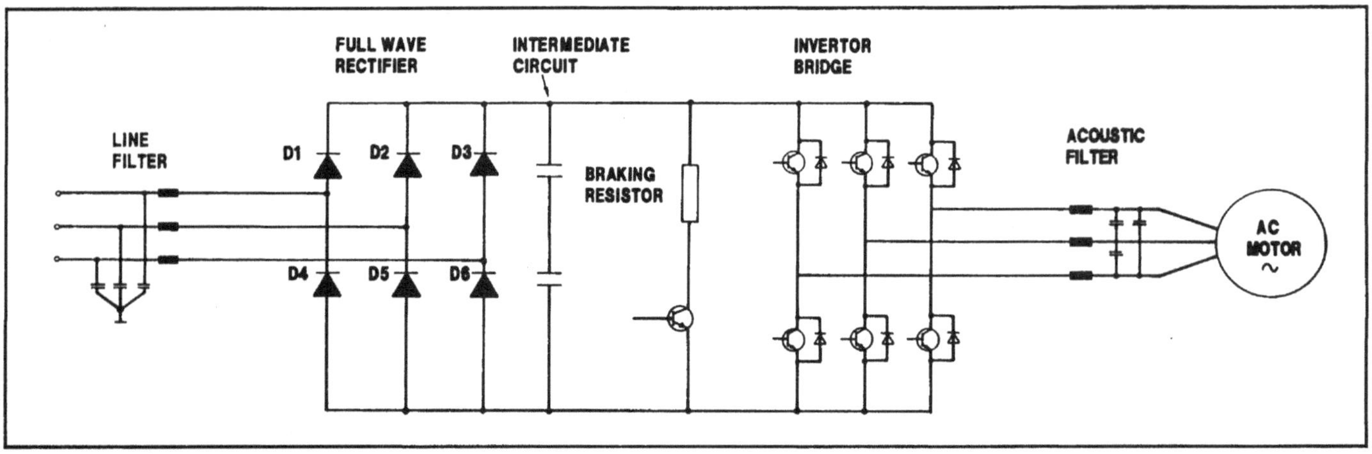

Figure 3: Circuit Diagram of VVVF Drive.

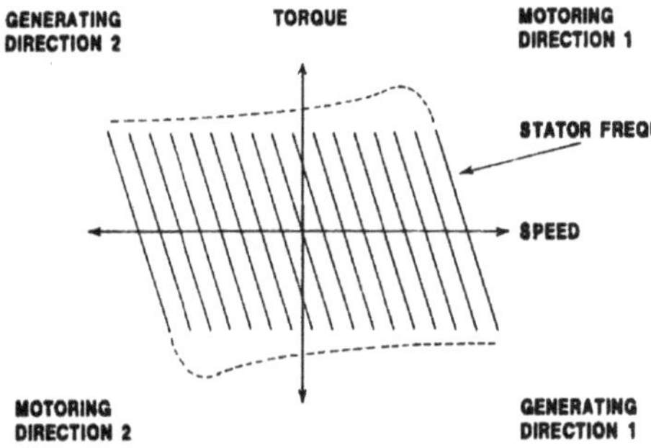

Frequency Controlled AC Motor.

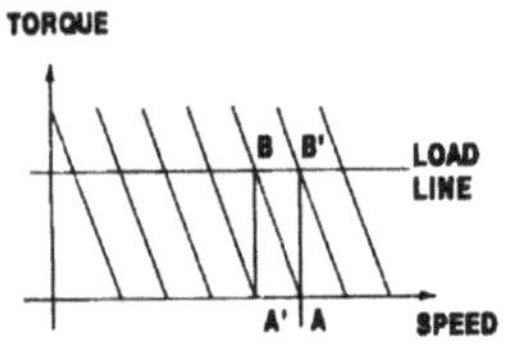

Principle of Load Compensation in VVVF Control.

Figure 4

illustrated on the torque speed diagram to the right of the figure.

With a light load the desired speed is shown at A. However, in a lift drive the load is variable and can also vary throughout a single journey. An increase in load results in a decrease in rotor speed to 'A'. The motor speed is returned to the desired speed by an increase in stator frequency to 'B'.

To maintain the linear relationship between the motor speed and the frequency, the motor excitation must also be kept constant. This is achieved by simultaneous control of the stator voltage.

The relationship is retained constant by an electronic regulator forming part of the drive system. As the rotating speed cannot exactly follow the speed reference, the regulation may be considered as a continuous operation of little regulation steps. Therefore, for any change in stator or rotor frequency the regulator produces an alteration in the stator supply voltage to retain the motor excitation constant. The voltage frequency curves of the drive are therefore a series of curves as shown in Figure 5.

At low frequencies the resistance of the stator must be compensated for by an increase in the voltage shown by the non-linear section of the voltage/frequency graph.

Looking at the individual elements of the VVVF drive system:-

The bridge and intermediate circuit functions are self explanatory. The inverter bridge comprises six power

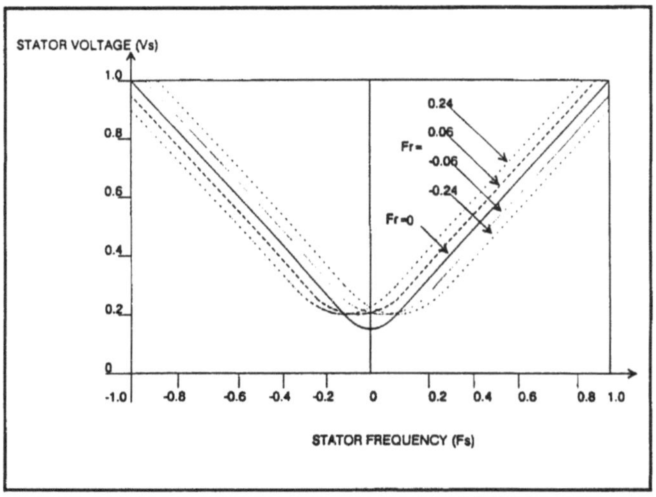

Figure 5: Frequency/ampltidue curves of VVVF.

transistor modules arranged in pairs. The transistor switching is controlled by the output of the aforementioned electronic regulator. (Figure 6).

The control sequence is based on a pulse width modulation technique. If the control of the pulses of Q1 and Q2, (which are controlled so that only one of them is on at any time), is as shown in the diagram the effective voltage output power will be approximately a sine wave of controlled amplitude and frequency. This is as shown imposed on the pulse diagram of Q1 and Q2.

The PWM switching frequency is limited by the maximum switching capabilities of the power semi conductors.

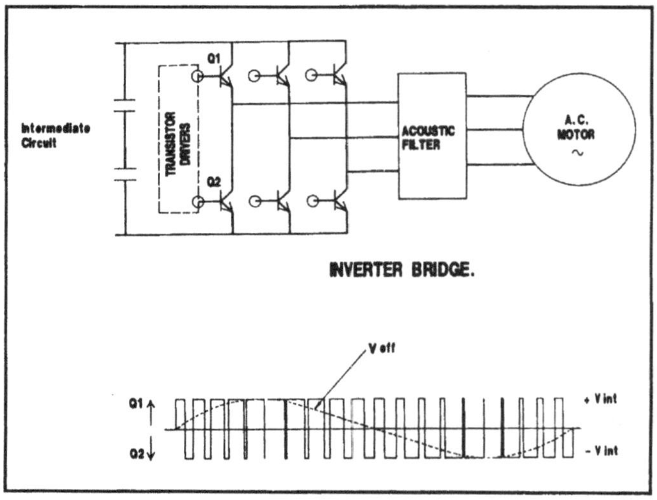

Figure 6: The Principle of PWM Control of the Inverter Bridge.

Current VVVF drives generally use power transistors especially designed for rapid switching operations however, their frequency is generally limited to a maximum of 2kHz. Power semi conductor development does promise higher switching frequency transistors which will provide superior VVVF drive characteristics in the future.

The drive output is filtered by a noise elimination network so that the 2kHz component does not impose any vibration on the motor or cause audible noise.

So what are the advantages of VVVF?

Power Consumption

The power consumption of VVVF high speed gearless installations is not significantly less than for a statically controlled dc drive. However, for low and medium speed VVVF geared installations the saving in power consumption is significant when compared to a conventional control system, which utilises voltage control to modify motor torque.

A comparison of the instant power is shown in (Figure 7).

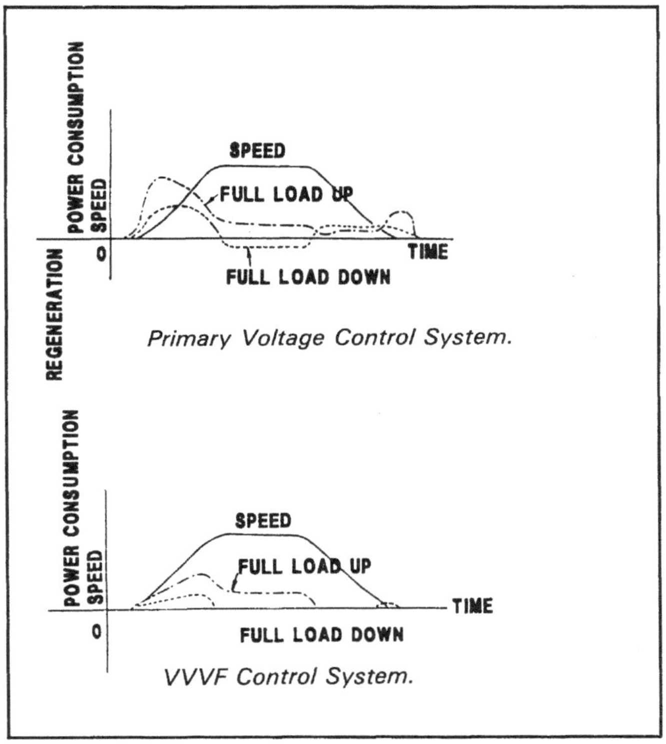

Figure 7

The voltage control system power consumption is shown for full load up and full load down travel. The decelerating lift provides DC braking by the direct current flow in the motor coil and it consumes relatively small amounts of power.

During rated load operation the power consumption increases towards the end of the later stages of deceleration because the car is controlled to approach the floor level at a slow approach speed which reduces the drive operating efficiency.

In the VVVF control system the power consumed is almost proportional to the mechanical output of the motor during acceleration. During the deceleration stages with rated load the motor operates as a generator and the regenerative power from the motor is fed back to the DC side of the drive.

The comparison of the power consumption graphs shows that the VVVF drive system requires approximately half of the power of a comparable installation using voltage control.

Reduction in Required Supply Capacity

The VVVF drive system operates at the point on the voltage frequency curves with minimal losses.

The power factor of the VVVF drive is considerably higher than for ACVV or DC static drives because the VVVF drive does *not* include phase control thyristors which have a particularly low power factor for low speeds. With the VVVF drive the power factor does not decrease quite so drastically as with other drive systems.

The VVVF system may therefore reduce the demand on the power supply due to improved efficiency and improved power factors.

VVVF overall power factor is approximately 0.9 lagging compared to the overall power factor of an ACVV or Static DC drive of 0.7 lagging.

For the VVVF system the reduction in supply currents compared to average ACVV systems for geared lift applications is approx 50%.

For Huddersfield Royal Infirmary

The VVVF drive provided a drive system that could be installed in place of the Ward Leonard drives without any requirement to upgrade the supply or cabling. Such upgrading would have been necessary with an ACVV system. In addition the drive system provides an efficient and optimum control of a simple squirrel cage induction motor with reduced maintenance requirements.

5. Conclusions

The concept of variable voltage variable frequency control has been widely utilised for fractional horse power drives however, the development of affordable power transistors capable of rapid switching rates has led to the application of VVVF drives for geared and gearless lift applications. These provide a superior ride quality and improved efficiencies compared with other drives and at increasingly competitive costs.

Currently VVVF geared lift drives are being installed in the UK in several commercial developments however, Huddersfield Royal Infirmary was the first UK hospital to have a VVVF lift drive installed (total of eight refurbished lifts so fitted by February 1991).

VVVF gearless drives are also a technically and commercially beneficial alternative to presently available drive systems.

A contract for the first application of a gearless drive in the UK has recently been placed for lifts in an R. W. Gregory & Partners designed project.

VVVF drives will become the optimum drive solution for all medium and high speed lift applications within the next five to six years (90% of all new lifts sold in Japan use VVVF drives). However, the rate of development varies considerably between Lift Makers.

Because of the rate of development, because of the highly technical nature of the options, because of the substantial costs and potential energy saving, but above all because passenger and operator safety is of paramount importance, the Authors believe that truly independent advice is essential. Whether such advice is obtained from the lift department of the Authors practice, or from one of their few competitors, does not invalidate the belief of the Authors.

Happy lifting!

Hospital Transport Systems General Background

by

W. Knicker, Dip Ing
General Hospital, Herford,
Nordrhein Westfalen, FGR

Chapter 1

1.1 The District General Hospital of Herford

In 1858 a small hospital, the Freidrich Wilhelm was opened and the records show that in its first year 17 patients left the hospital completely recovered. Over the years it was steadily extended until in the 1890s, due to space restriction in the town centre, a new hospital of 500 beds was built on the eastern side of Herford.

Exactly 115 years after the opening of the Freidrich Wilhelm ie in 1973, the new District General Hospital of Herford came into operation. Designed by Architect Peter from the design group Peter and Steffen of Frankfurt, it caters for about 700 beds in 18 wards and has all the usual facilities of a district general hospital. It is a teaching hospital of the Wilhelms University of Munster and therefore has a separate college in the grounds for approximately 50 students. A school of nursing is housed in the same building.

Building	Building Costs	Furnishing Costs
District Hospital	68,500,000 DM	12,300,000 DM
Staff 270 Accommodation (1 room/2 room/ 3 room appartments)	10,000,000 DM	1,000,000 DM
Childrens home (107 places)	2,000,000 DM	100,000 DM
Medical School	3,600,000 DM	300,000 DM

Table 1.1: Expenses for Building and Interior Decoration.

1.1.2 Energy Costs

Energy expenditure in 1988 reached about 1.5 million D-Marks. Electrical energy was the largest component used mainly for lighting but also for cooking in the diet kitchen and the bakery.

The boilers and steam generators in the boiler house are equipped with combi-burners which can burn gas or oil. Gas is the principal fuel and the contract is for an interruptable supply with 15 minute notice by telephone to change to oil. Such a contract avoids the high charges associated with periods of peak demand. The supplier, the town of Herford, passes on the rebate to the customer.

Energy			Energy Use	Energy Cost
Electricity	Light	Day	3,242,520 kWh	852,753,- DM
	Power	Night	1,987,120 kWh	
	Heating	Day	256,812 kWh	63,407,- DM
		Night	68,046 kWh	
Heating	Gas		1,722,961 m³	340,041,- DM
	Gas Rubbish Incineration		110,933 m³	38,104,- DM
Water			104,206 m³	145,181,- DM

Table 1.2: Expenses for Energy in 1988

The incinerator, however, can only use gas and is therefore more expensive to run at peak periods. For legal environmental reasons the operation of the incinerator must be discontinued after 1st April 1991.

1.1.3 Structural Considerations

Design studies commenced in 1966 and the building of the new hospital began in 1968. The site is sloping and soil tests showed that there was rock stone on the higher ground but on the lower part of the slope there was slate and clay. Expert advice from the soil laboratory indicated that the slate and clay would have to be removed completely. Although this would greatly increase the cost it provided the opportunity for a new sub-basement which could be used for installation of services and as a store.

Unfortunately the slate and clay was not completely removed and for financial reasons only a simple concrete base was installed whereas a pre-stressed concrete base was really required. Consequently after several years a major structural fault has occurred with the swelling of the clay and the base has to be rebuilt in large areas. There will be further reference to this later in the paper.

Chapter 2
Automatic Transport System for Good (AWT)

2.1 General Description

The hospital was built at a time of high industrial growth and acute labour shortages and this was one of the reasons for selecting a transport system for the sub-basement which would be as automatic as possible. It was decided that instead of the usual brigade of porters to transport goods an automatic conveyor system would require a few specialist electricians and mechanical craftsmen to maintain the system.

The transport system of Standard Elektrik Lorenz, SEL (the current licence is Schindler Aufrige Berlin) was selected and was sponsored by the Government of Nordrhein Westfalen. It is a type of conveyor system with coated rollers. Horizontal runs are installed mainly in the sub-basement linking all the important junctions and several elevators belonging to the system.

LE TRANSPORT DES MATERIAUX A L'HOPITAL

L'Hôpital Général de Herford a été daté d'un système méchanique de transport des materiaux, cette présentation est une revue de cette implantation, et des problèmes d'operation que se sont presentés, qui ont trait à l'entretien des équipments, et aussi des difficultés d'ordre structurel quand aux planchers dans les chambres, de machines, aux sous-sols. La résolution de ces difficultés avec les planchers coutera cher.

Containers are procured by Zarges and Gmohling in two different sizes to cater for all requirements. The container floors are double-walled and contain permanent magnets for encoding. The aluminium containers were produced to a hygienic specification and are washed and disinfected thermally after each round trip in the system.

The complete system operates under the supervision of the in-house hygiene department and so far all checks have been satisfactory. It is the author's opinion that the use of aluminium is one of the reasons for the good hygienic performance since metals are inherently bacteria free.

Prior to installation a detailed route plan was drawn up for the tower housing and wards and the podium containing the specialist medical departments. They form a 'distributed system' in that six Groups control the different section blocks.

The groups are as follows:-

Group 1 — Paediatric Clinic
1 Elevator
1 Remover (shifter)
Channel in/out system

Group 2 — Intensive care ward
Hydraulic elevator
Remover (shifter)
Channel in/out system

Group 3 — Laundry tilting device
Mainstock
Elevator tower block A
Three hydraulic elevators
Two removers (shifter)

Group 4 — Container station
Washing machine
Three hydraulic elevators
Channel in/out device

Group 5 — Elevator tower block B
Remover (shifter)
Channel in/out device

Group 6 — Tilting device for garbage containers
Channel in/out device
Routes

2.1.2 The Control System

SEL's basic idea was to build a conveyor system with coated rollers and belts and divide it blockwise like a railway system. This means that every block has to have a reading device and a decoder to determine the origin and destination of all passing containers. This information is put into the permanent magnets inside the double walled floors of the containers.

There are two different types of permanent magnet. One to record a fixed home address and container type and other weaker permanent magnets to encode the destination. A reading label starts the decoding procedure. During the system implementation and home address and container type are encoded permanently.

Each station in the wards or in the medical area has an address for permanent identification. The destination can be programmed by Keyboard or automatically in read/write devices. All the wards have only passive stations without facility for encoding. This is because of the frequent staff changes and the need to minimise the training to keep the system going.

The garbage container is first of all taken to the sub-basement by the elevator. The read/write device identifies and writes in as destination the garbage tilting device. From then on the container is routed automatically to the tilting device in front of the incinerator. After dumping the garbage the empty container is re-addressed by the read/write device to its new destination, the washing machine. On exiting from this machine it is re-addressed once more back to the home station.

Note:

Problems are now occurring with the use of relays and solenoids such as the pitting and fusion of contacts as the number of switching cycles reaches the limit of the useful life of such components. The downtime of the system is now fairly high and a great effort is required to keep the system from breaking down completely.

2.1.3 The Timetable for Transport

A timetable is needed to co-ordinate all the different movements in the system.

2.1.4 Staff Requirements and Emergency Cover

As mentioned earlier the hospital does not have a

Transport for	Time													
	7	8	9	10	11	12	13	14	15	16	17	18	19	20
Food		xxx -oo	x oo			xxx -oo	xx ooo	o		-oo			xxx -oo	x oo
Lab Test		xxx	-oo	ooo										
Laundry				xxx -oo	o									
Soiled Laundry		-x	xx -oo	oo								-x	x ooo	
Refuse			xxx -o	x ooo			-xx	xxx ooo	- ooo					
Pharmaceuticals							-xx	x ooo	o					
Stores								-xx	x ooo					
Sterile Materials	ooo	xxx												

Table 2.1: Transport Timetable.

Workman	Schedule			
	Normal Shift 7.00 to 16.00	Standby Duty 16.00 to 20.00	Early Shift 7.00 to 13.00	Late Shift 13.00 to 20.00
Electrician 1			x	
Electrician 2				x
Fitters	x	x		

Table 2.2: Staff Duty Roster

porterage staff and consequently the technical department has to think about emergency problems.

Under normal conditions one electrician and one mechanical fitter are on duty at all times. The working schedule shows how they work. Three electricians each work one week on early shift, one week on late shift and one week on normal shift. The working week for public sector workers is now about 38.5 hours. With that constraint it is very difficult to provide continuous cover between 7 am and 8 pm and it can only be done by balancing the hours worked over the 3-week cycle. We have operated that way since our hospital opened in 1973.

The fitters work during normal working hours and are on stand-by call as necessary between 4 pm and 8 pm when the transport system is closed down. They get a small extra payment for this and are not allowed to consume alcohol during stand-by duty.

Because of the great importance of the transport system, emergency instructions have been devised in several stages. Stage 1 comes into oepration if one of two elevators goes down. In this case most of the movements have to be conducted via the second elevator with additional assistance from the building and grounds staff belonging to the technical department. Further stages up to a complete breakdown of the whole equipment are catered for. In the latter case all the craft workers and some of the kitchen and ward staff have to assist to ensure that patients get their meals on time. Fortunately this has not happened so far. Transport by hand in emergency is carried out with trolleys from the cafeteria and all other movements with lower priority are left until later.

2.2 Stations with Encoders

2.2.1 The Central Pharmacy

All kinds of pharmaceutical products used in the hospital are produced and/or distributed from here. It is staffed by a pharmacy director, two pharmacists and three assistants.

Twice a week medical table water is suppled to all wards. Because of the enormous quantity this has been transported by hand for a long time, especially by community service conscripts. All additional goods in this area are suppled by the AWT equipment in half sized containers. By law they must have covers and be securely locked.

The Pharmacy has a keyboard at its terminal and can therefore send the container directly to the sender of the order. Orders are posted in every morning by the pneumatic post.

2.2.2 TheCentral Kitchen

The kitchen is staffed by a chef, a head cook, three cooks and two assistant cooks. It caters for all patients and some of the staff. There are normal menus and a diet menu and in addition seven special diets are served every day. The meals are put on trays with thermal covers to keep the food warm. The trays are loaded in special food containers and despatched to the consignee station by entering the code via the keyboard. Before starting a loaded container a plastic flap is clipped into the container's vertical opening.

The distribution of meals lasts for about 90 minutes and the receiving stations are supplied in rotation to avoid queueing.

Even before the meals service is finished provision is made in the control system to temporarily store used containers in the main container station until the washing up stage is reached, when all containers are sent to the kitchen again. Trays and dishes are sent along the washing street and the container is sent back to the container station via the washing equipment in the sub-basement. The china is then preheated in special containers.

2.2.3 The Incinerator

When the incinerator was installed it was a modern device complying with the current standards. However, the standards have been tightened up to such an extent for environmental reasons that we now have no alternative but to discontinue its operation on 1st April 1991.

The incinerator has a power rating of 14 50kw and can deal with about 325 kg of garbage per hour but the hospital will now have to pursue a new policy and sent all garbage to a large incinerator nearby. This will increase cost significantly because of the loss of heat recovery as well as the charges for transport and incineration. A major problem occurs with the hospital — specific waste which has to be delivered in one-way containers and is expensive to have incinerated. A new building complex is under construction and should be completed by the end of this year. It will contain a compaction machine, container store and a cooling cell.

2.2.4 The Laundry

Laundry from the wards in Hammerlit bags is loaded in containers with a blue coloured circle on the front. They are automatically routed to the laundry area where there is a special laundry tilting device. Empty containers are re-routed back the same way via the washing machine in the sub-basement. Great care has to be taken to prevent the staff from loading laundry into red marked containers which are routed automatically to the incinerator.

2.2.5 The Wards

Operation of the terminals in the wards is fully automatic. After coupling a container to the system, it moves away automatically and incoming containers either stop after leaving the elevator or move onto a special container carriage from where they can be brought to somewhere in the wards after decoupling. As mentioned earlier this method of operation requires only a very short staff training period.

Chapter 3 Maintenance

It is, of course, essential to have a planned maintenance system so that inspection, adjustment and repairs are carried out in an organised manner. In larger systems the data handling and scheduling are best performed by computer. It is the author's opinion based on his experience that in addition, regular brainstorming sessions with the maintenance staff can indicate probable faults that are otherwise unpredictable. This continuous analysis of weak points conducted in parallel to routine maintenance work can significantly increase the mean time between failures (MTBF).

Experience of the past 17 years also showns that it is necessary to distinguish between internal and external faults.

3.3.1 Internal Defects

Belt-tracking. Over the years it was noticed that the belts moved over to one side leading to fraying of the belt edge and several failures. We solved the problem by using crowned rollers and by making the bearings adjustable on one side.

Belt drive. We found that due to faulty design of the pulley arrangement V-belts bent in the wrong way and this led to stoppages. The construction was therefore re-designed completely using toothed belts on a drive system outside the belt.

Chain failure. The transportation chain in the washing machine for containers had no belt tensioning roller and temperature difference caused disruption. The problem has been solved by installing a belt tensioning roller and a new chain wheel to avoid slipping chains.

Control system. The relay system was rejected and a new microprocessor control system was built into the washing machine. Since that time there have been no problems with the control system.

3.3.2 External Defects

The distortion of the floor in the sub-basement due to the swelling of the clay sub-soil has caused secondary defects in the conveyor system. To solve this problem a great deal of money needs to be spent to renew the whole floor.

Use of incorrect china. Sometimes soup or milk has been delivered to the wards in incorrect containers and spillage has occurred which has damaged read/write logic components.

Incorrect load. The overfilling of plastic waste bags has resulted in containers jamming in tunnels.

Non-observance of colour coding. Laundry has been despatched in red-marked containers meant for waste with the result that laundry has been tipped in to the incinerator.

Chapter 4 Outcomes

4.1 Restoration with Government Help

Due to the floor problem in the sub-basement a complete retrofit of the transport system will be necessary. This will mean expenditure 50% over the budget and will need government subsidy — up to 1 Million DM from local government and the excess from Dusseldrof (the principal town of Nordrhein Westfalen).

4.2 Conclusions

Obviusly it is questionable whether we should spend a great sum of money to renew the system or revert to a manual porterage system which would give employment to some of the unemployed. On consideration there are some strong arguments for restoration.

- An effective transport system ensures that wards receive supplies when they are needed.
- It avoids the disturbance in the wards when porters pass through with trolleys.
- Ward staff are in control of the timetable and the whole logistic is performed with less effort.
- Waste is collected in plastic bags and is sent direct to the incinerator thus reducing the number of hazardous incidents.

So it can be said that the original concept of 1973 is still valid and the latest news is that the hospital has been informed that it will receive 6.8 Million DM for restoration. This is going to require a great deal of work from the technical staff.

Quality Assurance of Medical Equipment

by
Francisco Castella
Doctor Engineer
President of AEDIAH
(Spanish Association of Hospital Engineering and Architecture)

Introduction

For many years the working groups of the subcommission 62 of the IEC have been developing standards related to the electrical equipment and installations used in the medical practice; the work is followed in many associated countries, where similar groups are operating and collaborating with the IEC: ie in Spain the official organisation for standards, AENOR, has created the working group 62 for the study and application of the IEC 601 standards with the same objectives of improving the safety of the electrical devices used in the medical practice.

However, accidents still occur, risk evidently exist, and the fundamental question arises:-

1. Are the Current Standards Enough to Ensure the Safety Application of the Electromedical Equipment?

To answer the question and to debate aspects involved in the correct evaluation of the quality of the medical equipment, reducing the risks derivated from its application, a meeting of experts took place in February 1989, in Leiden, Holland, under the organisation of MTD (medical division of the research institute TNO); the meeting was sponsored by the DG XII of the European Community Commission.

Fourteen Countries were represented in this important workshop: a brief abstract of the meeting is presented, under my personal interpretation:-

- Accidents occur in the application of electromedical equipment in a significant proportion.
- The risk evaluated is high.
- Many defective equipments were in use during the inspection.
- The maintenance resources were insufficient.
- The design could be improved in many cases to prevent risks.
- The accuracy of the function was often neglected: simulators should be used for equipment adjustment.
- The current standards cover only a partial field of the possible causes of accident.
- The current standards often are referred only to parameters easy to control rather than to parameters essential for safety.
- The manufacturers influence in the publication of standards is superior to the users.
- The human factor is an important cause of accident.
- The instruction and training is insufficient: simulators again could help in this fundamental aspect.
- The design improvement should take in mind the human error and prevent it as much as possible.

The committee for concerted actions, however, considered that this kind of study and work, does not meet the objectives of basic research of the DG XII and by the moment and action indicated in Leiden has no continuity.

However, the importance of the ideas discussed and the transcendental objectives to reach in Safety, Accuracy and Reliability of the medical equipment, motivated me to follow in my country a study and audit to know the real situation of risk and to orient future actions toward the basic objectives above ennunciated.

2. Basic Principles of the Survey

2.1 Objective

Analyse the safety conditions, reliability and the degree of assistance quality that is expected from the examined medical equipment. Quantify and qualify the observed and measured defective conditions. Conclusions and recommendations.

2.2 Age

The technology advances very fast in the biomedical and electronic fields; usually a medical equipment should be depreciated very soon in three to five years. After this time the technical obsolescence advises for a reposition; however in our hospitals many aged equipments are still in use giving a poor quality of assistance when compared with the new models and modern performances.

The study tries to correlate the age with defective conditions.

2.3 General Condition

An aged equipment well maintained gives a quality of assistance very different from the assistance given by a degradated one. The survey qualifies the general condition of the equipment by visual observation, in three categories: B (well maintained) — R (regular) — M (bad).

On the other hand, we list the defects observed under this principle of general condition and we quantify them by category.

2.4 Localisation

It is normal that the equipments could have defective conditions after being used for a long time, nothing is perfect and everything needs some kind of maintenance. However we cannot admit that an equipment qualified as defective in a critical degree, be in normal use. So we take note that the place where we have found the equipment in question, randomly selected.

GESTION DE LA QUALITE DES EQUIPEMENTS MEDICAUX

Il y a un risque potentiel associé a l'aplication des equipements medicaux, en particulier ceux qualifié comme éléctromedicales et d'assistance vitale.

Les normes courantes couvrent seulement quelques aspects de la sécurité éléctrique, mais on oublie souvent des autres facteurs qu'on doit considèrer au moment de qualifier la qualité d'un equipment: la sécurité, la fonctionalité et la fiabilité.

Selon le type d'equipement et l'importance ou gravité du défaut dans chaque facteur analysé, nous pouvons évaluer le niveau de risque où au contraire le niveau de qualité.

En base aux considérations ennoncées, nous avons réalisé un examend'un echantillon de diffèrents equipements, choisis dans des hôpitaux du réseau de l'Institut Catalan de la Santé; les résultats analisés sont presentés avec des recommendations pour améliorer la qualité, la sécurité et la fiabilité des equipements medicaux.

2.5 Safety

Here we are very well guided by the standards of the IEC, which give all kind of details and precisions on the quantification of leakage currents, isolation parameters, etc . . . as well as on the procedure to measure.

That's only a routine to examine the corresponding parameters as per the IEC 601 standard.

The defective conditions will be listed, quantified and qualified. The criterium used is simple: we call m the minor defects, which need to be correct but do not constitute cause of equipment disconnection; we call M, the major defects, requiring an immediate repair in order to prevent risks; we call Cr, the critical defects which are dangerous for the health or the life of patients and require the immediate disconnection and separation of the equipment.

2.6 Functionality

An equipment can be safe according to theIEC standards as per the survey conducted according to the principle of safety described in the 25 paragraph; however the equipment could be unsafe when its accuracy is poor and does not give the performance and functions which we expect from it. Under this criterium we measure the parameters that come under the equipment specifications and we use simulators of the function, cardiac, pulmonar, etc . . . to contrast the equipment response and its accuracy.

We also list the defective conditions and we qualify them following the same criteria than in paragraph 2.5, let's say in m (minor) M (major) Cr (critical).

2.7 Documentation

An equipment can be excellent, with modern and efficient technology, well maintained, with quality, capacity and reliability; however all these qualifications can be ignored if there is not enough documentation or communication, and as a result the excellent capabilities are not known by the users and by technical personnel.

In many cases the operating manuals, maintenance manuals, technical description, etc . . . are often kept in a drawer or lost; nobody takes care of ordering the documentation in a proper way, ie by means of an equipment card, summary of characteristics, and guide to complementary information.

The survey analyses the available documentation and qualifies it as sufficient, not sufficient or inexistent.

2.8 Maintenance

This is a basic prinicple for the safety and reliability of the equipment. We know that in general the maintenance service has not enough resources; the personnel are often absorbed by the daily problems and are always busy on urgent work.

There is no time or organise, to prepare, to prevent . . . The Preventive Maintenance in many equipments (not in all) is a must. We qualify the maintenance service as sufficient or not and we note whether the audited equipment is subject to a program for preventive maintenance or is only subject to corrective repairs.

2.9 Environment

Some equipments need special conditions, ambient specifications, or some specific requirements in the electrical lines of grounding. For a good quality of assistance the environment must be also considered.

2.10 Instruction and Training

The final element of the chain is the user who applies the equipment. Here we must emphasise the essential importance of the human factor, with personnel educated, motivated and trained.

The survey examines the kind and degree of instruction and training received by the user.

Here again the simulators can help in training sessions.

Too many times however, the instruction received by the operator is very poor. This type of risk is often ignored but it is fundamental to take in account the possibilities of human errors or mistakes and this risk possibility we hardly recommend to minimise by an adequate design (preventing any possibility of error) and a complete education and training of the personnel.

The quality of the assistance expected from the equipment depends on this factor, more than usually suspected.

3. Survey organisation

3.1 Equipment Selection

First of all we want a sample as much representative as possible in order to can deduct valid conclusions.

We conduct the survey through five general hospitals of the Institute Catalan of Health.

Hospital Bellvitge — Barcelona
Residencia Valle Hebrón — Barcelona
Hospital Joan XXIII — Tarragona
Hospital Arnau de Vilanova — Lérida
Hospital Alvarez de Castro — Gerona

The types of equipments have been classified in the following categories:-

Respirators
Monitors
Defibrilators
Electrosurgery
Infusion pumps

The reason for this selection is the common aspect of vital assistance and the consequences of an error or defective condition for the health or life of the patients.

The first phase is to obtain from the hospitals an inventory list of those equipments.

Then, we have proceed to a random selection of the units in each list, proportionally to the weight of the specific type of equipment in each hospital and in the group, to obtain up to 400 units.

3.2 Auditor

The survey is conducted by a firm (Tecnocontrol, SA) with large experience in the maintenance of hospital equipment and installations, with personnel trained and qualified, and means to control measurements and performances.

The equipment used in this audit is the following:-

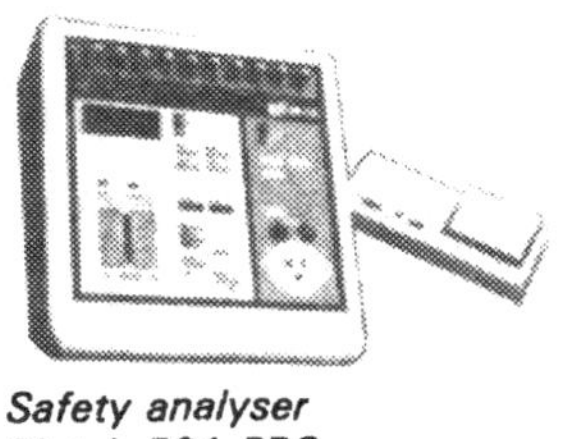

Safety analyser
Biotek 501 PRO

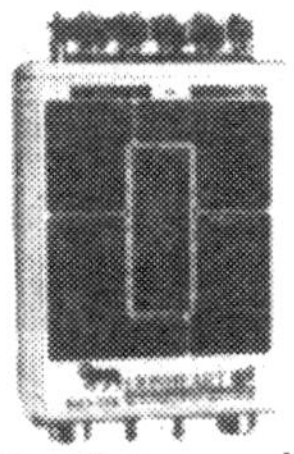

Ventilators verification
Biotek VT-2

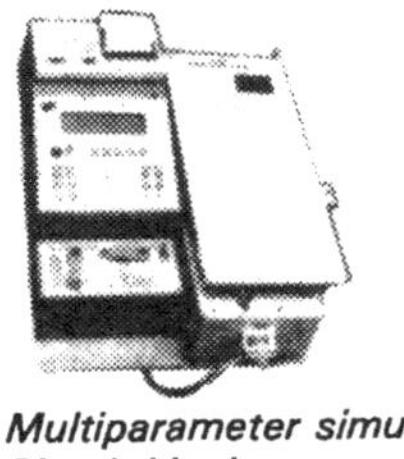

Multiparameter simulator
Biotek Lionheart

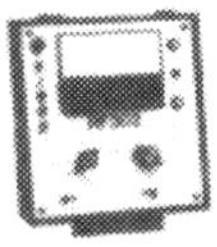

Electrosurgery analyser
Biotek RF 302

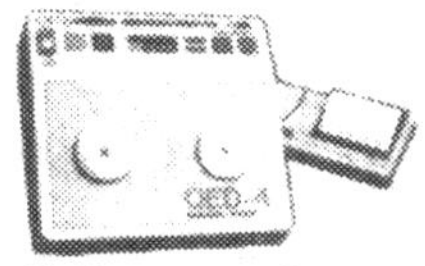

Defibrilators analyser
Biotek QED-4

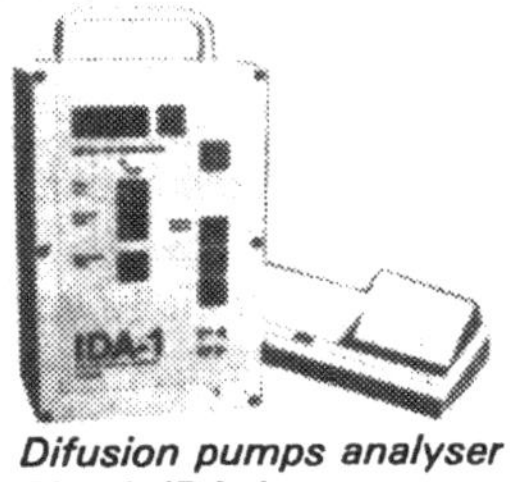

Difusion pumps analyser
Biotek IDA-1

The auditor has in each hospital a room where he checks the equipments piece by piece and where the analysing equipment will be installed, as a provision laboratory during the auditory work.

3.3 The Form

In order to have the survey and its results organised in an uniform system, an audit form has been issued, with the summary of inspections, qualifications and quantifications. The form is presented in the annex.

In addition, every type of equipment has its own form to note the measurements realised, and several of these forms are added in the annex.

3.4 The Computation of Results

A computer program has been adapted to introduce the data contained in the form. Different correlations can then be obtained.

Type of equipment — intervals of age
Total percentage of defects — age
— type of equipment
Percentage of critical defects — age
— type of equipment
Percentage of preventive maintenance
Percentage of complete instruction/training
Percentage of safety defects/functional defects

4. Results

The numeric results may vary from one country to other. The numbers obtained in our region and hospitals cannot be extrapolated to other countries; they reflect a particular situation in a concrete period of time. However they can be useful as a reference to compare other similar studies. We present them in a separate sheet not included in the Report of Proceedings book but distributed separately to the attendants to the IFHE meeting.

5. Conclusions

For the author, the conclusions are clearly defined in the following lines:-

The Quality of the application of the medical equipment requires the improvement and enlargement of the current standards, in order to cover.

- Intrinsic safety
- The accuracy of the function
- The instruction and training
- The reliable maintenance

This can be the objective of a concerted action amongst the national associations integrated in the International Federation of Hospital Engineering. If the Commission of European Communities did not consider this action, the IFHE can promote a working group composed by voluntary representatives of the 'A' members ready to cooperate and offer to the entire world a positive contribution to the objective of Quality Assurance Control of the medical equipment.

The study, the standards covering not only the electrical aspects (IEC) but much more risk factors, will be of interest of the national Health Authorities, who for sure will finance any cost incurred by the national assocation to do the work.

One non profit organisation, who can help and cooperate with IFHE, is ECRI (emergency care research) whose studies published in 'Health Devices' are known by all of us.

An internationally accepted 'Mark of Quality' is given by ECRI under the name of CITECH.

Introducing these concepts is not the work of one day. It requires time, work and dedication. Every association in its country may conduct a survey in a similar way we did, and the results compared. An executive committee of IFHE elected for this mission and objectives, should coordinate the actions and produce the fundamental document. This is the message, let's do it.

Annex

1 — General evaluation form sheet
2 — Measurements performed
3 — Data collection sheets examples

Annex 1

Institut Català de la Salut

FULL NÚM.

DATA

AVALUACIÓ D'EQUIPS MÈDICS

CARACTERISTIQUES TECNIQUES

EQUIP | LOCALITZACIÓ | CODI

ANY D'ADQUISICIÓ | EDAT

FUNCIONAMENT
☐ EN ÚS
☐ EN DESÚS
☐ EN REPARACIÓ

ESTAT GENERAL
☐ B
☐ R
☐ M

DEFECTES OBSERVATS. DESCRIPCIÓ — QUALIFICACIO m M Cr — TOTAL

DEFECTES DE SEGURETAT MESURATS SEGONS LES NORMES — QUALIFICACIÓ m M Cr — TOTAL

DEFECTES FUNCIONALS MESURATS — QUALIFICACIÓ m M Cr — TOTAL

DOCUMENTACIÓ
☐ SUFICIENT ☐ DESCRIPCIONS TÈCNIQUES ☐ FITXA
☐ INSUFICIENT ☐ MANUAL D'OPERACIÓ
☐ INEXISTENT ☐ MANUAL DE MANTENIMENT

MANTENIMENT
☐ PREVENTIU ☐ SUFICIENT
☐ CORRECTIU ☐ INSUFICIENT

INSTRUCCIO DE L'OPERADOR PER
☐ DEMOSTRACIÓ ☐ LECTURA DEL MANUAL ☐ PRÀCTICA

OBSERVACIONS GENERALS

Annex 2

Brief Specification of Measurements to be Performed

2.1 Electrical Safety Analysis
- Isolation resistances measurement
- Earth protection cables checking
- Earth leakage currents in normal conditions and in first defect condition
- Patient leakage currents in normal conditions and in first defect condition
- Auxiliary current to the patient by applying electrical tension

2.2 Electrosurgery Unit Analysis
- Power output measurement: variable load
  low load
  bipolar electrosurgery
- Low frequency output measurement
- High frequency leakage measurement

2.3 Defibrilator Analysis
- Power delivered measurement
- Wave configuration checking
- Synchronisation test

2.4 Infusion Pumps Analysis
- Flow measurement (instantaneous)
- Average flow measurement
- Volume measurement
- Pressure measurement

2.5 Respirators Analysis
- Flows measurement
- Pressures measurement
- Volume measurement
- Times measurement
- Ratios

2.6 Monitors Analysis
- ECG simulation
- Blood pressure simulation
- Respiratory rate simulation
- Temperature simulation

Annex 3

TEST DE SEGURIDAD ELECTRICA					
EQUIPO		CENTRO			
MARCA		N SERIE			
MODELO		N INVENTARIO			
CLASE	TIPO	FECHA	UBICACION		
TEST			ALIMENTACION	MEDIDA	UNIDADES
1	AUTO TEST ISA-470		NORMAL		
2	TENSION DE ALIMENTACION		NORMAL		
3	AISLAMIENTO	ALIMENTACION	NORMAL		
4		APLICABLES	NORMAL		
5	CONTINUIDAD CONDUCTOR TIERRA		NORMAL		
6	CORRIENTES DE FUGAS A TIERRA	CON ALIMENTACION	NORMAL		
			INVERSA		
7		SIN ALIMENTACION	NORMAL		
			INVERSA		
8	CORRIENTES DE FUGAS DE CHASIS	CON ALIMENTACION	NORMAL		
			INVERSA		
9		SIN CONDUCTOR DE TIERRA	NORMAL		
			INVERSA		
10		SIN ALIMENTACION	NORMAL		
			INVERSA		
11	CORRIENTES DE FUGAS DE PACIENTE	CON ALIMENTACION	NORMAL		
			INVERSA		
12		SIN CONDUCTOR DE TIERRA	NORMAL		
			INVERSA		
13		SIN ALIMENTACION	NORMAL		
			INVERSA		
14	CORRIENTE AUXILIAR DE PACIENTE	CON ALIMENTACION	NORMAL		
			INVERSA		
15		SIN CONDUCTOR DE TIERRA	NORMAL		
			INVERSA		
16		SIN ALIMENTACION	NORMAL		
			INVERSA		
17	TENSION DE ALIMENTACION EN PARTES APLICABLES	ALIMENTACION NORMAL	NORMAL		
			INVERSA		
18		ALIMENTACION INVERTIDA	NORMAL		
			INVERSA		

3.1 Electrical Safety Test

POTENCIAS Y FUGAS RF DE ELECTROBISTURIS					
EQUIPO	ELECTROBISTURI	CENTRO			
MARCA		N SERIE			
MODELO		N INVENTARIO			
CLASE	TIPO	FECHA	UBICACION		
			CARGA	ESU	RF-301
			OHMS	WATTS	WATTS
SALIDA DE POTENCIA	CARGA NORMAL	CORTE			
		CORTE			
		CORTE			
		CORTE			
		COAGULACION			
		COAGULACION			
		COAGULACION			
		COAGULACION			
	CARGA BAJA	CORTE	100		
		CORTE	100		
		CORTE	100		
		CORTE	100		
		COAGULACION	100		
		COAGULACION	100		
		COAGULACION	100		
		COAGULACION	100		
SALIDA BF		CORTE			
		COAGULACION			
FUGAS RF CHASIS	CORTE	CON CARGA			
		SIN CARGA			
	COAG	CON CARGA			
		SIN CARGA			
FUGAS RF PLACA DE PACIENTE	CORTE	CON CARGA			
		SIN CARGA			
	COAG	CON CARGA			
		SIN CARGA			
FUGAS RF ELECTRODO ACTIVO	CORTE	CON CARGA			
		SIN CARGA			
	COAG	CON CARGA			
		SIN CARGA			

3.2 Electrosurgery Power Output and Leakage Currents

The Safety of Electromedical Equipment

by
Dr Paolo Zavarini Eng
Responsible for electromedical and electronical hospital equipment USL 13 Ferrara, Italy

Introduction

The objective of this report is to pin-point useful methods to safeguard and prevent risks in medical environments.

From an analyses of existing publications and experiences achieved during different years of research work at the USL 31 of Ferrara, it is evident that the behaviour of the technicians and operators has played an important role in reaching adequate safety levels.

The Local Medical Unit 31 of Ferrara serves five towns providing assistance to a total population of 150,000 individuals. With 3,750 personnel, the Unit 31 accommodates 1,450 bed-places.

For over a decade, the Technical Assistance Service has been deeply concerned with the problems of safety, has gained more and more experience on the subject, is always on the look-out for possible conditions of risk, only to come-up with effective remedies.

Particular attention is being focused on such aspects as electrical, pollution, fire protection measures and mechanical problems especially in operating rooms, intensive therapy departments where the massive concentration of equipment and devices obviously increases the potentialities of risks.

It seems apparent that the education on safety encounters some difficulties in affirming itself in hospitals, or is simply not given the importance it deserves.

People continue to reason with ideas that belong to the past when it is necessary to keep up-to-date with today's constant advancements or the risk of being outraced by modern technological evolution and progress is inevitable.

Right from the start we were faced with several organisational problems, overcome some time after, caused by the shortage of skilled and professionally prepared technical personnel in the medical department.

Initial problems dealing with safety principally involved installations, utilities, pollution, fire precaution, machines, contamination risk to operating rooms due to the presence of anesthetic fly-away gases.

With this situation at hand, we endeavoured to cope and solve problems pertinent to safety by spotting possible hazards and by studying ways to affect them and correct the state of things.

Prevention was the next step.

Due to a lack of time and space it is feasibly impossible to discuss here all the arguments which, at one time or another, have received all attention and intervention.

It has therefore been decided to concentrate on one single topic concretely and extensively; namely electromedical equipment.

The Management: General Indications

The Public Health Service in Italy is the result of a series of laws, put together one on top of the other, originating as far back as the unification of the State of Italy.

Legislation 833 enacted 23 December 1978 marked the merging point in the organisation and evolution of the public health service.

Still, the reality is different today as it was then. Each USL (Local Sanitary Unit) can incorporate two organisations, each one capable of running the electromedical equipment in a correct and safe way.

Such organisational structure must be maintained in time.

The reality makes things difficult to accomplish as hinted below:-

(a) shortage of technical staff personnel professionally prepared to fulfill servicing needs directly; and
(b) guaranteed presence of technical staff personnel capable of meeting requirements, including machine maintenance (at least in part).

In this first case (a) the organisation is principally a technical-administrative force whose principal job is to maintain contacts with external, third, companies providing maintenance procedures, security tests, approves acquisition of new machines and performs periodic checks to ensure that safety levels are maintained in time.

The staff personnel working for the entire organisation do not have an easy job to carry out.

They must be endowed with professional knowledge and skill to accomplish various duties:-

(1) contracts for maintenance service drawn up with convenience in mind and according to the specific needs and requirements of the medical structure;
(2) ensure safety to the entire machine park; and
(3) handle new supplies.

Point (1) viz Contracts for servicing have to do with all technical-administrative aspects, taking into consideration circumstances as well as urgencies, convenience and the part of work commissioned to third companies.

The second point regards safety, made up essentially of two parts: purchase orders, require attentive investigation that existing norms and regulations are observed by manufacturers and that such conditions are naturally maintained in time by conducting periodic routine testing to important and distinctive parameters of the machine.

Finally, the third point deals with supplies: if a sound tie exists between medical and technical bodies, it is more likely that the choice of purchase is made in view of the parameters which each machine can actually offer, the results one purports to obtain in consideration of the use which the machine is designed for.

Getting back to case (b), where I'm personally involved, we are dealing with a complete organisation, made up of technical staff personnel permanently on premises.

LA SECURITE DES EQUIPEMENTS MEDICAUX

L'intention de cette revue est de préciser la technique à suivre pour éviter les accidents dans l'emploi des équipment médicaux. L'analyse des documents, et l'experience acquise a l'USL de Ferrara, on a pu conclure que la conduite des techniciens et du personnel affecté ont vue grande part à prendre pour achèver un niveau de securité adequat.

Eu particulier dans les salles d'operation, de soins intensifs, ou il y a une forte concentration d'équipment, électro-médicaux et donc un plus grand risque, la prévention des accidents due à l'électricité, la pollution, l'incendie, et a l'action mechanique est extrémement importante.

Il y a aussi les difficultés qui peuvent survenir quant on essaie de perfectionner le personnel employé à ces équipments modernes, ainsi que le manque d'agents qualifiés, en face des attitudes et pratiques traditionelles.

L'auteur presente les procedures pour l'identification des problèmes de securité et l'action à prendre pour les éviter.

USL 31: Experience and Management

After Legislation 833 came into force, in addition to the S. Anna, F. lli Borselli, S. Giorgio Hospital, the technical Service of Ferrara was put in charge of the various medical surgical care centers located in the territory.

Points of analyses for the electromedical equipment were as numerous as the factors which concern them:-

(1) maintenance (preventive, corrective);
(2) electrical safety of the machine (for patients, operators and environment);
(3) plant safety and installation;
(4) correct use (in connection also with the environment); and
(5) analyses of the various parameters.

Service Equipment

For many medical departments, service calls to machine are part of everyday urgencies and for this reason they must be viewed as one of the primary duties which the management of a hospital structure operating for years must be in the position to satisfy.

Our department meets this need in two ways:-

(1) by availing itself of the support of an electronical service within the department itself, capable of offering, professionally qualified expertise to meet the various needs, rapidly and efficiently (prompt intervention, co-operation with medical staff etc); and
(2) dependability provided by third companies which, on request, assist us with cases of repair where, for instance, spare parts or electric flow diagrams are absolutely required to get the machines running again.

Technical staff personnel must have good training basics, keep constantly up-to-date with technical advancements to better understand and solve specific problems and technical queries which could arise.

This is achieved by selecting personnel with the right background and knowledge which practical experience can only improve.

Emerging new technologies obviously represent a challenge for continuous enhanced education, establishing a correct relationship between manufacturing companies and/or suppliers and the technical service itself could be mutually helpful.

Participation at technical courses arranged by manufacturing/supplier companies are essential and mandatory for a proper up-dating in this field of developments.

They can infact offer the possibility to gain an almost perfect knowledge and understanding of machines, of their operational principles, and correct methods of use resulting in adequate management, effective prevention of technical inconveniences and an overall greater safety.

In case staff personnel are unable to fulfill these needs satisfactorily, recourse is made to third companies, under different forms of service contracts:-

(a) full risk, whereby the Service Company assures consistent and continuous equipment operation and performance.

An unlimited number of service calls and technical interventions are envisaged and eventually spare parts included. However, all parts and accessories better known as 'consumables' are not contemplated in the contract.

(b) general contracts, most varied; some may include spare parts, others foresee unlimited service, specific servicing or on request only, etc.

It can be said that almost half of the service duties carried out on machines installed at the Centre during a year were handled by staff personnel of the USL 31 (about 4,500), with considerable savings in terms of money and time of machine arrest.

Periodic testing to equipment calls for an efficient maintenance program, set-up systematically, which replaces worn-out parts, regulates calibrations whenever and wherever necessary, etc.

Safety

For some years now the question of safety of electromedical equipment conforming to IEC 601-1 Standards (equivalent to Italy's CEI 62-5) has assumed great significance.

Particular safety regulations exist in connection with: bedstead equipment, high frequency electrosurgery equipment, cardiac defibrillators with built-in monitor, shortwave therapeutical equipment, electrocardiographs, infusion pumps, microwave equipment therapy, patient monitoring systems, hemodialysis equipment, lung ventilators, equipment for anaesthesia, neonatal incubators, apparatus for ultrasound therapy, neuromuscular stimulators, equipment for clinical laboratory analyses, pacemakers, X-ray equipment.

An accurate study of specific norms and regulations for safety has contributed to the developments of suitable methods to obtain testing acceptance and periodic routine checks to machines.

Such a task however encountered many difficulties, firstly because we had to change to standards from a situation which existed and was functioning for years.

This is also why talk about modifications and patch-up jobs to machines was heard; normal consequences of a restriction in costs which do not take into account conditions for safety management of all components and parts which may come into contact, even if only superficially, with patient and/or operators.

The presence of electricity on patients already in precarious health conditions, and in many cases contemporaneously connected to more than one device by means of probes or catheters, can represent a potential hazard.

Low frequency currents (ten microampere) can have lethal consequences on patients a thousand times more vulnerable as compared to a normal individual.

In order to better understand how electrical contact can affect a person I will proceed to analyze two general situations macroshock and microshock.

Macroshock arises from the passage of electrical current applied between two hands, where one hand is externally exposed to a conductor momentarily under tension (ex framework of machine with failure at earth connection), and the other hand is in contact with an earth conductor.

Under such circumstances just a proportion of the current which passes from one hand to the other crosses the heart.

Such condition may occur in any environment where the electrical equipment has isolation failure at earth or due to accidential failure.

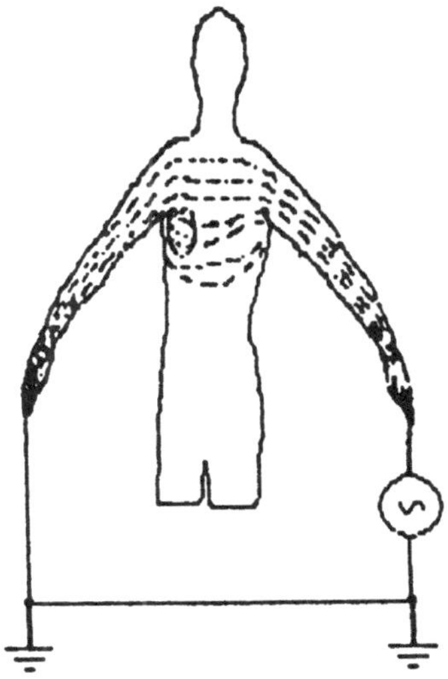

Microshock may arise in condition where the patient is connected to an electrode (catheter) in direct contact with the earthed heart.

Should accidentally, the patient come into contact with a framework under tension, the electrical current flowing between the two points will concentrate at the heart.

Direct stimulation may result.

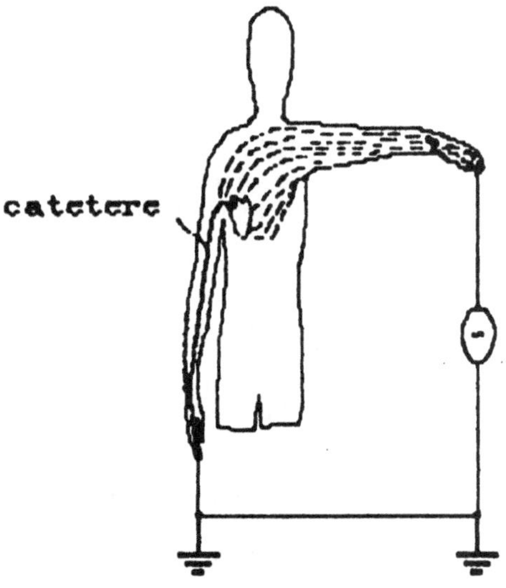

It is necessary to analyse the magnitude of the current that flows in order to understand the risks of ventricular stimulation involved in both cases indicated above.

The hazard current threshold for macroshock is about 200mA, whereas for microshock 20 microA is considered dangerous.

Electrical installations and medical equipment must therefore be engineered and constructed using particular safety expedients and precautions.

Before describing the testing procedure which equipments undergo, let us look at two important classifications:-

(1) Classification of the location where the equipment will be installed and will operate (hospital room, ambulatory, laboratory, intensive care department operation room etc).
(2) Classification of the equipment according to the type of standards, general or particular.

An identification card for each single equipment is kept by our service department, noting:-

- trademark;
- manufacturer/supplier;
- serial number;
- inventory;
- allocation;
- classification; and
- type.

In-coming supplies are checked to assure that order requirements are met and that all necessary documentation has been regularly included (hand-books, technical manuals, approved standards certificate, operational diagrams, warranty etc).

A study is made to correctly interpret meanings and practices of symbols found on machines.

Tests and practical operational trials are then conducted on instruments and constructional component parts:-

- main power switch;
- fuses;
- checking against human errors during use; and
- checking the state of supply cable, plug and relative compatibility with the electrical system.

Instrumental inspection is then carried out to verify that:-

(1) the resistance value of the earth cable (referred to class I equipment) does not exceed standard values imposed;
(2) leakage currents;
    - to earth;
    - in the chassis;
    - in the patient; and
    - ancillary equipment connected to the patient.

Another important control regards alarm warnings. In accordance with standards, they must be checked for presence and performance.

As concerns equipment with specific requirements described earlier, it is necessary to fulfill specific controls and measurements such as: high frequency leakage current and electrosurgery power, test of power-energy generated for defibrillators, adequate construction and presence of all necessary alarms.

The Technical Service of the Local Medical Unit USL 31 of Ferrara together with its electronical Dept takes care of this control.

Equally important, it supervises over safety levels, sees that they are maintained in time for the entire lot of machines, by effecting necessary periodic controls at least once a year for electromedical equipment.

It may be decided to put a machine out of use if it does not fall within safety levels and no modification is possible.

The electronic department operates with the aid of computers which are indispensable for the input of test data, for the management of general files and records relative to the equipment, as reminders when periodic safety checks are due, to verify servicing performed by staff personnel as well as by outside companies.

All this falls under the subject of management which controls maintenance costs for each single machine in time, and shows convenience of repairs brought to machines, residual costs etc.

Conclusion

The organisation within a complex structure as that of the Public Health Service is a difficult affair especially as concerns technologies.

A method of information must exist which permits us to analyse and evaluate the true efficiency of the machine, its method of use and safety, to gain new technologies or replace old ones based on certain economical aspects: Estimated value of the single equipment up-dated yearly, method of amortisation at constant quotas, calendar schedule of programmed maintenance calls, expiration of warranties, safety standards.

We have sought useful indications to establish a purchasing policy which keeps a 'watchful eye' on prices, obtained through standard contracts, setting-up criteria to evaluate machine potentialities and effective performances, service costs involved, and organisational impact on the users.

When it comes to safeguarding, for so many important parameters, the professional expertise of a 'pool' of qualified personnel within the medical structure becomes essential.

In addition to an organisational structure and safety methods summarised earlier, a constructive relationship between the electronic personnel and the medical staff is equally important; nothing must be left to chance, the very best use must be made of all resources available, all precautions for prevention must be adopted for greater life saving.

Systems of Security and Methods as Applied to Hospital Environments

by

J. H. Gibbons IEng, FSERT, MIHospE
West Berkshire HA

Until recently security was one of the Cinderella departments within most hospitals, and at best not much more than lip service was attached to it.

I feel that this attitude stems from the fact that in the past hospitals were much more disciplined. 'The Matron' had her eagle eyes on the staff, the doctors, the patients and visitors. The results of misdemeanours were dealt with more severely. No matter what or where things went wrong Matron was behind you.

Hospitals had an in-built discipline; they were much more revered and respected than now, and people generally were more honest.

Post-war hospital development has seen a mixture of upgraded workhouses with bits added on as required and finance allowed, to a variety of building developments from single storey buildings with or without link corridors through to multi-storey blocks, some with 17 or more floors.

The element of security that such diverse building patterns require is quite challenging and is on a par with airports, docks, railway stations and the channel tunnel.

Crime Prevention

Security

Territorial Defence — Security of buildings, departments, wards and the site.

Intruder Deterrent — Burglar alarms.

Protection— Staff, patients, visitors, property etc.

Whatever you call it, why do we need it? A quotation that I feel to be appropriate is 'Society prepares the crime; criminals commit it'.

A classic example of this may be seen in the supermarkets where shoppers gaily wheel their trollies round with the purse or wallet lying on top in full view. Or they have handbags open swinging on their arms displaying the housekeeping cash — often called 'the little old lady' syndrome, why I know not. It applies to all persons regardless of age.

They have unwittingly prepared the crime. The criminal, you may rest assured, is not far behind.

From now on the term 'Hospital' will include clinics, surgeries, community nursing, home care patients, domicilliary outpatients, ambulance services etc.

Walking round hospital buildings and grounds I see many examples of the 'little old lady' syndrome. Typically some of them are:-

(a) Staff and patient changing rooms — unlocked and doors wide open — lockers badly sited and used.
(b) Personal items — keys, wallets, bags, lying on tables whilst queueing for a coffee. Yes, it does happen.
(c) Cars parked with contents on the seats; an open invitation to the criminal.

Incidentally, cars parked out of sight behind a building are an even better invitation. Apart from the contents, you may find your wheels missing, even your engine!

The success of crime and the success of protection from crime is very dependent on personal attitudes. Health Authorities and hospitals would be well advised to invest in staff indoctrination in crime prevention, with particular emphasis on their own department, ward, clinic etc.

With high staff turnover this may present difficulties, but staff training on simple crime protection may well save the necessity for costly security systems.

Security within hospitals should mean just that. Every ward, department, office, staff accommodation, should be looked at in depth and a security cost-effective rating given to it.

Each department has a value which may for example include:-

(a) an asset value;
(b) the building and its fabric, and services supplied to it;
(c) contents such as medical, laboratory or other equipment; and
(d) a contribution value, ie its value to the overall health care system.

What is the cost to the service if your department is out of action due to theft, vandalism, break-in, fire, flood etc?

How much value or worth this is to the hospital or health service will influence the budget allocation for security which, in turn, will influence the type of system to be used.

Typical areas of importance will include:-

(1) patients, personnel;
(2) property, building etc;
(3) stores and contents;
(4) linen, laundry and clothing;
(5) catering dept food and equipment;
(6) drugs — pharmacy, path labs, wards;
(7) offences against the person ie assaults and violence, abduction, assassination, industrial action;
(8) road traffic within NHS premises;
(9) vehicle security — cars, lorries, ambulances;
(10) fraud — financial and contract;
(11) physical security of the hospital;
(12) computer security, programmes etc;
(13) security of information;
(14) security of cash; and
(15) security in mental and psychiatric hospitals (a) high security wards, (b) regional secure units.

It is obvious from the above list, which is not complete, that well planned professional systems are going to be the

SYSTEMES ET METHODS DE SECURITE EN MILIEU HOSPITALIER

Jusqu'à récemment, la prévention des délits et actes criminels en milieu hospitalier représentait bien le moindre des soucis des responsables. Il est vrai que précédemment, une discipline stricte régnait dans les hôpitaux. L'infirmière-chef (the 'matron') surveillait de près tout le personnel, les médecins, les patients et les visiteurs. Toute faute, si minime soit-elle, était sévérement sanctionnée. Rien ne lui échappait.

Les hôpitaux avaient une sort d'auto-discipline. Ils étaient bien plus respectés et le public était plus honnête.

Les hôpitaux qui se sont développés après la guerre varient, depuis les 'workhouses' (sortes d'asiles pour pauvres) auxquels s'ajoutaient des parties annexes ici et là à mesure que les finances le permettaient, jusqu'à toute une série de bâtiments d'un seul étage avec ou sans couloirs de communication, ou multi-étages (17 ou plus dans certains cas).

Avec une pareille variété, les problèmes de sécurité sont bien réels et peuvent aisément se comparer à ceux des aéroports, des chantiers navals, des gares ou même du tunnel sous la Manche.

Cet article traite les nombreux aspects des problèmes de sécurité en milleu hospitalier.

most cost-effective approach. Your local DIY kit spells disaster in these situations.

Health Authorities are recommended to approach more seriously the total security concept. Guidelines and recommendations have been published by the NAHA England and Wales, and by the Department, viz the NHS Security Manual 1984, Losses Theft and Security in the NHS 1982, and DHSS Security Circular LAC (84) 1.

Guidelines and recommendations do not in themselves solve problems, neither do they identify them. Perhaps ones first awareness that a problem may exist is by the number of complaints from staff or heads of departments.

Maybe audit deficits or irregularities are a clue. Your stores and stock controls may well throw up clues; so may your supplies and purchasing procedures. The list is as large as the number of problems.

Awareness that all is not well in your department should not be passed over and left until it is serious. This does not mean that you immediately apply for a budget to procure a security system. Until you have identified the real problem and its root cause, the type of system required, if indeed one is required, will be an unknown factor. First look inwards at your department, the staff, including yourself, the departments' working methods and procedures.

Are they security orientated? Are they open to abuse? ie can they be fiddled?

Staff morale — is it good? If not, why not? Personal animosities, dislikes, hatreds etc.

The general working environment — is it safe and secure for persons in it? If not they are unlikely to behave in an appropriate manner.

In consultation with your staff a fairly simple working procedure may be implemented.

Crime Prevention and Personal Security

Perhaps you could look at:-

(1) Methods of protecting staff and personal property. The NHS as a body does not accept responsibility for loss or damage of personal property. However under the Health and Safety Act they are obliged to ensure that safe and secure facilities are provided for use by staff.
(2) What is the probability of staff being assaulted, in any way, in your department?
(3) Physical attack and armed raiders. It would appear that hospitals are not immune from such incidences.

Staff who become victims of crime at any level suffer emotional upset and will require support in the knowledge that follow-up investigations will be carried out. In severe cases the victims may require counselling. Do not underestimate the effect that even petty crime will have on your staff. The air of suspicion that lingers in a department is very demoralising, both individually and as a body.

Many Authorities and hospitals now realise the importance and cost-effectiveness of a total security commitment, and either set up a department in its own right, or incorporate it as part of Health and Safety or Risk Management.

In either case the following is usually included:-

(1) An effective corporate policy and general organisational procedure.
(2) A security department with good operational and management procedures.
(3) Incident reporting procedures by the staff and procedures for calling the police.
(4) Crime prevention training.

The Security Manager should be responsible for producing security passes and identity badges and ensure that the security policy and procedures are carried out within budget allocations.

Security

What do we mean when we use this word? The Shorter Oxford English Dictionary gives the definition as:-

> The condition of being secure; the condition of being protected from or not exposed to danger; freedom from doubt; freedom from care, anxiety or apprehension; a feeling of safety.

Chambers Dictionary gives it as:-

> A feeling or means of being secure; protection from espionage, carelessness etc; a pledge, a guarantee, a right conferred on a creditor to make him sure of recovery.

Are we not in danger of using the word 'security' when we really mean protection, defence, or deterrents against crime, vandalism, personal attack etc? When analysing problems you will find that your choice of words will affect your approach to, and the analysis of, the problems.

The cost of making anything 'secure' is quite high. Whereas the cost of protection and deterrent is relatively inexpensive. It may even be more cost-effective and equally as 'crime preventive'.

To compress as much as possible into the available time I will discuss equipment hardware in parallel with examples of probable uses in some hospital departments.

Intruder Deterrent and Protection

Wards are one of the areas most difficult to control. Generally they are open plan, may have more than one point of access and are freely accessible to staff and visitors. To attempt anything more than basic precautions may give patients the impression of being in an institution rather than a hospital. Problems here are associated with:-

(a) The patient. If there is any known threat to them or the patient is a VIP who may be vulnerable to unwarranted attention, they should of course be in rooms where the necessary precautions are more easily implemented.
(b) Patients generally are responsible for their own personal effects. Valuables or cash, if they must be brought into hospital, should be locked in the ward safe.
(c) Bedside lockers are provided for patients' use and loss or theft from them is very low in the statistics.

If necessary, alarm devices are available for use with lockers, but they may cause more problems than they solve.

Should patients received unwelcome visitors, or consider that they are under threat, the nurse call system may be an effective way of calling for help.

On the other hand staff may be more vulnerable and open to attack than patients. In this situation it will be necessary to look at staffing levels and to discuss ways of alerting other staff for assistance ie panic buttons located at convenient points; personal attack alarms. Patients should also be encouraged to summon help.

I am talking here of a general ward with free and open access. Hard and fast rules are difficult to apply and implement. Nursing management should discuss problems with their staff, and if necessary a consultant may be called in.

Accident and Emergency Department

Departments such as these are usually the only ones open to the public at night. It is important to plan security so that trespassers, drunks, junkies and other persona non grata do not gain access to the main hospital or sensitive areas such as patients records, path labs pharmacy etc via this department.

Where, for numerous reasons, to impose a physical barrier such as a locked door between the A & E and other parts of the hospital may not be acceptable, surveillance by closed circuit television may assist in identifying trouble. It will of course require someone to watch the monitor screen or screens. Two-way radios, attack alarms and security guards are other methods that may be appropriate to this particular problem.

Vehicle access control on the approach to the A & E doors may be considered. A pressure pad or inductive loop is buried in the approach road. When an ambulance passes over this point its approach is indicated to the reception area and electronically controlled doors are unlocked. Once the patient and crew pass through the doors either the reception desk will activate and lock the doors again, or a PIR detector will sense that they have entered and automatically re-lock them. Alternatively, on departure the ambulance may pass another set of buried detectors which cause the A & E doors to close and lock. An extension of this would, by means of transponders in the ambulance, record the code for that vehicle, its time of arrival and departure. Vehicles other than ambulances would sound an 'alert' rather than an 'alarm' at the reception desk, with or without visual warning, enabling appropriate action to be taken.

Access Control

As its name implies enables the control of access to areas, buildings, car parks, hazardous areas etc by a variety of methods usually by electronics, but mechanical methods may be used.

In addition to intruder alarms and security lighting access control is amongst the most useful forms of security systems within a hospital.

There are numerous types, all of which are designed to allow access to controlled areas only to authorised persons:-

(a) digital keypad coded locks;
(b) magnetic swipe cards;
(c) smart cards;
(d) weigand cards;
(e) voice recognition;
(f) fingerprint pattern recognition;
(g) eye retina pattern recognition;
(h) door 'phones; and
(i) door T/V 'phones.

Two other methods now at the trial stage are the use of digitised frame store technique to store a photo-image of the face and compare this with the T/V scan of the person requiring access, and a system that will scan non-invasively the vascular blood flow, analyse the cell structure, and compare that with previously stored data. Other methods of biological sensing are under development.

I must not digress!

Whichever system is used, the object is to allow only authorised persons, vehicles or property to proceed through the controlled area.

Methods of alarms and systems management depend on the level of security required, the system design, and management protocol.

Security Lighting

This plays an important part from dusk till dawn in areas such as car parks, public and staff areas, walkways, passageways, internal and external pathways that may be classified as risk areas for staff and patients.

Lighting may be planned as zones (areas). Each zone may be a system in its own right. Alternatively they operate on a zonal entry/exit sequential basis; in which case zones are arranged to illuminate a given area in front and behind a body moving from one zone to the other. Detectors sense a body entering and leaving a zone and switch lights on for a pre-determined time, after which, if no movement is detected they switch off. The zones are, of course, bi-directional.

Levels of lighting required will be governed by the area and site to be illuminated. Remember that the brighter the light, the darker the shadows, and of course, the risk of dazzle.

Lighting is an effective deterrent against the opportunist or petty thief, who relies on concealment and a fast in-and-out technique. Delay his movements and light up his area of activity. It may well save several hundred pounds worth of damage to your property, even if the contents amount to very little.

Psychiatric Hospitals

These create a different criteria in that the patients may be a bigger threat to the safety of staff than to security. Patients, their behaviour, conduct and well-being is the remit of the nurses and nursing heirarchy.

Safety of the staff and protection of the patient (or should it be the other way round?) is the responsibility of the Health Authority. Generally psychiatric hospitals and mental illness units manage day to day running without serious incidents. Where a number of disturbed high risk patients exists in any one hospital it is usual to contain them in one or two wards classified as high risk, or secure, wards or units.

The equipment in such areas may comprise:-

(a) panic alarm buttons in specific areas;
(b) alarm buttons integrated with a group call paging system;
(c) personal attack alarms of the radio frequency type routed to a central panel; and
(d) personal attack alarms based on ultrasonic or infra red transmissions. These, although not ideal, have their uses when linked with a radio system forming part of an incident location method.

Such systems are used to summon help and will only be as effective as the management protocol.

Any device that hangs around the nurses neck, including jewellery, should be banned, particularly in high risk areas.

High Security and Regional Secure Units

In addition to personal attack alarms for staff these will incorporate security fencing and gate or gates surrounding the entire site. Closed circuit TV at the main gate, main door, and other strategic points inside and outside buildings; infra red night TV cameras; site floodlighting to enhance normal background levels.

Fencing

The construction, design and installation of security fences and gates is well documented in Home Office, DHSS and BSI publications. Protection and detection against attempts to cut through or scale the fence may make use of:-

(a) microphonic cable, which is a sensor cable installed on the fabric of the fence, which acts as a tuned mircophone reacting to any impact movement of the fence, however slight;
(b) taut wire is a mechanical device detecting the deflection or cutting of wires held under tension between fence posts, coupled to an acoustic sensor and possibly a broken circuit detector; and
(c) microwave curtain, an invisible pattern of microwave energy is generated by a transmitter and field pattern disturbances are detected by a receiver.

Vertical and horizontal coverage is good. Other methods such as geophones, electrostatic sensors, electromagnetic buried lines and pressure tubes are outside the scope of this paper, but do have uses in high risk areas and other Government and Military establishments.

Closed Circuit Television

This, using slow scan frame store (or frame comparison) techniques, is very useful to scan large areas. It does not require an operator to continuously watch a screen; an alarm will be raised when changes are detected between successive frames, or every third, fourth, fifth frame etc, however it is set.

Internal Intruder Detection

Within any hospital there will be areas where only authorised staff should be permitted at any hour, day or night. To cover such situations a combination of a simple access control door lock or door phone, coupled with correctly selected and correctly placed PIR (passive infra red) detectors will cover most internal requirements for administration, outpatients, physiotherapy, works department, boiler house, plant rooms etc.

PIR's work on the principle of heat detection and the changing radiated heat pattern given off by a moving body. The area covered is a function of the lens used in the detector and the detector element itself.

The market is becoming so full of a variety of this type of detector, many of which boast at least three or four different freznal type lens configurations, which may be changed by the user or installer, that it is not surprising that problems arise due to bad positioning, incorrect lens configuration for the design requirements, false triggering etc.

Having said that, a well-planned system using PIR works very well and is an improvement on older methods.

System Management

I have spent some time giving a very brief overview of some of the uses for which security components may be used. However there is little point in designing and installing any system when no thought has been given to the management of it. An alarm sounds, lights flash, and, as is the case when bells clang outside the High Street bank, nothing happens. It rings for hours. Eventually a keyholder arrives to re-set the alarms. Much the same is happening in hospitals. Some may even switch systems off because they forget code numbers, or lose a swipe card. I have seen doors wedged open because it is not convenient for staff to use the system.

Appoint a security officer. Ensure that the system is designed to meet *your* requirements, and that it will respond to *your* problems, and that people will use it. Manage the system properly. Tell people in no uncertain terms exactly what they must do when an alarm sounds, or what will happen if they abuse or mis-use it.

I had originally intended to be more technically orientated and describe the technological aspects of equipment and systems design. This I soon discovered was developing into a complete one-day session. It was therefore necessary to carry out some drastic surgery for transplanting in the future.

Summarising the main points of this paper:-

(1) It is vital to discuss with staff at all levels the importance of security awareness in the form of crime prevention at their place of work.
(2) Set up a working party to examine problems.
(3) Ensure that you understand fully the problems and their causes.
(4) Plan a system that gives you the protection required.
(5) Ensure that staff and management are aware of the consequences of implementing security procedures.
(6) Look at the existing equipment market and be prepared to consider the interfacing of different types to meet your requirements.
(7) You may wish to support your project in part or in total with the services of an independent consultant.

In conclusion may I suggest that where data highways exist, consideration be given to intergrating the systems within the data network. It may be linked to energy management and fire alarm highways.

Piped Medical Gas Services

by

S. Phillips
Groote Schuur Hospital,
Cape Town, South Africa

In the continual changes of health care and technology it would be worthwhile to reflect on medical gas services and allied equipment as used in the past 20 years. Most anaesthetic machines have now lost the gas cylinders, (and only retain the oxygen cylinder) for emergency purposes. We have seen the greatest change with the oxygen/air blender which has transformed the gas services to the intensive care unit. In the same period we have grown from a small oxygen, nitrous oxide, and vacuum service in theatres, and now add low and high pressure medical air, entonox, carbon dioxide, and the more recent Draeger Scavenger System.

Having been involved in the planning, design and commissioning of the Medical Gas System, at the New Groote Schuur Hospital, it may be desirable to give a short overview of the building itself. The construction was carried out on a sloping site, which has 13 levels at one end and 10 at the other.

There are five levels which are windowed, and these are the nursing and medical wards. Between each of these levels is an interfloor where all services (M&E, air conditioning, medical gas, etc) are run. The ward areas are dry wall construction, and all services either drop or rise from the interfloor as desired, such services being in the dry wall, or in an horizontal trunking which contain the bed head services. The lower levels of the building are taken up with stores distribution, cleaning services, plant rooms etc.

Now let us consider the safety features of the medical gas services, and the best area to commence would be the Gas Bank. A decision was taken in September 1988, at an SABS meeting, to extend the Pin Index Coding of medical gas cylinder to all sizes of cylinders. This is indeed a giant step forward, from two points of view.

The first being the extension of a safe code which has applied to the small gas cylinders used on anaesthetic machines, this code being formulated in the USA in 1953, and introduced into South Africa in 1970. The second major safety feature is that we will no longer have two different valves on, oxygen cylinders in the hospital environment, (as exist at present) and all cylinders will be pin indexed. This from a gas bank installation is of paramount importance, as it prevents the interchange of oxygen and air cylinders, (and from personal experience of witnessing air cylinders connected to an oxygen bank, giving a hospital oxygen purity of 63%), this can no longer happen. From the designers approach we can now house all cylinders or gas banks in the same room, because the interchange of such cylinders is prevented by the Pin Index Coding.

All the gas lines that reticulated from the gas bank, are individually painted, colours which have been accepted for a number of years.

It is agreed that from an international view, and the colour codes in South Africa, problems of identity could arise with other countries, but the earlier ISO/South Africa code of 'Colour Banding' has not been found to be acceptable in the Cape Province, as clarity of identification in maintenance is deemed to be very important. The medical gases are reticulated at the following pressures: Oxygen 450Kpa, Nitrous Oxide 360Kpa, Vacuum 15/24inHG, LP Air 420Kpa, HP Air 700Kpa, Entonox 350Kpa and Carbon Dioxide 300Kpa.

The compressor plant room, is the next important one to be considered, and a very successful form of installation introduced in 1968, has been incorporated in the New Groote Schuur Hospital. There are eight Ingersoll Rand (Model 10T3 NL) oil free compressors, running as four duplex units. From the layout diagram you will see the simplicity of the installation, in particular the filter/drying process. All compressors have a two cubic metre storage receiver, and are cycled to run consecutively. When attempting to cycle the compressors with electrical controls, a very complex systems of relays is required.

With however the pneumatic system as illustrated, any multiple of compressors can be installed or additions made, without any need for major electrical switchboard changes.

The cycling of the compressors is controlled by the 'Mercoid' pressure switch on the receiver which determines the on/off running of the plant to the required differential. For instance, when Plant A starts running, (to replace the differential now used) a pneumatic signal (50Kpa) is switched onto Plant B delivery regulator, thus receiver B now supplies the hospital. When Plant A stops the pneumatic signal to regulator B will remain 'locked in' until the mercoid on/off control on Plant B makes and starts the B compressors. At that time the Plant B mercoid will exhaust the signal on its own regulator, and apply a further pneumatic signal to Plant C, which will then start delivery air to the hospital.

The overall feature of this installation, is primarily the complete dryness of delivered air.

From the stop/start compressor principle most of the condensate falls out in the receivers, and with the use of the 'Van Air' (Model D16) deseccant dryers only delivering air from the individual plant in use the delivered air has so far always passed the necessary bacteria testing which is regularly carried out. You may feel that the overall cost of such an installation, is high but this is not the case. From a maintenance view point, any plant can be taken out of service, for whatever reason, and the only need for attention would be to disconnect the pneumatic signal device from such plant under maintenance, and the remainder of the whole installation functions normally.

Let us now move into the user areas where medical gas services are required. Operating theatres are no doubt the priority, and the multiplicity of such services must retain the overall safety features. The normal anaesthetists need of oxygen, nitrous oxide, vacuum, low pressure air, carbon dioxide, and scavenging, are all positioned on the wall installation, in both theatre and induction rooms. There are ceiling pendants which carry these same services, but the medical gas services are not now duplicated on opposite walls in the designated theatres.

For the surgeon, separate vaccum outlets are installed, with further outlets for high pressure air, this being used for power tools etc. A ceiling pendant is also provided for the surgeon, with the vacuum and HP are being fitted to the pendant. The provision of HP air is always kept away from the anaesthetic gases are installed. All services are individually valved in wall mounted boxes outside the theatre, which from a maintenance aspect is most important.

From the safety aspect we have installed in the New

GAINES TECHNIQUES POUR LA DISTRIBUTION DES GAZ MEDICAUX

Une revue historique de développement des équipment des gaines techniques, et des procedures pour l'emploi des gaz médicaux pendant les 20 annees passées, et une discussion le l'application de nouvelles methods pour ces gaz à l'hôpital, Groote Schuur, Cape Town, Afrique du Sud.

Hospital the updated configuration for medical gas outlets, and this is a giant step forward. All the outlets are of different configuration, with the safe gases adopting the 14mm probe dimension, and the toxic gases the 12mm dimension. This therefore ensures the added safety feature, that if by any means the configuration was overcome, then with a 12mm probe inserted into the 14mm outlet, only a safe gas could be delivered. The installation of piped medical gases with all the safety standards that are incorporated, unfortunately does not prevent the wrongful connection of any probe to a designated service, and this factor still remains the greatest single hazard to medical gas services.

In moving to the ward areas, the bed head trunking accommodates all the necessary nursing services. Many attempts have been made to a suitable bed head trunking, and in the case of the New Hospital a three sectioned aluminium extrusion was designed. The lower section is used for medical gas at a height of 1.5m, AFL, the centre section for Low Voltage circuitry (communications — nurse call etc) and the upper section for switch socket outlets. The trunking can accommodate six gas services, and all are provided with isolating valves except the medical vacuum. The beauty of this trunking is the facility for extension or alteration of the services without the need for chasing walls, or running surface pipework etc. A recent addition of extra oxygen and vacuum outlets to those installed was carried out in two hours, without any other disruption to the remainder of the ward.

The appendix drawings give a layout of the ring main pipework for the various services, but the vacuum service is provided from the three towers on the roof of the main building, on each phase of construction (as earlier explained).

Two vacuum plants were provided in each tower, and from this plant room a vertical ring main drops down into the building to the fifth level where a horizontal line completes the ring. The vacuum plants are time clock controlled (through the building management system) and each plant runs for a two hour period. A 'baffle' receiver is positioned on the fifth level, and if the plant 'on run' is not able to cope, then the fifth level control will start the second plant in the same plant room. All the plants therefore run for four hours each daily, and ample facility exists to carry out maintenance.

An equaliser pipeline connects the three plant rooms at the 13th floor level, and a further equaliser is provided on the seventh level (theatres). This equaliser is valved at all interconnections to facilitate isolation of any area that may be desirable.

Many changes will also be made in the future, and it would indeed be a major advance if the use of air separation plants could be used for medical oxygen provision.

The handling of cylindered gas is very expensive, and with the overall demand from the user to piped gas services, it is most desirable to consider on site plant which will provide the necessary gas services (ie Oil Free compressors). Many of the hospitals in South Africa are remote from gas production centres, and many problems could be eliminated with on-site plant. A further major consideration to gas services must be to prevent wastage, and particular reference is made to the Oxygen/Air blender, which has a created leak, for balance of the delivered oxygen concentration. This should be looked at because it has been recorded on many cases of paediatric care that approximately 60% of the input gases were wasted to atmosphere.

The overall cost of medical gas installation is always a large factor, but it is of great importance that the safety features of such installations are not jeopardised by any economy. The demands of the health care user of gas services must always be met with the greatest safety standards prevailing, and to give the end user the peace of mind that these gas services cannot fail.

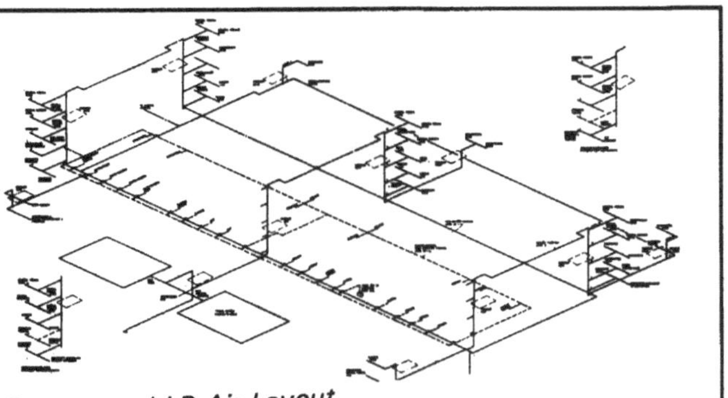

Oxygen and LP Air Layout.

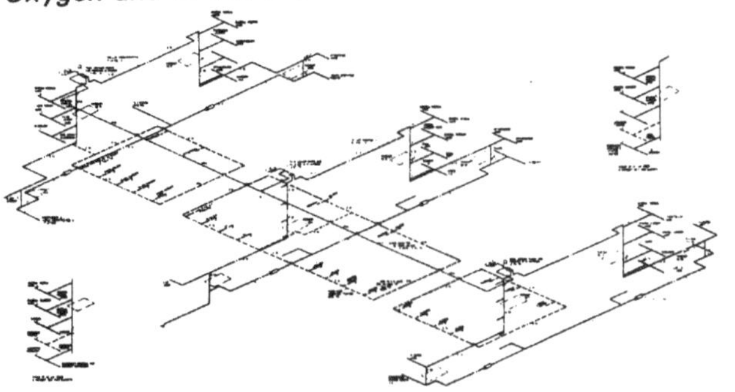

Vacuum Layout.

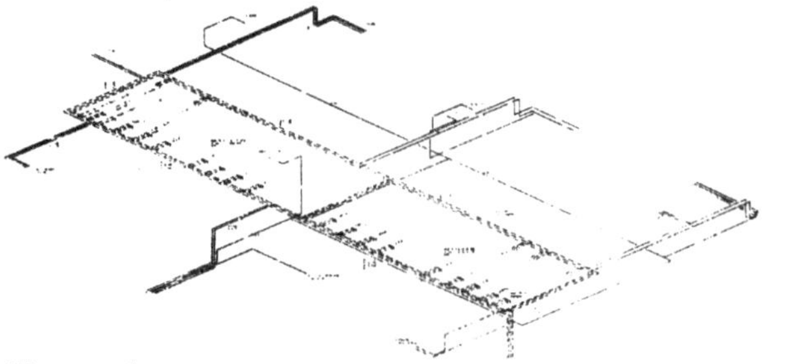

Theatre Layout.

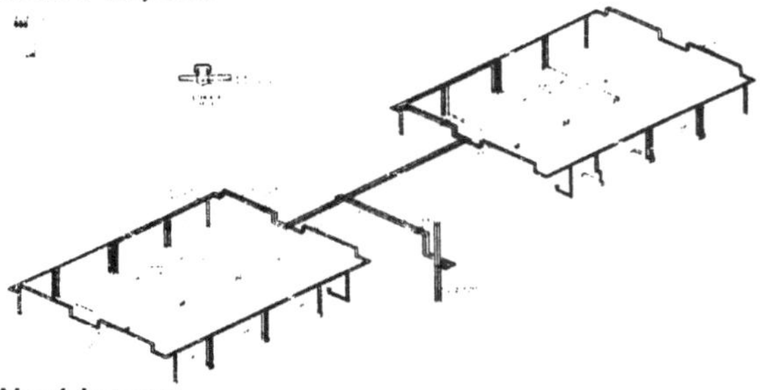

Ward Layout.

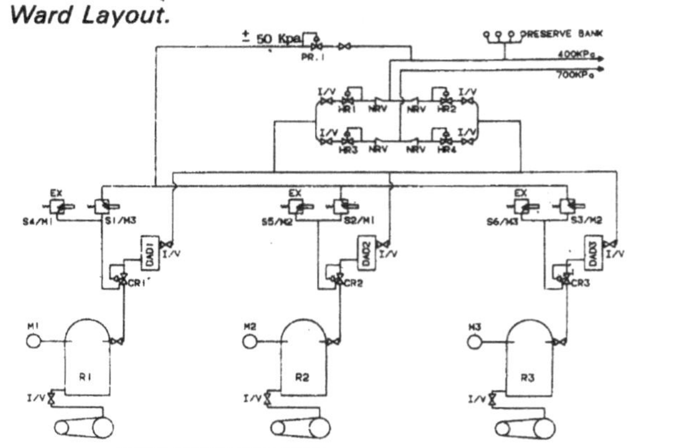

MEDICAL AIR COMPRESSOR SYSTEM

RUNNING SEQUENCE CONTROL

1. ALL RECEIVERS SET BY MERCURY SWITCH TYPE CONTROL TO CYCLE BETWEEN 850KPa AND 1100 Kpa
2. ALL CONTROL REGULATORS (C.R.) SET AT 800 Kpa
3. WHEN MERCURY SWITCH 1 "CLOSES" A PILOT SIGNAL OF 50 Kpa IS APPLIED TO CONTROL REGULATOR 2. THIS SIGNAL NOW MEANS CR2 IS FEEDING AT 850 Kpa AND RECEIVER 2 IS SUPPLYING THE SYSTEM.

   WHEN MERCURY SWITCH 1 "OPENS" THIS CONTROL SIGNAL IS "LOCKED IN" AND RECEIVER 2 CONTINUES TO SUPPLY THE SYSTEM UNTIL MERCURY SWITCH 2 OPERATES.
4. WHEN MERCURY SWITCH 2 "CLOSES" A PILOT SIGNAL IS NOW APPLIED TO CR3 AND THE "LOCKED IN" SIGNAL TO CR2 IS EXHAUSTED BY SOLENOID S5.
5. THIS SEQUENCE CAN BE MADE FOR A MULTIPLE OF COMPRESSORS. MONITORING IS BY MEANS OF "RUNNING TIME CLOCKS" TO EACH INDIVIDUAL COMPRESSOR. NO FAILURE OF ANY SECTION OF THIS SYSTEM CAN RENDER COMPLETE FAILURE, AND ANY INDIVIDUAL ALARMS WOULD BE INSTALLED, FOR LOW PRESSURE INDICATION IN RECEIVER, INDICATING PLANT FAILURE. THESE ALARMS WOULD BE SET AT 820 Kp ON SEPARATE MERCURY SWITCHES.

LEGEND

R1.2.3	- AIR RECEIVERS
DAD	- DESSICANT AIR DRYER
CR1.2.3	- CONTROL REGULATOR
I/V	- ISOLATING VALVE
M1.2.3	- MERCURY SWITCH CONTROL
S1.2.3	- PILOT SOLENOIDS
S4.5.6	- EXHAUST SOLENOIDS
PR.1	- PILOT REGULATORS
HR1.2.3.4	- HOSPITAL SUPPLY REGULATOR
NRV	- NON RETURN VALVE

SEQUENCING SYSTEM FOR MEDICAL AIR COMPRESSORS LAYOUT AND FUNCTION

Prevention of Airborne Transmission of Infection Past, Present and Future

by

F. H. Howorth
OBE, FRSA, FIPI, PPIHospE
Oulton Research Laboratories
Chorley, Lancashire

History

That air is a vehicle which transports infective organisms in the operating theatre and elsewhere was first identified by Lister (1827-1912), then in 1919 by Huxley and Howorth, F. C., over exposed fermentation processes and subsequently in 1961 by Charnley and Howorth, F. H., in the operating room.

IN 1962 Howorth donated a prototype ultra clean air (UCA) enclosure to Wrightington hospital for Charnley to use during hip joint replacement. Because of its appearance, it was known as 'the greenhouse' and during the 933 hip joint replacement operations done there, it became apparent that the lower the number of colony forming units (CFU) in the air around the wound, the instruments and everything which is to come into contact with the wound, then the lower is the incidence of wound sepsis[1].

Clinical trials conducted jointly by the British Department of Health and the Medical Research Council[2] showed that there is a linear relation between CFU in the air and wound sepsis whether antibiotics are used or not. In order to prevent peripheral entrainment of extraneous contaminants and their inward dispersion to the UCA zone (Figure 2) the first two generations of Charnley Howorth UCA systems had transparent side walls extending down to 150mm (6in) above the floor.

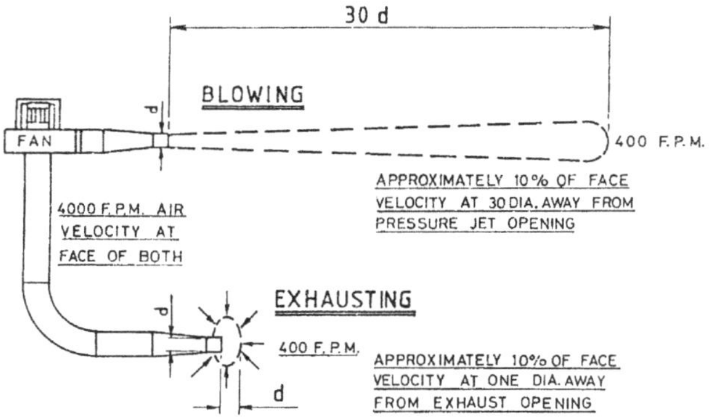

Figure 1: Ratio between sucking and blowing air.

The third generation overcame the problems of peripheral entrainment and inward dispersion of contaminants by establishing a downward and exponentially curved outward UCA pattern from below partial walls extending down to 2m (6ft 6in) above the floor. This was achieved using a regressively graded air flow diffuser which allowed the gentle pull of the re-circulation inlets to induce a slow outward air flow[3].

Present

Based on the monitoring results of performances of various types of UCA systems and observing the very local pull provided by air suction (Figure 1) the fourth generation of UCA systems, the Omniflow, has been designed and developed at the Ollerton Laboratories.

The Omniflow requires no side panels and may be installed either below or level with the false ceiling. Its downward and outward UCA flow pattern is not dependent on the pull of re-circulation inlets; it is positively projected to oppose the peripheral entrainment and inward dispersion of extraneous contaminants.

The omnidirectional downward and outward air flow pattern is achieved by locating rows of air projector apertures all around the perimeter of the central downward air discharge area. From these rows of air outlets, the UCA is projected radially at a higher velocity and in this way positively opposes the entry of airborne contaminants (Figure 3).

The Omniflow UCA system can operate with either integral or remote fans and because there are no partial side walls so operating lights, cameras, image intensifiers etc can move freely. A streamlined lighting system is located on all four sides of the Omniflow, this provides good background lighting for the whole of the operating room.

The Omniflow UCA projector has variable air flow control and so it is able to accept either bio filters or HEPA filters. It is, therefore, applicable not only to surgery, but also to pharmaceutical and microelectronic processes where air cleanliness standards are currently much higher than those suggested for surgical operating rooms[4].

The Future: A Discussion

As patients and their lawyers become better informed about airborne infection during surgery[4] as well as the problems which can be created by the excessive use of antibiotics, then the operating room and its supporting services will be expected to conform to those standards which are laid down for all items which invade the body[4].

Because of this, together with the number of hospitals experiencing a shortage of funds, it would seem logical to have a small, mobile UCA supply unit which can protect all sterile items when they are exposed and ready for surgery as well as protecting the wound and the surgeons gloved hands which, during an operation, are sticky and, therefore, arrest any CFU in the ambient air[5].

To satisfy this requirement a smaller version of a UCA

PREVENTION DE LA TRANSMISSION DES INFECTIONS PAR VOIE AERIENNE — HISTORIQUE

Au cours des trente années depuis le moment où John Charnley a découvert que l'infection des blessures était souvent due à la transmission aérienne de microbes infectieux, l'auteur a mis au point trois générations d'equipment pour le maintien d'une ambiance sterile. Il s'agit ici d'en faire la description ainsi que de certaines de leurs variantes.

A partir de cette mise au point, de nouvelles dispositions de construction sont définies. Le système OMNIFLOW reprśente la quatrième génération de ce développement.

L'entrainement périphéral et la dispersion interne des contaminants externes sont examinés dans l'article, ainsi que l'interrelation des flux d'air, de la recirculation et contrôle climatique.

Outre les systémes ultra-aseptisés de circulation d'air, il est aussi question d'un nouveau système du evacuation corporel, décrit et illustré ici, qui donne à l'utilisateur confort et liberté de mouvements.

supply trolley which is currently produced for pharmaceutical applications, is being developed for surgery at the Ollerton Laboratories. This is an air projector with similar, non-entrainment characteristics to the new Omniflow (Figure 4).

Like all horizontal flow systems it should be positioned near to the operating table so that there are no emitters of bacteria (people) able to move between the UCA source and the clean zone.

Instruments etc exposed ready for use are available on trays on and around the sides of this UCA supply trolley. The dominant UCA flow extends over the operating zone and a lower UCA flow passes over the much smaller zones where the instruments etc are exposed in their trays or trolleys.

As with the Omniflow, this UCA trolley accepts either bio or HEPA filters and has a variable air flow facility and is plugged into a standard power socket. Depending on the type of air filters used, both the Omniflow UCA ceiling system and the UCA supply trolley showed during validation tests, air cleanliness zones of a size suitable for their applications in compliance with the appropriate international standards[4].

It is the first requirement of a hospital that it shall do the patient no harm and certainly all forms of prevention of bacterial infection are better than attempted cure by antibiotics.

References

(1) Charnley, J. Post-operative infection in total prosthetic replacement arthroplasty of the hip joint. Brit, J., Surg 1961 Vol 59-9.

(2) Lidwell, O. M., et al. Effect of Ultra Clean Air in operating rooms on deep sepsis of the joint after replacement. Brit Med J 19823 July 285, 10-14.

(3) Howorth, F. H. Prevention of Airborne Infection during surgery. ASHRAE Transactions 1985 Vol 91 pt1.

(4) US Fed Std 209D. British Std 5295/89 EEC, GMP 1989.

(5) Howorth, F. H. Prevention of Airborne Infection during surgery. 1985 The Lancet Feb 16 PP306-388.

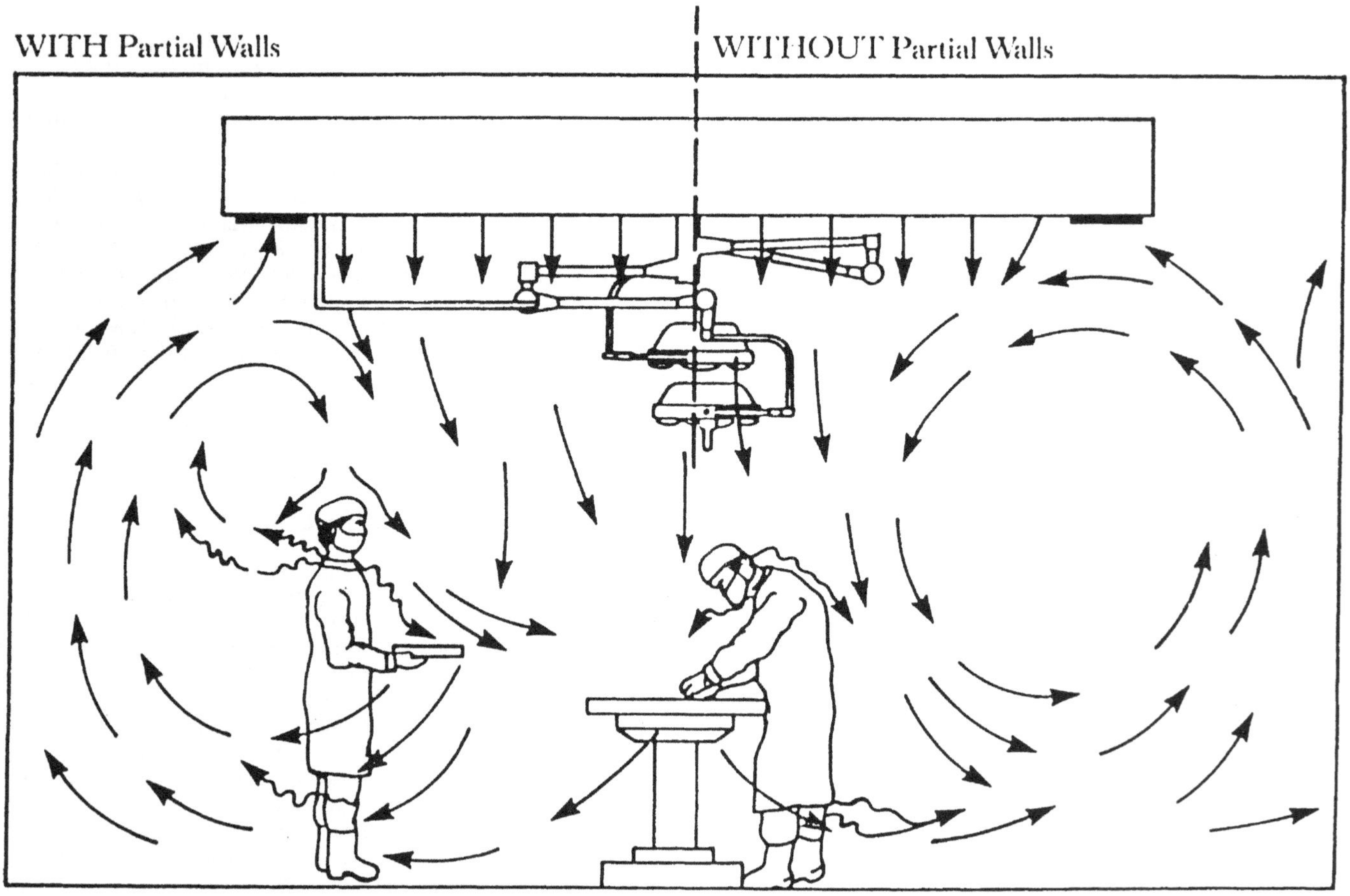

Figure 2: Airflow patterns from uniform discharge velocity downflow systems showing peripheral entrainment and inward dispersion of extraneous contaminants.

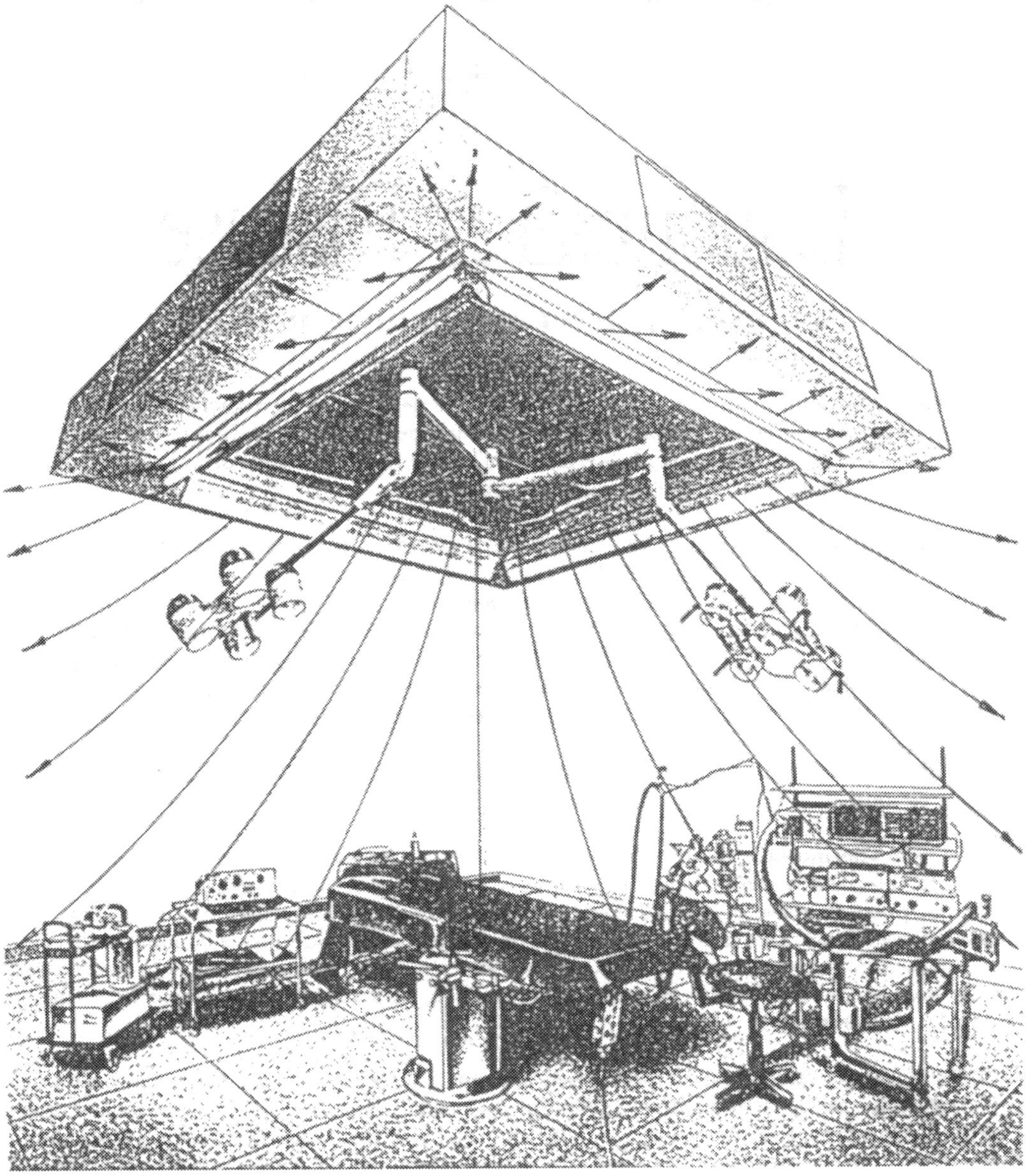

Figure 3: Omniflow ultra clean air projection pattern.

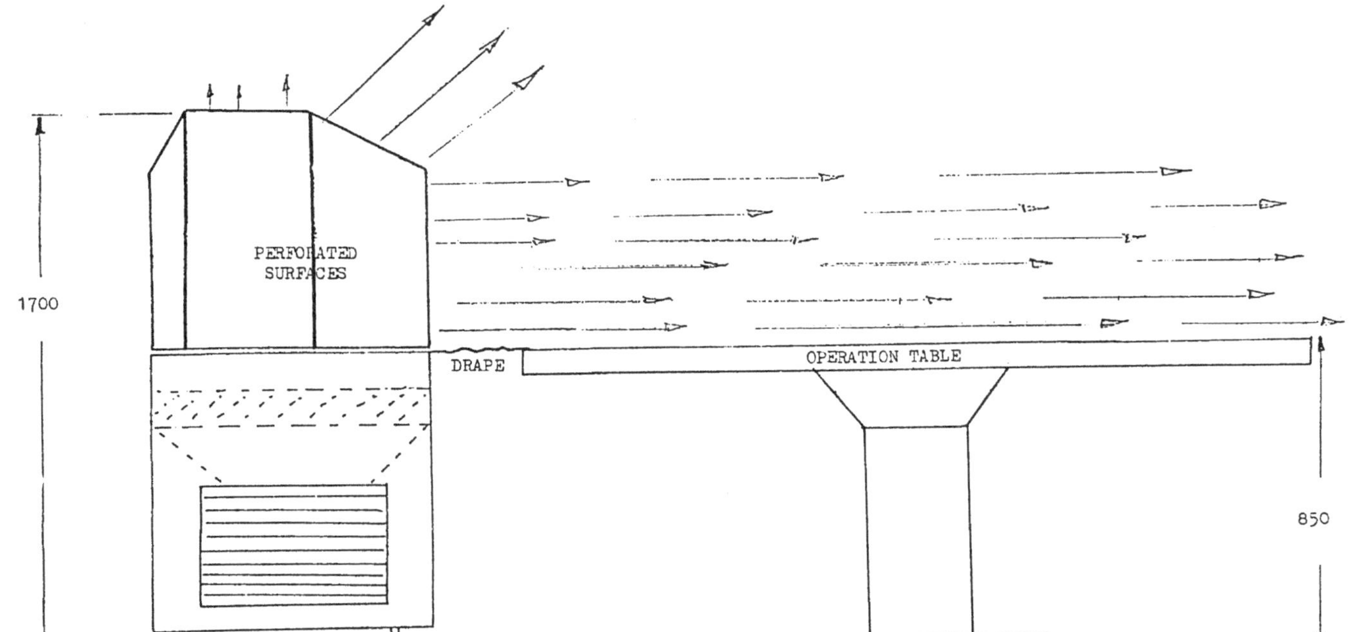

Figure 4: Ultra clean air supply trolley.

Legionnaires' Disease — Aspects of Prevention

by
Dr A. E. Wright
TD, MD, FRCPath, DPH, DipBact (Lately of PHLS)

Engineers and Medical Microbiologists have always found common ground especially for example in the fields of ventilation systems in operating theatres and biological safety cabinets. This work demands a knowledge of the science of aerobiology as does a study of legionnaires' disease.

In the years following the war aerobiology was more fashionable than it is now and papers were published showing good epidemiological evidence of the spread of diseases such as foot and mouth disease over long distances. The outbreak of legionnaires' disease associated with the BBC in London confirmed the role of the aerosol spead of this disease. What are the requirements for such a spread to take place and what action can be taken to prevent such spread? A considerable amount of energy is required to produce an aerosol. In a wet cooling tower this energy is provided by gravity aided by a fan as a forced draught. The cooling tower water is broken up into droplets which may escape through an inefficient drift eliminator into the surrounding air. There the larger droplets fall to the ground whilst smaller droplets remain suspended for a while. If the ambient temperature and the relative humidity are suitable these droplets evaporate slowly becoming, as they do so, very much smaller and lighter. They are now capable of remaining suspended in the air for very long periods and are carried in the wind to be perhaps eventually inhaled by some unfortunate individual. If the cooling tower has been neglected these fine droplets may incorporate fungal spores, viruses and even legionellae and other bacteria. In the absence of sunlight these organisms may remain viable for some time and if inhaled in a large enough dose may cause disease in susceptible humans. This then, is the concept of an aerosol, a term originally thought to have been coined by Professor Donnan when studying phosgene gas in World War 1.

The Health and Safety Commission recently issued a Consultative Document[2] which outlined possible legal aspects of the prevention of legionnaires' disease. Whatever the fate of this document the Code of Practice incorporated would be difficult to enforce but could be useful as a guideline to hospital engineers faced with a plethora of advice from other sources. It does however suggest that 'if it is reasonably practicable, the use of equipment which can create a spray of contaminated water should be avoided or abandoned.' This would seem to advocate the end of wet cooling towers in spite of the fact that epidemiological evidence supports the contention that such towers properly maintained are not a source of legionella. The point that is missed here is that if properly looked after they are efficient, cheaper to run and many claim more flexible, compact and quieter than alternatives.

If you accept a need for such cooling towers what are the features on which you should concentrate to make them efficient and safe? It is important that when a contract is granted to a firm to maintain cooling towers the hospital authority should make it clear exactly what objectives are sort. To this end the Expert Committee on Biocides in their Report[3] gave as an Appendix a list of questions which should be asked and answered. They included a request to the maintenance firm for a clear statement as to who in the firm will be taking responsibility, how often he or she will visit, what chemicals will he need at what concentration and where is the evidence that they are effective. Biocides are invariably used in this situation but it is not always understood that they are not designed to kill all bacteria, algae, fungi, yeasts and protozoa. Indeed no such agent exists. A biocide will, if properly used, prevent the multiplication of many such agents and will usually do so by intermittent dosing of a system depending on its volume, the losses occurring from the system and the strength of the biocide. However efficient the biocide it will not be effective if the system is not kept mechanically clean. This involves a weekly inspection and a twice yearly thorough cleansing and treatment. Even with this rigorous regime it is not suggested that cooling towers will be free of bacterial growth but any organisms present should only be in small numbers. Total bacterial counts together with pH ranges and a measure of total dissolved solids should be followed over a period to establish base lines. Any deviation from these being an indication for action to be taken. Testing for the presence of legionella is not usually advocated on a routine basis because of the delay in receiving results but might be done during a commissioning stage. The development of monoclonal antibody techniques which detect the presence of legionella very rapidly might result in this view being revised in the future.

Which Biocide should you use? The Biocide Committee was criticised for not being specific enough in recommending a 'best buy'. Clearly however, a league table could only have been produced on the basis of laboratory findings and this would not necessarily have been applicable to the conditions applying in the field. A list of biocides which are in use together with published reports on their efficacy was given in the report. In all cases one must ensure that the dose used is adequate and hence it is imperative that the total capacity of the unit is measured accurately. When the biocide is introduced the system must be operated so that thorough mixing takes place and contact with all parts of the system maintained for the requisite periods. Factors such as the hardness of the water, ambient temperature and pH may all affect the efficacy of the biocide. In the case of chlorine the degree of acidity is of primary importance. Chemicals used to prevent corrosion and scaling must be compatible with the biocides employed. Considerations which are indirectly important concern the safety of personnel and the toxicity of biocides when released into the drainage system.

Chlorine, usually in the form of sodium hypochlorite (NaOC1), is widely used because it is relatively cheap. It should however, be remembered, that it is highly reactive and an oxidising agent and functions most effectively in the absence of organic matter, ammonia, ferrous and manganous salts. All these may neutralise chlorine before it is free to act on micro-organisms. A very good reason for keeping the plant free from slimes and organic debris.

Many chemicals and particularly the quaternary ammonium compounds are incompatible with chlorine and

MALADIE DU LEGIONNAIRE — MODES DE PREVENTION

La prévention de la maladie du légionnaire repose avant tout sur une bonne connaissance de l'aérobiolgie. L'article décrit la formation d'un aérosol en faisant référence aux refroidisseurs humides.

Il est question du rôle par les nettoyants mécaniques, et l'utilisation des produits chimiques et des biocides contre les risques des aérosols dangereux est également passée en revue.

Il faut s'attendre á de nombreux progrès dans ce domaine.

this biocide will also react with nitrites often used as corrosion inhibitors. Extensive studies of industrial cooling towers both here and in the United States of America give conflicting reports on the efficacy of chlorine to inhibit legionellae. Failure has often been attributed to a residual biofilm harbouring the bacteria and sometimes associated with materials such as rubber grommets. If these are replaced with approved fittings the cleaning is adequate, chlorine is effective.

For routine cleaning levels of 15 mg/l for a period of 4-6 hours is usually recommended but in an emergency, levels of up to 50 mg/l have been used. Such levels are difficult to attain and sustain.

Other biocides often used include the halogenated biophenols, Bronopol and Quaternary Ammonium compounds amongst many others.

Water maintenance firms often have their own formulae and may use biocides in rotation.

Are biocides the only answer? We do not have sufficient evidence to suggest that biocides can be replaced in water systems to control legionella. Certainly in domestic hot water systems biocides have no place and water should (like food) be kept either very hot or very cold. Research is being done into a system in which cooling tower water is continually abstracted from the system, heated to a temperature of over 70°C and then returned, clear of pathogenic organisms, to the tower. Heat is always the best method of killing micro-organisms and this method shows much promise. Another procedure which may prove useful is based on electronically released copper and silver ions. These, in the correct proportions, act synergistically to disinfect the circulating water and are also said to be effective in removing biofilm.

In conclusion, wet cooling towers can be maintained safely by scrupulous attention to mechanical cleanliness, by the use of chemicals to prevent scaling and corrosion and by the use of biocides to control the growth of micro-organisms.

References

(1) Norris K. P. and Harper G. J. 1970. Windborne Dispersal of Foot and Mouth Virus *Nature* 225, 98-99.

(2) The Control of Legionellosis: Proposals for Statutory Action. 1989 Health and Safety Commission.

(3) Report of the Expert Advisory Committee on Biocides 1989. Department of Health HMSO London.

Hot Water Service Systems and Risks of Legionnaires' Disease

by
Ing E. van Olffen
Tebodin, Curacao, Parera, PO Box 2085, Willemstad,
Curacao, Netherlands Antilles

Legionnaires' disease is the name of an infection from the legionella bacteria caused by the services within a building. It was first recognised in July 1976, when outbreak occurred among delegates attending the American Legion Convention in a hotel in Philadelphia. About 182 of 4,000 delegates became ill and 29 (= 16%) of these died. Possibly taking a shower by the first of them was fatal. After several months scientists reported the isolation of the aetiological agent. Because of the occurrence the bacterium was named: Legionella pneumonia.

It is sure that outbreaks as in Philadelphia did not happen in 1976 for the first time. For example in 1965, there was another outbreak in Pontiac, this time not in form of pneumonia but in a form of high fever, well known by the name of 'Pontiac Fever'. Of 170 delegates 49 became ill, caused by a bacterium from the same family.

The diagnosis of Legionnaires' disease is a very difficult one. It has been admitted by officials, that at least 6% of diagnosed pneumonia, are in fact Legionella pneumonia.

Legionella pneumophila is one member of a large genus of Legionellacae. There have been reported 24 other species of legionella and at least 41 serogroups of Legionella pneumophila have been described until now.

Members of the family Legionellacea — including Legionella pneumophila serogroup 1, are commonly found in water systems, both natural and man made.

You may be thinking now, Legionnaires' disease is very rare and that these cases only happen in the United States. However the answer is: 'No'! It is very active here too, possibly in your hotel, hospital or even at home. A newspaper report from the 'Frankfurter Allgemeine Zeitung', Germany, tells us about investigations in the sphere of Legionnaires' disease: In Western Germany alone, 6,000 to 7,000 people become ill by legionella and 900 to 1,200 people die every year! Hot water service systems are assigned as the most important cause.

Sheet 1

(Infection Route)

Legionella bacteria are found in water. They presumably enter the water from the atmosphere. The infection route is through inhalation of aerosols, contaminated with bacteria. Air mixed with aerosols may be inhaled, when you are taking a shower or anywhere where aerosols (very fine liquid drops) in combination with air are found. Do not forget whirlpools etc!

Legionella Bacteria

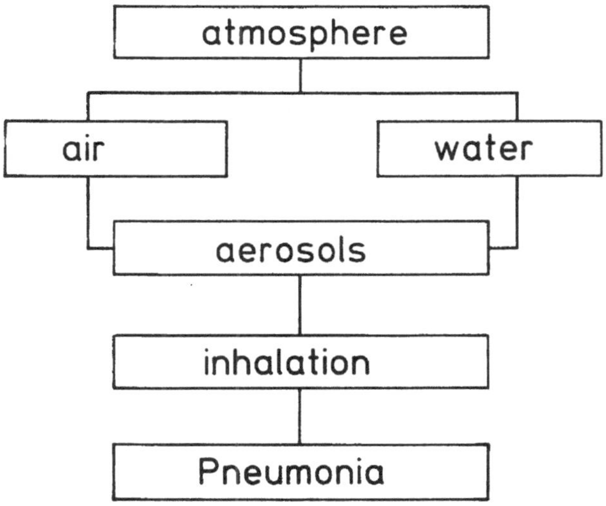

Sheet 1.

Sheet 2

(Combination of Circumstances to Increase Risks of Legionnaires' Disease)

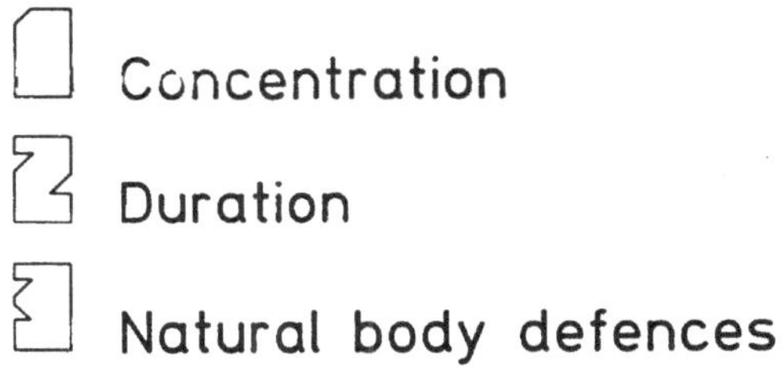

Sheet 2.

The risk increases with the number of inhaled bacteria. So there is a combination of concentration of bacteria and duration the person stays in the contaminated zone. Important also is the natural body defence. Legionella pneumophila is an ordinary bacterium and can be eliminated by a Normal Body Defence. Highest danger is for individuals who are specially susceptible. Children will be seldom infected. The risk for individuals increases over 50 years of age. There is no proof of people who are infected by

PREVENTION DE LA MALADIE DU LEGIONNAIRE CAS DE CONTAMINATION PAR LES SYSTEMES DE CIRCULATION D'EAU CHAUDE

La présence de bacilles legionella dans les systèmes de circulation d'eau chaude et froide dans les bâtiments hospitaliers a été constaté dans environ 70% des cas.

Les bactéries survivent et se multiplient à un maximum dans l'eau lorsque les températures sont situées entre 35 et 45 degrés Celcius.

On estime que les bactéries pénètrent dans le système par les conduites d'eau froide, dans la mesure où l'eau du robinet contient parfois de petites quantités de legionella.

Au cours des dernières années, l'auteur a mis au point un système de circulation d'eau chaude qui supprime les risques de legionella ainsi que de brûlures accidentelles. Ce système se base sur le fait que les bactéries de legionella ne résistent pas aux températures de plus de 65 degrés Celcius. Au lieu de mélanger l'eau du robinet chauffée à plus de 65 degrés à de l'eau froide, l'eau du robinet est refroidie par un échangeur de chaleur. Ce refroidissement ne représente pas de perte d'énergie, dans la mesure où celui-ci s'effectue par l'eau froide qui coule en même temps dans le calorifère. Cet effet de pasteurisation fait fonctionner avec succès les systèmes de plusieurs hôpitaux hollandais.

drinking contaminated water. There is also no record of person-to-person spread of infection.

The incubation period for humans (= the time between exposure to the organism and development of first symptoms) is usually 3-6 days, but may range from 2-10 days.

Sheet 3

(Presence of Legionella in Buildings)

Building	Service	Number of establish-ments sampled	Proportion of establishments in which positive traces of *legionella* were found (%)
Hotels	Hot and cold water	104	53
	Cooling water systems	9	67
Hospitals	Hot and cold water	40	70
	Cooling water systems	13	38
Business premises	Hot and cold water	17	75
	Cooling water systems	24	54
Residential establish-ments	Hot and cold water	3	67

Sheet 3:

This table from Technical Memorandum number 13 of 1987 of CIBSE (Chartered Institution of Building Services Engineers) shows the result of investigations of outbreaks of Legionnaires' disease in several buildings. Domestic hot water services in large buildings such as in hotels and hospitals are considered to be the most likely source. In this paper I will exclude cooling towers because of the simple fact I haven't yet any experience.

However the proportion of positive traces of legionella in hot and cold water service systems is alarming!

Sheet 4

(Analysis for Presence of L. by C. Winston May 1988)

SOURCE	ALL SITES			HOSPITAL SITES		
	SAMPLED	POSITIVE	% POSITIVE	SAMPLED	POSITIVE	% POSITIVE
CALORIFIERS	362	61	17%	62	11	18%
SHOWERS	339	27	8%	31	13	41%
HOT DOMESTIC SOURCES OTHER THAN SHOWERS	1535	88	6%	146	23	16%
COOLING TOWERS	567	29	4%	33	-	-
ALL OTHER SOURCES	1171	15	1%	111	4	4%
TOTALS	3974	220	5%	383	51	13%

Sheet 4: (Detection Level 40cfu/litre).

This quite recent table shows that showers in hospitals are most hazardous and alarming. I think just showers are infected, because of the addition of cold water. I will consider this point later.

Sheet 5

(The Increasing Risk for Multiplication of Legionella)

This figure, published in the same publication of CIBSE, as mentioned before, gives a very good picture of the increasing risk of multiplication of legionella bacteria. Especially at temperatures between 35 and 45°C and bacteria will multiply rapidly. The doubling time will then increase to about 120 minutes. Of course there are also the influences from breeding-grounds, pH etc. Over about 50°C the multiplication stops, but the bacterium does survive at higher temperatures. Over 55°C the bacteria will die successively and at 70°C the bacteria will die immediately. Below 37°C the multiplication rate decreases and can be considered insignificant below 20°C and at much lower temperatures the bacteria can remain dormant. They will return to active multiplication whenever more favourable temperatures occur.

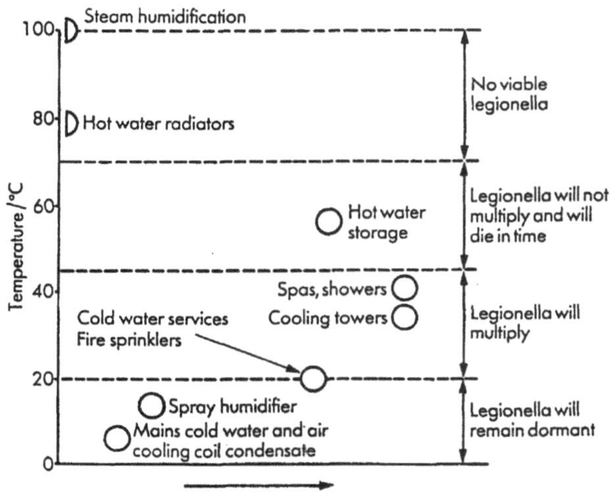

Sheet 5.

Did you ever try taking a glass of cold drinking water in a hospital?

Why are showers, especially in hospital sites, so hazardous?

Look at the point of 'cold water services' in this diagram! That's why I looked for a solution to the problem.

Increasing the temperature of your hot water system is no guarantee what so ever for excluding any risk of Legionnaires' disease and you will increase the risk of scalding. Scalding by liquids, especially by water, is the worst of all.

To kill the bacteria before water is added to your hot water service system, it is necessary to heat the water over 70°C. This temperature is however too risky to add to your system. Normally we mix the hot water with cold water to reach the required temperature. By adding cold water we introduce water which is presumably contaminated with bacteria in a system with a perfect temperature to multiply.

The simple solution is: Do Not Mix Your Hot Water But Cool It by a heat exchanger, as shown in the next diagram.

Sheet 6

(Diagram — Hot Water System)

The principle of the system is a central mixed hot water service system, which will not be supplied with cold water but with cooled hot water, which is cooled in a heat exchanger without any loss of energy. The cooling water is the water which flows to the calorifier at the same moment that draw-off takes place.

The principle of this system is like a process of pasteurising. Dead bacteria usually don't multiply.

A problem might be the way how to heat your hot water service system when no draw-off takes place. Therefore I designed a special connection between the hot water system and the calorifier. The most important feature of this connection is, that there is a continuous flow of your circulation water of the hot water service system returning to the calorifier so that the water in the service system will be continuously pasteurised.

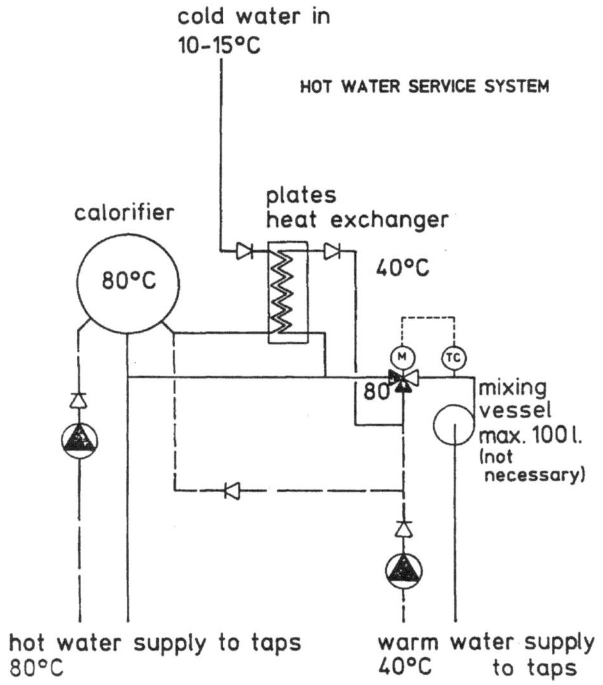

Sheet 6.

Sheet 7

(Isometric Diagram)

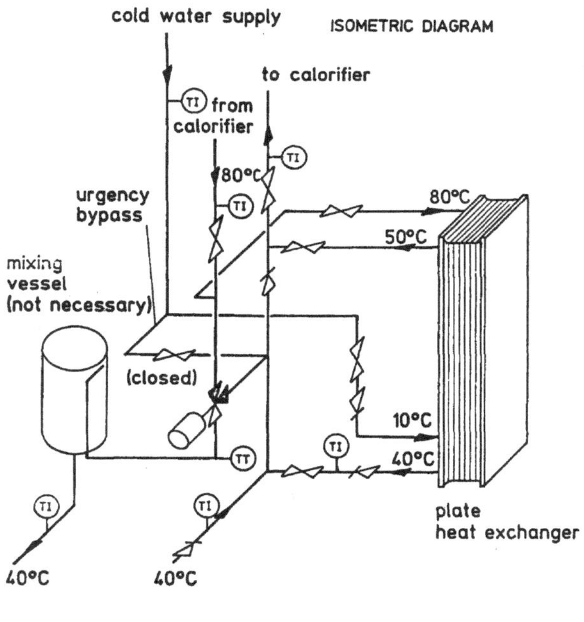

Sheet 7.

This isometric disgram shows the same system as mentioned before and shows the way the system could be installed.

Sheet 8

(Basic Diagram for a Complete Hot Water Service System)

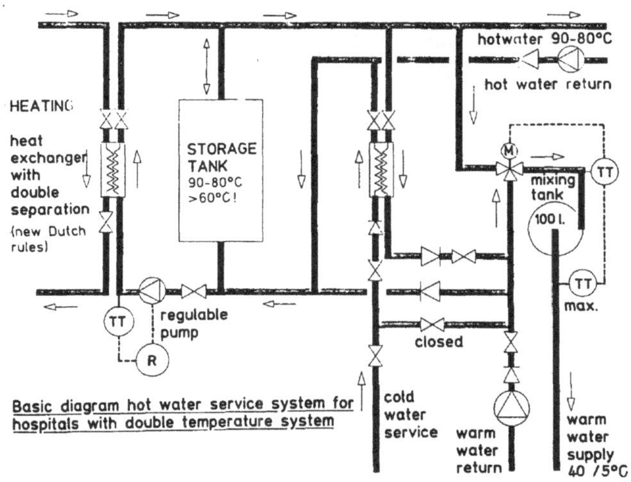

Sheet 8.

This diagram shows the complete hot water system as it has been installed in the hospital in the town of Oldenzaal. This system has operated since December 1987.

Two heat exchangers are used. The hot water is generated outside the calorifier. The system makes a double separation between the heating medium and drinking water possible, which is a new regulation in the Netherlands. It is also possible to run with a minimum temperature difference between the heating medium and the hot water service temperature. For different sections in hospitals, water between 80 and 85°C will be required. This system has been installed at Oldenzaal, Netherlands and has operated successfully since 19 December 1987.

The Summary of Experiences

In Germany it is officially recognised that legionella bacteria enter the hot water service system through the cold water system. The pasteurising process I showed you is a very simple, effective and inexpensive way to exclude any risk of Legionnaires' disease in your hospital.

Several hospitals installed the system for a longer period. No legionella have been found in their system until now. However, the first years I hadn't any proof with contaminated hot water systems.

In the Netherlands two hospitals had hot water service systems contaminated with legionella. After installing this simple pasteurising system the hot water systems in both hospitals are completely free of legionella.

The system, as shown today, has the following features:-

(1) guaranteed thermal killing of legionella bacteria without any extra energy consumption;
(2) low costs;
(3) low energy costs because of low temperatures in your hot water service system;
(4) no risks of scalding;
(5) simple installation; and
(6) suitable for existing hot water service systems.

Air Flow Control Systems for Hospitals and Hospital Laboratories for the 1990's

by

Dr Merlon E. Wiggin
and
Robert H. Morris
Isocon Ltd, One Bootleg Alley,
PO Box 672, Greenport, New York 11944

Today there is an increasing need for the maintenance of air movement relationships within specific designated areas of hospitals and hospital laboratories. With the recognition that air movements can, and does, affect patient care and patient well being, it is now becoming increasingly well recognised that the types of air flow controls that have been associated with research laboratories are appropriate to be adapted for specialised areas in hospitals as well.

The extent of the areas of hospitals that should have air flow controls is indicated in the 'Guidelines for Construction and Equipment of Hospital and Medical Facilities', published by the US Department of Health and Human Services. This Guide includes in it a table of 'ventilation requirements for hospital areas effecting patient care'. In this table, 31 areas are designated to have a required air movement direction between its area and adjacent spaces; 27 of the areas do not permit air to be recirculated by means of room units; and 24 require all air to be exhausted directly outdoors. Table 3 from these Guidelines, with its applicable notes, are included as Addendum No 1.

Now that we have all recognised the importance of controlling the air flow between spaces, what is the best way to insure and maintain its accomplishment? In the past some have simply felt that we can just install a few commercial type volume boxes, and we can be assured that the air is always flowing in the right direction. It is not that simple or easy.

The difference in air volume and its inherent velocity pressure is very small, and because of this control is difficult. To best illustrate this, let's take a typical sized room that is 5m × 5m × 2.5m, 67.5m^3, that has its air systems designed for 15 air changes per hour, and we want to maintain this room at a negative pressure to its corridor. The negative pressure to be maintained has been selected as 10 to 12 Pa and leakage around the door at this pressure has been calculated to be approximately .025m^3/sec. The required air supply is .425m^3/sec, and the required exhaust is 0.450m^3/sec. As it is impractical to expect any system to control the exhaust flow at exactly 0.450m^3/sec, an acceptable range is established, and for this example we will use $\pm$ .005m^3/sec, or 0.445 to 0.455m^3/sec of exhaust air flow that needs to be maintained.

Using the exhaust 0.445 to 0.455m^3/sec and the duct size, we calculate the range of flow velocity that is required to be maintained. For this example, at 0.445m^3/sec is 2.19m/sec, and at 0.455m^3/sec is 2.25m/sec. Now, the velocity pressure for each of these two volumes — for the 0.445m/sec it is 2.9 Pa and 0.455m/sec it is 3.1 Pa, and the difference between these two is 0.2 Pa. With this being the difference in velocity pressure we must have a control that will maintain this small variation, or on a basis of percent we need to control the air flow at a $\pm$ 2%.

Needing to control an air flow at a $\pm$ 2% is difficult enough without adding variables such as filter loading, two-speed fans, doors opening and closing, drifting of the control devices, turning hoods off and on, day/night set-back, and so forth.

One of the first decisions that an engineer has to make if he is to accurately control air flow is to select industrial quality air flow control equipment and linear, or nearly linear, dampers. And thirdly, in my opinion, electronic controls.

There are two basic methods of maintaining differential space pressurisation of rooms. The first is by sensing, measuring, and comparing by static pressure sensors the room versus the corridor. And the second is by an accurate air flow measuring devise such as an Ambient Mass Flow Sensor that will measure the change in air flow mass.

The development of Electronic Controllers, coupled with temperature compensated drift-free and dynamic stable transducers, has simplified and improved the ability to control air flow direction within designated areas. A typical flow control diagram using static pressure differential is depicted in Figure 1. The air supply of this space is monitored (in this case emphasise monitoring only) to an air flow measuring device which is helpful to determine the approximate volume of the air in the room, and is also helpful in balancing the systm. Static pressure is monitored within the space and compared with the static pressure in the corresponding space, usually the corridor.

These two readouts are sent back to a pressure differential transmitter, which in turn, is used to control an electronic damper actuator, which maintains the correct amount of air being exited from the room. These systems have the capability to hold the static pressure within 1.25 Pa.

These systems do, however, depend on the stability of the corridor or other reference data, which can often result in noisy signals. With the development of the self-calibrating ambient mass flow sensors with an accuracy of $\pm$ 1.5% of range, and utilising a three-mode controller which includes proportional band, reset rate, and derivative (inverse), it is possible to accurately control air flow to a room or area, compare it to the room's exhaust flow, and maintain a space differential pressure. An example of this for a positive pressurised operating room with unoccupied set-back is depicted in Fig 2. In this example, an air flow tube through the wall with its own air flow velocity sensor is used for

SYSTEMES DE CONTROLE DE CIRCULATION D'AIR POUR LES HOPITAUX ET LES LABORATORIES D'ANALYSES MEDICALES — NOUVELLE REGLEMENTATION

Il est reconnu que les mouvements d'air ont un effet indéniable sur les soins et le confort des malades. De ce fait, le contrôle des mouvements d'air en milieu hospitalier représente un problème tout à fait actuel.

Les recommendations émises par le Département des Soins de Santé (Construction et Equipements des Hôpitaux et Services Annexes) des Etats-Unis cite 31 domaines spécifiques qui requièrent des contrôles de mouvements d'air et 24 domaines spécifiques qui requièrent l'évacuation de l'air vers l'extérieur. Dans la mesure où la santé des patients est en jeu, fiabilité et efficacité des systèmes sont de rigueur.

A cause des difficultés associées à la mesure et au contrôle de faibles différences de niveau dans les mouvements d'air, il est nécessaire d'utiliser des équipements de contrôle de qualité industrielle. Les capacités et les applications de ces niveaux de contrôle sont passées en revue en détail; et des exemples spécifiques les illustrent.

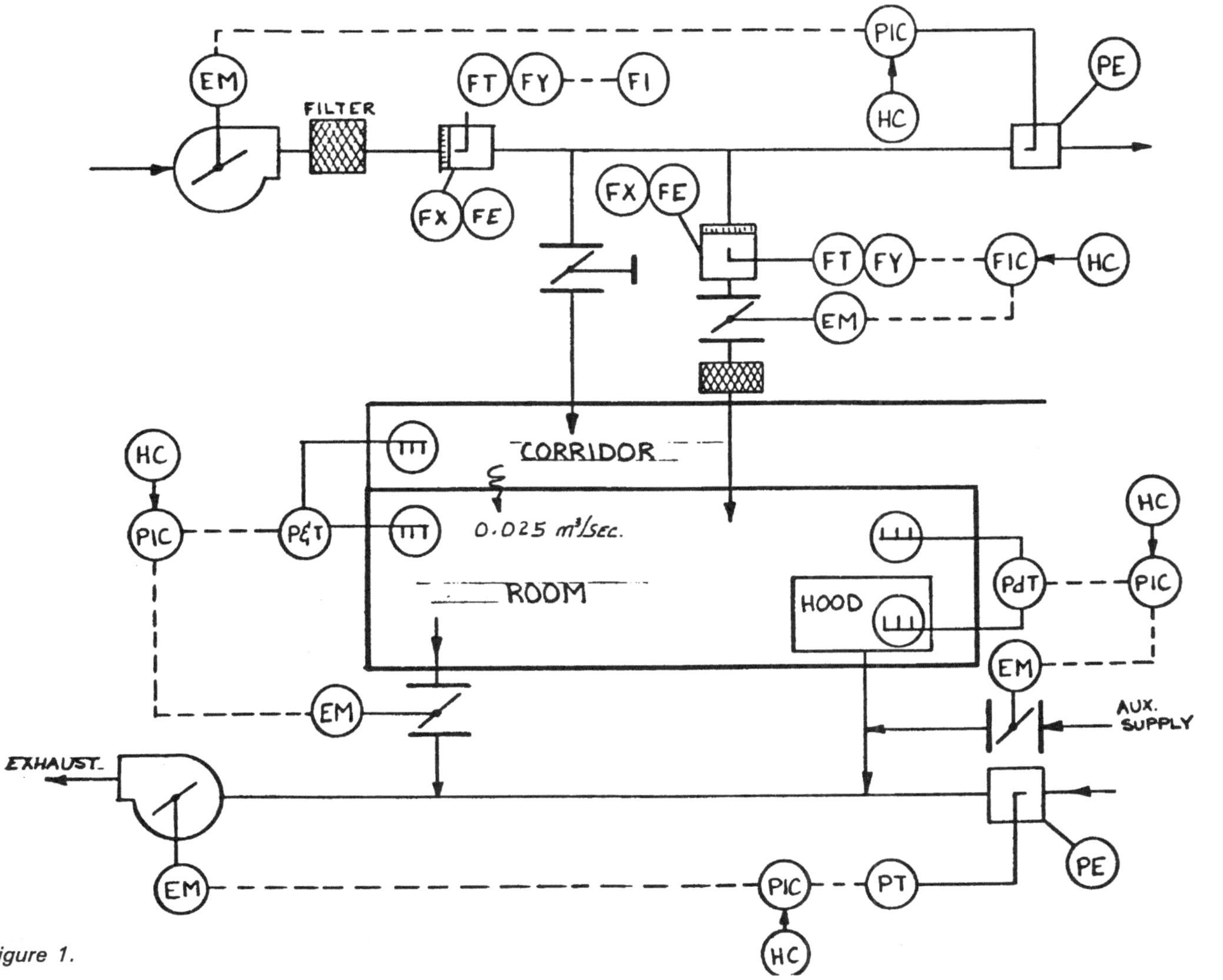

Figure 1.

space pressure override as a back-up to the volumetric control system.

Even though it is a subject unto itself, at this point I would like to just mention about the importance of inverse derivatives as the type of controller action that is used in air flow and pressurisation control processes. Air flow is typically noisy. By that I mean, not sound noisy, but signal variations because the air flowing in a duct is highly turbulent and regardless of the air flow measuring means, this turbulence results in signal pulsations (noise) which are amplified into control signals by pressure transmitters.

The following figures are from 'Process-Control Systems, Application/Design/Adjustment' by F. Gregg Skinsky, Senior System Consultant, the Foxboro Company, and they very accurately depict the input and output differences between derivative and inverse derivative types of control (Fig 3 and Fig 4).

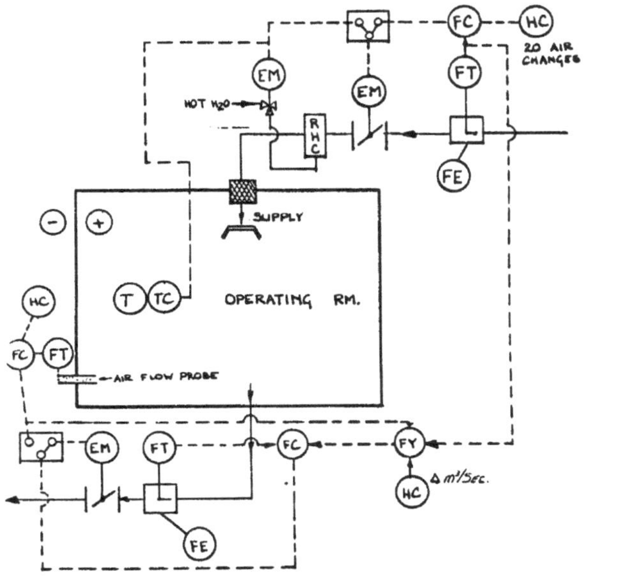

Figure 2: Variable volumetric air flow control with space pressure override.

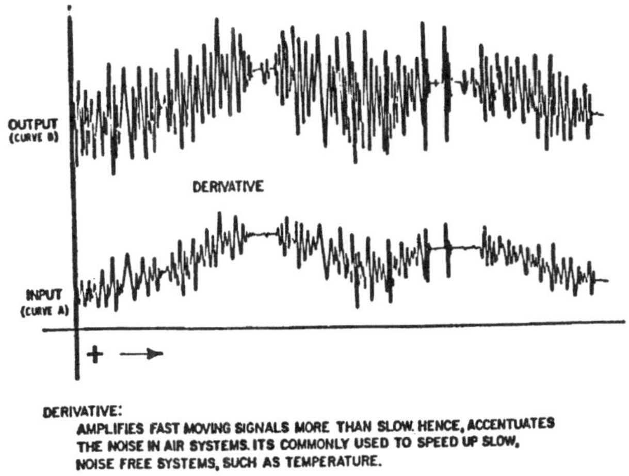

Figure 3.

Another important aspect of air flow control for hospitals in the 1990's is the face velocity control for fume hoods. With the newly developed electronic control for fume

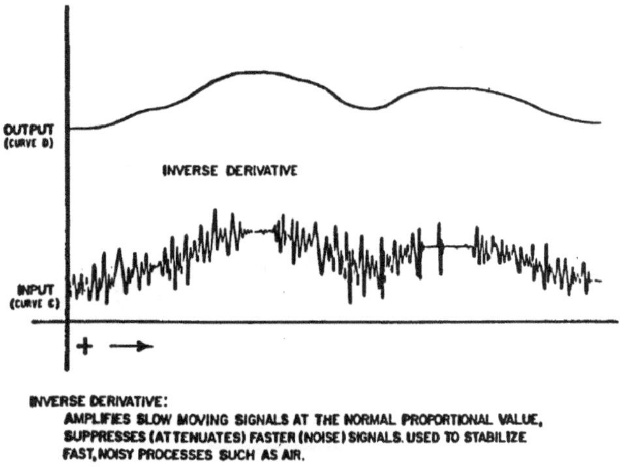

Figure 4.

hoods, it is possible to control face velocity within ± 0.025m/sec within normal sash position ranges. This not only insures the safety of the hood, but also can be a significant energy saver.

When this system is tied in to and is made part of the electronic flow controls for the air supply in a room, it is possible to maintain air flow between spaces, even with variable exhaust flows through a laboratory fume hood. An example of this control arrangement for a hospital laboratory to be maintained at negative pressure and contains fume hoods is shown in Fig 5. It is also strongly urged that any fume hood installations installed have their performance vertified by the ANSI/ASHRAE 110 Standard, keeping in mind that a laboratory fume hood is a personnel safety devise, and should be treated and tested accordingly.

The control of air direction can, in my opinion, only be insured by the use of industrial quality controls. How to define industrial quality has often been an elusive one. To assist in this effort we have developed some standards that we feel can be used in the specifying of this level of controls. These are contained in Addendum No 2.

In conclusion, if we are to seriously design air flow systems to control and maintain positive air flow direction, for designated hospital areas, then specific application of industrial type controls such as the above will be necessary.

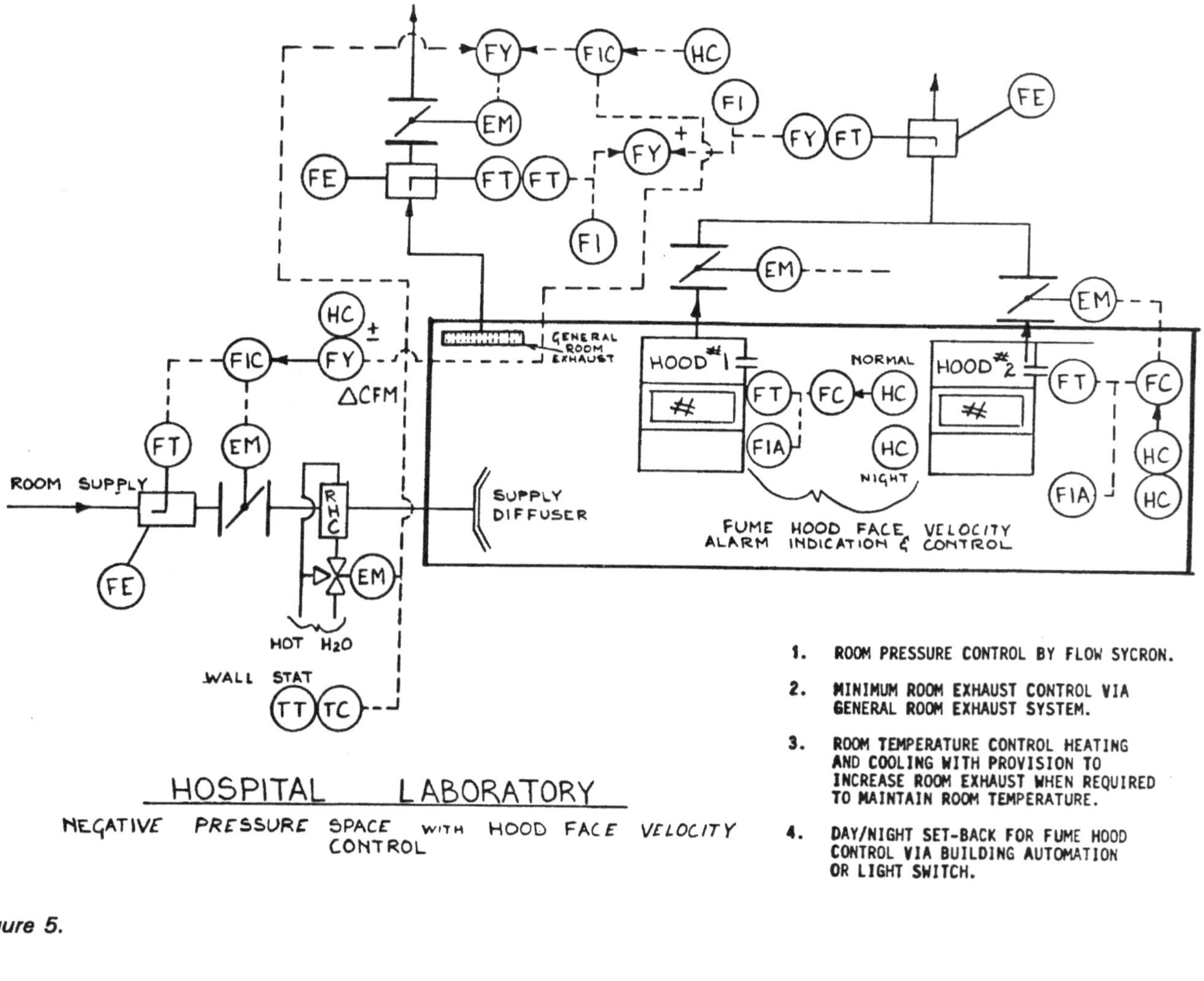

Figure 5.

ADDENDUM NUMBER 1

Area designation	**Air movement relationship to adjacent area[2]**	**Minimum air changes outside air per hour[3]**	**Minimum total air changes per hour[2]**	**Recirculated by means of room units[4]**	**All air exhausted directly outdoors[3]**	**Relative humidity (%)[4]**	**Design temperature (degrees)[7]**
Operating room[14]	Out	3	15	No	—	50-60	70-75
Delivery room[14]	Out	3	15	No	—	45-60	70-75
X-ray card, cath, and invas, spec, proc[15]	Out	3	15	No	—	45-60	70-75
Newborn nursery	—	1	6	No	—	30-60	75
Recovery room[14]	—	2	6	No	—	30-60	70
Intensive care	—	2	6	No	—	30-60	70-75
Isolation room[10]	In	—	6	No	Yes	—	70-75
Isolation alcove or anteroom[10]	Out	—	10	No	Yes	—	—
Patient room	—	—	2	—	—	—	70-75
Labor delivery rooms (LDR)	—	—	2	—	—	—	70-75
Patient corridor	—	—	2	—	—	—	—
Examination room	—	—	6	—	—	—	75
Medication room	—	—	4	—	—	—	—
Pharmacy	—	—	4	—	—	—	—
Treatment room[8]	—	—	6	—	—	—	75
Trauma room[9]	Out	3	15	No	—	45-60	70-75
X-ray room, and nonivas, spec proc[15]	—	—	6	—	—	—	75
Physical Rx							
Hydrotherapy	In	—	6	—	—	—	75
Treatment room	—	—	6	—	—	—	70-75
Soiled utility	In	—	10	No	Yes	—	—
Clean utility	—	—	4	—	—	—	—
Autopay room	In	—	12	No	Yes	—	—
Darkroom	In	—	10	No	Yes	—	—
Non refrigerated body-holding room[12]	In	—	10	Yes	Yes	—	70
Toilet room	In	—	10	Yes	Yes	—	—
Bedpan room	In	—	10	Yes	Yes	—	—
Bathroom	—	—	10	—	—	—	75
Janitors closet	In	—	10	No	Yes	—	—
Steriliser equipment room[12]	In	—	10	—	Yes	—	—
ETO-steriliser room[13]	In	—	10	No	Yes	—	75
Soiled linen and trash rooms	In	—	10	No	Yes	—	—
Laboratory							
General[15]	—	—	6	—	—	—	—
Nuclear medicine[15]	In	—	6	No	Yes	—	—
Pathology	In	—	6	No	Yes	—	—
Cytology	In	—	6	No	Yes	—	—
Biochemistry[10]	Out	—	6	No	—	—	—
Histology	In	—	6	No	Yes	—	—
Microbiology[14]	In	—	6	No	Yes	—	—
Serology	Out	—	6	No	—	—	—
Glass washing	In	—	10	—	Yes	—	—
Sterilising	In	—	10	—	Yes	—	—
Food preparation center[11]	—	—	10	No	—	—	—
Ware washing	In	—	10	No	Yes	—	—
Dietary day storage	In	—	2	—	—	—	—
Laundry general	—	—	10	—	Yes	—	—
Soiled linen (sorting and storage)	In	—	10	No	Yes	—	—
Clean linen	—	—	2	—	—	—	—
Anesthesia gas storage[14]	—	—	8	—	Yes	—	—
Central supply							
Soiled room	In	—	6	No	Yes	—	—
Clean workroom and sterile storage	Out	—	4	No	—	(max) 70	75

From: Guidelines for Construction and Equipment of Hospital and Medical Facilities 1987/1988 Edition
Published by: US Department of Health and Human Services, Public Health Service, Health Resources and Services Administration

(1) This table covers ventilation for comfort, as well as for asepsis and odor control in areas of acute care hospitals that directly affect patient care. Areas where specific standards are not given shall be ventilated in accordance with ASHRAE Standard 62-1981. 'Ventilation for Acceptable Indoor Air Quality Including Requirements for Outside Air'. Specialised patient care areas including organ transplant units, burn units, specialty procedure rooms, etc, shall have additional ventilation provisions for air quality control as may be appropriate. OSHA standards and/or NIOSH criteria require special ventilation requirements for employee health and safety within health care facilities.

(2) Design of the ventilation system shall, insofar as possible, provide that air movement is from 'clean to less clean' area. However, continuous compliance may be impractical with full utilisation of some forms of variable air volume and load shedding systems which may be used for energy conservation. Areas which do require positive and continuous control are noted with 'out' or 'in' to indicate the required direction of air movement in relation to the space named (this designation was previously described as 'positive' or 'negative' pressure). Rate of air movement may, of course, be varied as needed within the limits required for positive control. Where indication of air movement direction is enclosed in

parentheses, continuous directional control is required only when the tool is in use or where room use may otherwise compromise the intent of movement from clean to less clean. Air movement for rooms with dashes and nonpatient areas may vary as necessary to satisfy the requirements. Additional adjustments may be needed when space is unused or unoccupied and air systems are shut down or reduced.

(3) To satisfy exhaust needs, replacement air from outside is necessary. Table 3 does not attempt to describe specific amounts of outside air to be supplied to individual spaces except for certain areas such as those listed. Distribution of the outside air, added to the system to balance required exhaust, shall be as required by good engineering practice.

(4) Because of cleaning difficulty and potential for buildup of contamination, recirculating room units shall not be used in areas marked 'No'. Isolation and intensive care unit rooms may be ventilated by reheat induction units in which only the primary air supplied from a central system passes through the reheat unit. Gravity-type heating or cooling units such as radiators or convectors shall not be used in operating rooms and other special care areas.

(5) Air from areas with contamination and/or odor problems shall be exhausted to the outside and not recirculated to other areas. Note that individual circumstances may require special consideration for air exhaust to outside, eg, an intensive care unit in which patients with pulmonary infection are treated, and rooms for burn patients.

(6) The ranges listed are the minimum and maximum limits where control is specifically needed.

(7) Dual temperature indications (such as 70-75) are for an upper and lower variable range at which the room temperature must be controlled. A single figure indicates a heating or cooling capacity of at least the indicated temperature. This is usually applicable when patients may be undressed and require a warmer environment. Nothing in this document shall be construed as precluding the use of temperatures lower than those noted when the patients' comfort and medical conditions make lower temperatures desirable. Unoccupied areas such as storage, etc, shall have temperatures appropriate for the function intended.

(8) Number of air changes may be reduced when the room is unoccupied if provisions are made to insure that the number of air changes indicated is re-established any time the space is being utilised. Adjustments shall include provisions so that the direction of air movement shall remain the same when the number of air changes is reduced. Areas not indicated as having continuous directional control may have ventilation systems shut down when space is unoccupied and ventilation is not otherwise needed.

(9) The term *trauma room* as used here is the operating room space in the emergency department, or other trauma reception area that is used for emergency surgery. The first aid room and/or 'emergency room' used for initial treatment of accident victims may be ventilated as noted for the 'treatment room'.

(10) The isolation rooms described in these standards are those that might be utilised in the average community hospital. The assumption is made that most isolation procedures will be for infectious patients and that the room should also be suitable for normal private patient use when not needed for isolation. This compromise obviously does not provide for ideal isolation. The design should consider types and numbers of patients that might need this separation within the facility. When need is indicated by the program, it may be desirable to provide more complete control with a separate anteroom as an air lock to minimise potential for airborne particulates from the patients' area reaching adjacent areas. Certain types of patients such as those with organ transplants, burns, etc, may require special consideration, including reverse isolation for which the air movement relationship to adjacent areas would be 'out' rather than 'in'. Where these requirements are reflected in the anticipated patient load, ventilation shall be modified as necessary. *Variable exhaust that allows maximum room space flexibility with reversible air flow direction would be useful only if appropriate adjustments can be assured for different types of isolation procedures.*

(11) Food preparation centres shall have ventilation systems that have an excess of air supply for 'out' air movements when hoods are not in operation. The number of air changes may be reduced or varied to any extent required for odor control when the space is not in use. See section 7.31D(1)(p) of this document for designation of hoods.

(12) A nonrefrigerated body-holding room would be applicable only for health care facilities in which autopsies are not performed on-site, or the space is used only for holding bodies for short periods prior to transferring.

(13) Specific OSHA regulations regarding ethylene oxide (ETO) use have been promulgated. 29 CRF Part 1910.1047 includes specific ventilation requirements including local exhaust of the ETO steriliser area. Also, see section 7.31D(l)(r) of this document.

(14) National Institute of Occupational Safety and Health (NIOSH) Criteria Documents regarding Occupational Exposure to Waste Anesthetic Gases and Vapors, and Control of Occupational Exposure to Nitrous Oxide indicate a need for both local exhaust (scavenging) systems and general ventilation of the areas in which the respective gases are utilised.

(15) Large hospitals may have separate departments for diagnostic and therapeutic radiology and nuclear medicine. For specific information on radiation precautions and handling of nuclear materials, refer to appropriate publication of National Radiation Safety Council and Nuclear Regulatory Commission. Special requirements are imposed by the US Nuclear Regulatory Commission (Regulatory Guide 10.8-1980) regarding use of Xenon-133 gas.

(16) When required, appropriate hoods and exhaust devices for the removal of noxious gases shall be provided (see section 7.31(D)(1)(o) and NFPA 99).

ADDENDUM NUMBER 2

SUGGESTED OPERATIONAL REQUIREMENT FOR INDUSTRIAL QUALITY OF CONTROLS — PNEUMATIC OR ELECTRONIC

1. System Air Supply

System Static

Pressure transmitters

Range — not more than three times design duct static
Span — fully adjustable within the specified range of the transmitter
Accuracy — 1.5 to 2.0% of span
Repeatability — within 0.5% of output
Hysteresis — non-measurable
Linearity — 1.0% of span

Controller — three mode — proportional + reset + derivative (inverse)

Loop — closed
Proportional band — 0.5 to 40%
Reset rate — 0.2 to 75 per minute
Hysteresis — .008% of span
Inverse derivative — 0.5 to 18 minutes
Repeatability — .05% of span

Fan control — variable speed drive — 6 to 66 HZ

2. Room Differential Pressure Control

Static Pressure

Transmitter

Range — not more than three times the design space static pressure
Span — fully adjustable within the specified range of the transmitter
Accuracy — 1.0% of span
Repeatability — 0.1% of output
Linearity — ½% of span

Controller — three mode — proportional + reset + derivative (inverse)

Band — .25% to 40%
Accuracy — 0.05% of span
Repeatability — 0.2% of span

3. Space Volumetric Control

Flow Measuring Device (FMD)

Turndown — 5 to 1
Accuracy — within 2% of design flow with straight duct sections not more than 2 duct diameter upstream and ½ duct diameter downstream

Square Root Extractor
Accuracy ± 0.5% of span
Transmitter or Transducer
Range — not more than 3 times the velocity pressure signal produced by the flow measuring device
Span — fully adjustable within the specified range of the transmitter
Output — 3 to 15 PSI or 4 to 20 mADC
Accuracy — ± 0.5% of span
Repeatability — within 0.1% of output
Controller
Band — .25% to 40%
Reset Rate — .08 to 75 repeats/minute
Repeatability — .05% of span

4. Fume Hood Control
Static Pressure
Transmitters — Temperature Compensated — Drift Free
Span — 0 to 20 Pa
Accuracy — 0.25 to 0.5% of span
Repeatability — 0.15% of span
Controller — three mode — proportional + reset + derivative (inverse)
Span — 0 to 20 Pa
Accuracy — 0.15% of span
Volumetric
Transmitter — mass air flow — temperature compensated — drift free
Accuracy — ± 2%
Controller — closed loop — three mode — proportional + reset + derivative (inverse)
Accuracy — ± .02m/sec
Flow Measuring Station —
Average mass flow within 2% of the design including a 5 to 1 turndown

ADDENDUM NO. 3

DEFINITIONS

Range: Determined to be not more than three times the design signal.
Span: Range of instrument or control device adjustable within the specified span. A smaller span is critically important, especially with velocity pressure.
Accuracy: Expressed as a percentage of span. A 2% accuracy of 500 Pa span versus a 20 Pa span equates to a ± 0.55m/sec versus a ± .05m/sec. Pressure control of a space would be impossible with the higher span.
Repeatability: Amount of deviation in the output signal compared to a return to the original input signal.
Hysteresis: The distortion of the output signal which occurs because of increasing and decreasing input signals.
Linearity: Expected deviation of output signals from the theoretical straight line signal.
Inverse Derivative: A control mode that permits the controller to be tuned to the dynamics of air flow (without its noise) and eliminates most hunting and instability.

Sterilisation in UK Hospitals

by
N. Cripps
Regional Steriliser Engineer
West Midlands Regional Health Authority

Historical Review

Some of the ealiest writings contain references to techniques for preserving food by removing foul odour and taste. These references recognise that washing food containers is inadequate and an additional process is required. In the Old Testament Book of Numbers there is reference to 'flaming' cooking vessels as a means of cleaning them. Another classical reference is Aristotle recommending to Alexander the Great the practice of boiling his armies' drinking water.

In the 17th and 18th century empirical research methods were slowly replaced by scientific methods. At this time there was a gradual realisation that visible living matter was implicated in spreading disease and some experiments accidentally discovered materials which are still used for disinfection.

The increasing pace of technical change in the early years of the 19th century led to the significant development of the microscope and steam pressure vessels. Work during the latter half of the 19th century led to discoveries that hot air, irradiation and aldhydes have some use as disinfection and sterilising agents.

In 1832 a Manchester physician William Henry used a primitive steam pressure vessel to process clothes worn by sufferers of typhus and scarlet fever. Henry demonstrated that clothes subjected to this steam process could be worn by others who did not then contract these diseases. Louis Pasteur also used a pressure vessel with a safety valve for sterilisation.

When the National Health Service was formed in 1948 a bewildering assortment of sterilisation and disinfection processes were in use. Detailed investigations[1][2] highlighted a number of deficiencies and urged the use of properly controlled, central sterilisation facilities rather than numerous small sterilisers and disinfectors in wards or operating theatres.

Processes

Figure 1 indicates the processes commonly found in the National Health Service. Ideally equipment should be 'single use', that is sterilised by the manufacturers, kept sterile in its packing and discarded after use. Some equipment is too expensive to use only once and the Health Service undertakes cleaning, decontamination and re-sterilisation to make the equipment fit for re-use. To prevent re-used equipment transmitting infection between patients and effective, a reliable reprocessing system is required.

Most pathogens are made safe by hot water, 80°C for 1 minute, 71°C for 3 minutes are typical time temperature relationships,[3]. For sterilisation, dry saturated steam is required, typically 134°C for 3 minutes or 121°C for 15 minutes. Some equipment will not withstand these high temperatures and cold chemical processes are available. Low temperature steam with formaldehyde and Ethylene Oxide are chemical processes suitable for equipment that will withstand some heat.

The most common faults occurring during equipment processing are:-

(1) failure to clear;
(2) inadequate disinfection or sterilisation processes;
(3) recontamination of the goods after processing;
(4) failure of disinfection or sterilisation because:
    (a) the equipment is broken down; and
    (b) the disinfecting/sterilisation agents are not safety encapsulated within the pressure vessel or container.

Cleaning

Standard time temperature relationships associated with decontamination processes assume the goods are 'clean'. Processing dirty equipment is likely to lead to a process failure.

The normal practice is to wash equipment before subjecting it to a terminal disinfection or sterilisation process. A number of manufacturers supply washing machines which include a final rinse which is intended to disinfect the load. This type of machine is specified by the National Health Service[4]. Equipment requiring disinfection only, such as anaesthetic circuitry need not be subject to a further process and washing machines used for this purpose require monitoring including a permanent record of the disinfection process. There is a conflict between the need to avoid handling contaminated equipment and loading machines to ensure they clean safely and efficiently. Unfortunately the conventional washing machines require the load to be handled before it is decontaminated.

There are systems using mesh type theatre instruments baskets which can be efficiently processed through washing machines with the instruments remaining on the tray avoiding the need for staff to handle instruments by transferring individual instruments from the theatre tray into the washer/disinfectors loading system. There are only a limited number of applications of these systems but its use is expected to increase.

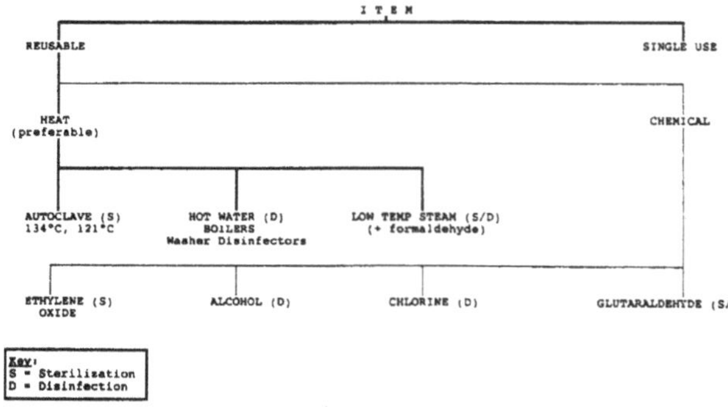

Fig. 1

LA STERILISATION DANS LES HOPITAUX BRITANNIQUES

Les méthodes de stérilisation et de désinfection visant à conserver la nourriture existent depuis l'antiquité. Les micro-organismes ont eux été découverts au XIXeme siècle, ainsi que la pression de la vapeur, ce qui a amené d'importants progrès dans le domaine de la stérilisation. La vapeur demenure la méthode la plus utilisée. La stérilisation elle-même en constitue qu'une partie d'une opération globale de nettoyage, comprenant la prévention de recontamination et les mesures de sécurité quant à la manipulation des produits chimiques utilisés dans cette opération. Les stérilisateurs achetés dans le commerce varient du simple au très complexe, les prix variant proportionellement. Les utilisateurs potentiels devraient s'assurer que le stérilisateur de leur choix correspond bien à leur besoins. Cet article passe en revue ces problèmes et fait état des progrès actuels dans ce secteur.

While it is preferable to decontaminate equipment in a washing/disinfecting machine this is not at present possible in all departments, particularly small clinics located a considerable distance from a sterile service department. A recent survey in the West Midlands Region indicate that 15% of equipment decontaminated with Gluteraldhyde is not pre-cleaned. This is unlikely to be successful because glutaraldehyde is a fixative, which will make subsequent cleaning much more difficult and the dirt will impare contact with the de-contaminating property of the fluid.

Effective Disinfection and Sterilisation

There have been a number of reported instances where a sterilising failure has led to the death of numerous patients[5]. Disasters invariably lead to improvements. Machinery manufactured and maintained to British and Health Service Standards[4][6][7] has resulted in significant advances in quality control techniques. There is however a need for vigilance as steriliser engineers continue to report equipment or operating practices which are unsafe and require substantial modification.

Dry saturated steam is the preferred method of sterilisation, it is very effective, has fast process times and can be physically monitored. Chemical and gas methods are much slower and are not usually capable of physical monitoring.

There is a requirement for an automatically controlled process, high standards of monitoring and an interlock which prevents the load being removed until the operating cycle has been satisfactorily completed. A separate steriliser is required for goods to be used on a patient and other materials such as discard from laboratories.

For effective steam sterilisation air must be removed from the load and chamber. Small plastic items containing discarded material, paper, linen and wrapped theatre instruments tend to retain air during sterilisation and active air air removal systems are employed which involve vacuum pumps and diluting residual air with steam. Less complex air removal systems and sterilisers can be employed for the sterilisation of unwrapped theatre instruments and utensils.

Simpler, less expensive sterilisers are available including modified domestic pressure cookers which operate as sterilisers and open boiling vessels for disinfection. These are particularly useful in countries where there is insufficient expertise to maintain complex equipment and they can be heated by direct firing. The users of such equipment need to be carefully instructed on their safe operation. In the UK careful consideration must be given to their compliance with statutory requirements.

Hot Air

Hot air is a gas sterilisation process which is capable of physical monitoring. Compared with steam the process times are long, usually between 3 and 5 hours. From time to time inexpensive hot air sterilisers are marketed principally for 'high-street' practitioners. Tests on one steriliser of this type revealed that disinfection was not achieved when the steriliser was operated in accordance with the manufacturers recommendations for sterilisation. In addition inexpensive hot air sterilisers do not usually incorporate an interlock to prevent the load being removed before the process is complete. Such equipment must be used with caution and does not comply with National Health Service requirements[7].

Low temperature steam and formaldehyde is regarded by some authorities as providing a marginal sterilisation process [8]. In the West Midlands a number of formaldehyde sterilisers have been commissioned but they have been rarely used. Hospitals prefer to forward their heat sensitive goods to one of the Regional Ethylene Oxide facilities or use liquid sterilising processes.

Liquid chemical sterilisation is often employed for heat labile equipment especially for fibre-optic instruments. These instruments are expensive and are decontaminated within the clinic because there is insufficient equipment available to compensate for the time of transportation to a central sterilisation facility. Fibre-optic instruments often contain narrow lumens which are difficult to clean and penetrate with the liquid sterilising agents. Debris and air bubbles are particularly effective at preventing adequate surface contact resulting in failure to decontaminate. Immersion times in glutaraldehyde, a commonly used material, are 10 minutes for disinfection 3 hours for sterilisation. A number of washer disinfector machines are now available for fibre optic instruments and these have advantages over hand washing and simple immersion in liquid techniques[9].

Numerous pharmaceutical and food products are damaged by prolonged exposure to heat. The European Pharmacopoeia[10] permits the use of Fo as an alternative to standard sterilisation time/temperature relationships. Fo is a calculation based on time and temperature giving a measure of the heat absorbed by the load. Within the Health Service the prinicpal applications for Fo are the sterilisation of culture media and heat labile pharmaceutical preparations. While simple temperature measurement and calculations by microprocessor enable Fo to be determined, to validate the process considerable microbiological analysis is required.

Recontamination

It is important sterilised/disinfected items are not recontaminated before use. Wrapped loads must be dry when removed from sterilisers. Wrapping materials are invariably designed to provide a bacteria proof barrier and high quality storage is required to maintain this essential property. Goods should not be stored where they are subject to damp, rodent or insect infestation.

Goods should always be re-packed and re-sterilised where packaging is damaged or there is any suggestion that recontamination may have occurred.

Reliability and Safety

Disinfection and sterilisation prevents the transfer of disease. Machines used for this purpose must operate reliably to ensure the appropriate products are available when required. An urgent case cannot wait for the steriliser to be repaired.

Vessels are subject to considerable pressure during steam sterilisation and effective pressure release devices (safety valves) must be fitted. Door interlocks must be provided to prevent uncontrolled discharges from pressure vessels. The principal interlocks being:- (a) a device directly connected to the chamber atmosphere, to prevent the door opening when there is pressure in the chamber and; (b) a temperature measuring device not located in a local container which prevents the door opening when contained fluid loads are above 80°C.

Many substances used for sterilisation and disinfection are harmful. Gluteraldhyde, Formaldehyde and Ethylene Oxide are all subject to occupational exposure limits and come within the scope of Control of Substances Hazardous to Health (COSHH) legislation[11]. Such materials must be contained to prevent them being hazardous to the staff. Residual material must be removed from the load to make it fit for use on a patient.

Ethylene Oxide has the added problem of being an explosive gas when mixed with air at concentrations greater than 3%. This gas requires careful handling; it should only be installed at Regional Centres where specialist expertise is available[7][12].

Enclosed drains and good local extract ventilation are required for Formaldehyde and Ethylene Oxide Sterilisers.

Local extract ventilation is also required where gluteraldhyde is used.

Gluteraldhyde is used in a wide variety of applications and there is evidence its use is sometimes inappropriate. The recent West Midlands Regional Survey indicted that its use could not be justified or was very questionable in 47% of departments reporting use of the chemical.

Some traditional methods of handling gluteraldhyde could be improved. Figure 2 illustrates a process of cleaning and disinfecting a fibre optic instrument. The process results in considerable spillage and vaporisation of gluteraldhyde.

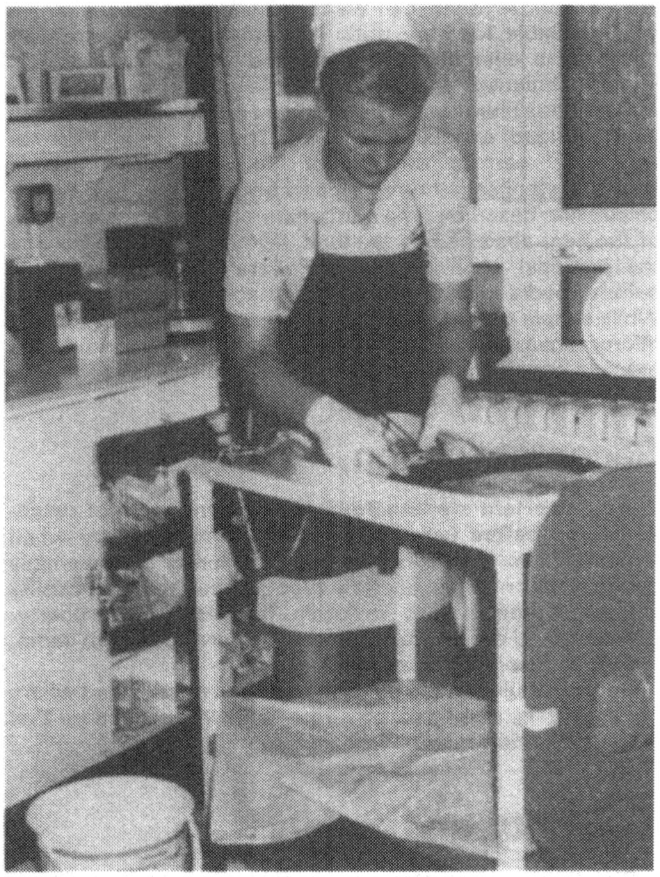

Fig. 2

The Future

The trend towards single purpose disinfection or sterilisation equipment will continue especially for the preparation of culture media and re-cycling fibre-optic equipment. There should be further applications of recent developments associated with using fans in the chamber of sterilisers processing contained fluids which has resulted in significant reductions in cycle time and improved product quality: Microwave radiation has been suggested as a means of sterilisation or a means of improving the Ethylene Oxide process[13].

These developments are being observed with interest.

References

(1) Central Sterile Supply Departments, Interim Report of Joint Committee, HM(62)59, Department of Health 1962.

(2) Central Sterile Supply Department, Reported the Joint Committee (Collingwood Report), HM(67)13, Department of Health 1967.

(3) Sterilisation and Disinfection of Heat Labile Equipment, Working Party Report No. 2, Central Sterilising Club 1986.

(4) Specification for instrument washing machines, West Midlands Regional Health Authority and Common Services Agency (Scotland), 1989.

(5) Report of the Committee appointed to inquire into circumstances including the production, which lead to the use of contaminated infusion fluids in the Devonport Section of Plymouth General Hospital, Her Majesty's Stationery Office, 1972.

(6) British Standard 3970, 1966 (issue of a revision is imminent), British Standards Institution, 1990.

(7) Sterilisers, Hospital Technical Memorandum No. 10, Department of Health (HMSO), 1980.

(8) Problems with low temperature steam and formaldehyde sterilisers; Cripps, Deverill, Ayliffe; Hospital Engineering, 1976.

(9) Control of Hospital Infection, A practical handbook; Lowbury, Ayliffe, Geddes and Williams; Hall and Chapman, 1981.

(10) European Pharmacopoeia, Current Edition.

(11) The Control of Substances Hazardous to Health Regulations 1988, (COSHH) Statutory Instruments 1988 No. 1657, Health and Safety Commission, 1988.

(12) The Health Services use of Ethylene Oxide Sterilisation; Ayliffe, Cripps, Deverill and George; Proceedings of a Symposium, October 1982, Central Birmingham HA.

(13) Optimisation of the Ethylene Oxide Sterilisation Process; Mathews, Samuel and Gibson; Journal of Sterile Service Management, June 1989.

Gas Sterilisation in the Medical Field

by
Dr E. Fischer-Bothof
DMB-Apparatabau, Saarbruecker, Allee 3, PO Box 130202,
6200 Wiesbaden 13, FGR

The introduction of highly sophisticated equipment as the heart-lung machine, electronic controls in intensive care, instruments made of plastics and other thermosensitive material into the medical field caused a dramatic search for non-thermic methods of sterilisation. Without a reliable method of cold sterilisation the revolutionary break-through in medicine runs the risk of ending in an impasse. Liquid microbicidial agents were excluded because of the well known problems of air-bubbles in tubes and insufficient moisturing of surfaces. The frantic chase for a suitable gaseous agent converged finally on ethylene oxide.

In view of the wide spread uneasiness concerning ethylene oxide it seems necessary to recall the reasons which decided the final choice of this agent for cold sterilisation.

First of all it must be kept in mind that a microbicidial agent has to destroy living proteins. Therefore any disinfectant per definition is harmful to human beings.

Non-thermic sterilisation is based, in contrast to thermic sterilisation as a physical process, on a chemical reaction of the agent with the protein. For this kind of sterilisation an agent is needed with an extremely high reactivity to reach a complete transformation of the protein of the germs. Furthermore this reaction has to be performed in an acceptable time.

Even more important is the capacity of penetration. Gas sterilisation has to deal with complicated narrow-lumen tubing systems, with endoscopic instruments of labyrinthine interior and with plastic surfaces. These surfaces tend to craze and present microscopic crevices. With all these objects the microbicidial agent must reach the deepest recess. This can only be done with an extremely high penetration power.

Ethylene oxide accomplishes perfectly these requirements and there is no other agent with nearly comparable properties.

It is only the other side of the same coin which creates an ill-considered fear in people, not realising that there is no harmless disinfectant.

The high reactivity of ethylene oxide cannot be restrained to proteins. Among other things it reacts also with oxygen which means ignition. Ethylene oxide is even so reactive that it can react with itself, it polymerises.

But the problem of ignition and polymerisation can easily be controlled by technical means. In a mixture with inert gases as $CO_2$the ignition area is considerably reduced and especially the lower ignition point is raised substantially. The mixture of 15% ethylene oxide and 85% CO_2 as an example has an ignition range between 21 and 49%. With such a mixture polymerisation is not possible. If in addition the interior of the steriliser casing is permanently ventilated any risk can be excluded.

Furthermore the reaction of ethylene oxide with the protein of the germs means that the same reaction takes place also in the human cell. Ethylene oxide is therefore toxic.

Fortunately the level of the lethal dose is rather elevated and the symptoms of intoxication are well noticeable and progressive. In the last 30 years there have been no intoxication with permanent damage in the medical field even under conditions which cannot be compared to the actual technical standards.

The mechanism of chemical sterilisation means interference with the structure of a living cell. It is therefore obvious that every chemical disinfectant must have a cancerogenic potential. In view of this fact discussions about the reliability of the latest animal tests concerning the cancerogenic potential of ethylene oxide or their significance for man are idle talk.

The cancerogenic potential cannot be excluded regardless which chemical disinfectant is used. Chemical sterilisation implies the absolute necessity to avoid any permanent exposition of the staff to small concentrations of the microbicidial agent.

This fact is connected with another property of ethylene oxide, its outstanding capacity of penetration. Unfortunately this penetration is not limited to the depth of crevices, but ethylene oxide penetrates also into the interior of the material itself. The desorption of these residues is a very slow diffusion process. The parameters of this diffusion process are the gradient of concentration, temperature and a constant related to the material. As we have only a very restricted range of influence on these parameters we must optimise these conditions. This is only possible in the sterilisation chamber itself and not in those so called ventilation cabinets. This imperative requirement is even more important in order to avoid any exposition of the staff transporting contaminated material from the steriliser to the degassing locker.

As gas sterilisation is a chemical reaction it is obvious that this sterilisation is a most complicated process with several parameters to comply with. It cannot be compared to steam sterilisation which is based on just one parameter that is temperature. Furthermore there is a strong interdependence of the parameters. Therefore a manual operation of the process must be excluded even in case of a fault in the automatic control. For the same reasons it is of vital importance that the automatic control system should be regularly maintained and calibrated.

As ethylene oxide is a dangerous product, a steriliser using this compound should be equipped with a suitable system of safety devices. There must be a reliable automatic leak control which controls the tightness of the whole system before the admission of gas. The interior of the steriliser casing including the cylinder compartment must be ventilated permanently. This ventilation must be automatically controlled and the whole process must be stopped if the ventilation fails. In addition the area of the door gasket should be sucked off. The door of the chamber must be locked in order to avoid any opening during the process including a sufficient desorption period. As the duration of the desorption depends considerably on the form and kind of material the desorption period must be determined by testing or related to the most unfavorable material.

Pure ethylene oxide with an ignition range from 2.6 to 100% in mixture with air should not be introduced into a

L'EMPLOI DES GAZ STERILISANTS EN MEDECINE

L'auteur met en valeur la raison pour le choix de l'oxyde d'ethylène commes agent froid pour la stérilisation des équipements medicaux complexes; il present les exigences de ce choix.

Il continue par vue présentation des proprietés de ce gaz suscitant des craintes de son emploi, et il dresse une perspective les vrais dangers et des modalités d'emploi et de securité nécessaires. En conclusion, il affirme que si ces conditions de securité sont satisfaits le personnel opère en toute securité et que c'est le gaz le plus fiable pour le malade.

hospital. Safety mixtures with inert gases should be used.

For the exchange of cylinder the steriliser should be equipped with a discharge of the flexible hose connecting the cylinder with the steriliser to avoid the exit of gas caught between the cylinder valve and the high pressure valve in the steriliser.

Beside personal safety it is important that the parameters of the sterilising cycle are exactly controlled and monitored and the process interrupted if any of the conditions are not met.

If all these requirements are met the sterilisation with ethylene oxide is not a hazardous enterprise but a safe operation for the staff and the most reliable gas sterilisation for the sake of the patient.

CFCs: The Way Ahead for Refrigerants and Sterilisation Mixtures

by
T. S. Barclay
Product Manager
BOC Limited — Special Gases

Introduction — Refrigerants

Prior to the 1920's, the refrigeration industry had developed using ammonia, methyl chloride, sulphur dioxide and carbon dioxide. With the coming of national and even transcontinental food distribution, a new refrigerant was sought that combined high performance and chemical inertness with low toxicity and flammability: although the refrigerants of the day possessed some of these characteristics, none possessed all.

In 1928, Thomas Midgely, while working for the Frigidaire Division of General Motors Corporation, was given the task of developing a new refrigerant with all these key properties. In a matter of days, Midgely had discovered the first of a class of compounds that came to be known as chlorofluorocarbons, or CFCs. As the name suggests, these compounds consisted of an alkane chain in which the hydrogen atoms are either partially or wholly substituted by fluorine or chlorine atoms.

A systematic numbering system was developed for these new refigerants based on a 3-digit number which denotes the number of carbon atoms in the molecule less one, the number of hydrogen atoms plus one and the number of fluorine atoms present. Figure 1 shows how this convention leads to the numbering of refrigerants 11, 12, 22 and 115. (nb R115 is used in a mixture with R22 to form R502. This refrigerant is widely used in industrial and commercial refrigeration).

In 1931, the first of Midgely's new refrigerants, R12, was launched commercially; this was quickly followed by a second refrigerant, R11. A number of related compounds were also identified, which contained other halogens: these were called halons.

Introduction — Ethylene Oxide

At about the same time Midgely was engaged in this research, Schrader and Bossert were carrying out research into the properties of ethylene oxide, EtO, which had been discovered by Wurtz in 1859. Although by the late 1920's it was known that EtO possessed pesticidal properties, Schrader and Bossert demonstrated that it was also a powerful bacteriocide.

EtO was shown to have advantages over steam and dry heat sterilisation methods since, unlike these techniques, it was suitable for use with a wide range of heat sensitive and thermal insulating materials. Also, not only does it possess excellent penetrative properties but also leaves no residue film on equipment, unlike some other sterilising agents such as formaldehyde.

REFRIGERANT	CHEMICAL FORMULA		CONVENTION: [No.C−1][No.H+1][No.F]
R11	CCl_3F	1xC,3xCl,1xF	R [1−1][0+1][1]
R12	CCl_2F_2	1xC,2xCl,2xF	R [1−1][0+1][2]
R22	$CHClF_2$	1xC,1xH,1xCl,2xF	R [1−1][1+1][2]
R115	$CClF_2-CF_3$	2xC,1xCl,5xF	R [2−1][0+1][5]
R502	All '5' series refrigerants are mixtures and are assigned an arbitrary number.		

Fig. 1 — Refrigerant Numbering System.

Interest in EtO as a sterilising agent increased and in 1949, Phillips and Kaye published a series of four papers setting out the parameters necessary for achieving sterility of bacterial spores using EtO.

The mechanism of this bacteriocidal activity was not fully understood; despite this, EtO found widespread use as a sterilant. (It was later shown that EtO and similar alkylating agents disrupt the normal metabolic and reproductive processes of the microbial cell by reaction with sulphyl, amino, carboxyl or hydroxyl groups within the cell. Figure 2 illustrates this mechanism).

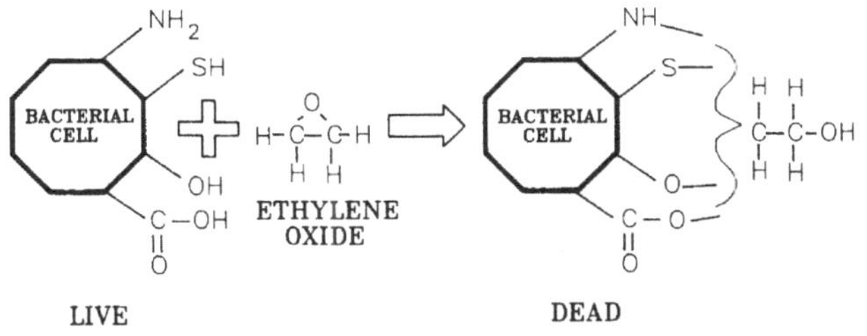

Fig. 2 — Theoretical Reaction of Ethylene Oxide on a Bacterial Cell by Alkylation.

EtO/R12 Sterilisation Mixtures

Although seemingly ideal as a sterilising medium, EtO does have one major drawback: it is flammable in almost all concentrations with air. Therefore, a diluent carrier gas was sought that was both readily miscible with EtO and which quenched its flammability, without impairing its excellent penetrative properties. The common refrigerant of the day, R12, was identified as being the most suitable since not only did it possess the key characteristics already mentioned but also formed perfect mixtures with EtO due to

LES CFC ET L'AVENIR POUR LES REFRIGERANTS ET LES STERILISANTS

A cause des effets néfastes des réfrigérants CFC sur la couche d'ozone de la terre, des accords internationaux ont abouti au Protocole de Montreal, qui prévoit un remplacement progressif de ces substances dans la mesure où les réfrigérants sont souvent employés dans la composition des stérilisants, le Protocole a des implications évidentes.

Des mélanges de remplacement beaucoup moins nocifs pour l'atmosphère ont été découverts, et ceux-ci devraient être commercialisés dans les années qui suivent. En attendant, il devrait être possible de remplacer le R12 (réfrigérant le plus commun dans la composition des stérilisants) par un autre réfrigérant en usage, qui ne serait pas inclus dans le Protocole.

the polarity of the R12 molecule. Figure 3 shows a comparison of the physical properties of EtO and R12.

	R12	EtO
Chemical Formula	CCl_2F_2	C_2H_4O
Molecular Weight	120.92	44.05
Specific Volume (20°C, 1 atm.)	198 ml/g	557.1 ml/g
Boiling Point (1 atm)	−29.79 °C	10.5 °C
Freezing Point (1 atm)	−158 °C	−112.5 °C
Density, liquid @ 20°C	1.33 g/ml	0.872 g/ml
Density, gas (20 °C, 1 atm)	5.06 g/l	1.795 g/l
Specific Gravity (Air = 1)	4.2	1.49
Critical Temperature	112°C	195.8°C
Colour	colourless	colourless
Flammability	non flammable	flammable limits: 3 – 100% by vol.
Odour	odourless in moderate conc.	sickening odour at moderate conc.

Fig. 3 — A Comparison of R12 and Ethylene Oxide.

Unlike other possible diluents such as carbon dioxide, R12 and similar refrigerants have low, positive vapour pressures; this is advantageous to their introduction into the sterilisation chamber. In addition, since EtO and R12 form perfect mixtures, the ratio of EtO to R12 remains constant throughout use, unlike other possible mixtures in which the ratio of EtO to diluent varies with use, thereby impairing process control.

For all these reasons, the use of EtO/R12 mixtures increased throughout the 1950's and 60's: they came to be used in an increasing range of applications including the sterilisation of medical and cosmetic products and for the sterilisation of spices.

Refrigerants and The Environment

While the use of EtO/R12 was becoming more widespread, questions were being asked about the ultimate fate of CFCs after release to the atmosphere. It was well known that CFCs are largely chemically inert and studies showed them to have long atmospheric lifetimes (typically 60-400 years).

In 1974, Molina and Rowland of the University of California began a study into the environmental impact of CFCs after release to the atmosphere. Their findings proposed a link between the depletion of stratospheric ozone (more commonly termed 'the Ozone Layer') and the presence of chlorine monoxide radicals produced by the breakdown of CFCs under the influence of the Sun's ultraviolet radiation. One such radical is capable of catalysing the breakdown of 10,000 ozone molecules!

This hypothesis had implications of a global scale since it is the stratospheric ozone layer that is responsible for absorbing much of the Sun's UV radiation. Without this fragile layer, more UV light would reach the Earth's surface, resulting in damage to crops and to the photoplankton at the base of the food chain. In addition, it is estimated that an increase in UV levels of just 1% could lead to a three-fold increase in the incidence of skin cancer.

The US authorities were quick to note Molina and Roland's findings and responded by prohibiting the use of CFCs in aerosols for all but essential (medical) uses. In Europe, the use of CFCs as aerosol propellants continued, largely unabated, despite the lower cost of many hydrocarbon alternatives.

The Montreal Protocol

By 1987 there was mounting international pressure for the use of CFCs to be regulated on a worldwide scale. Although, at the time there was no conclusive proof linking CFCs and the depletion of statospheric ozone, it seemed prudent for concerted action to be taken.

In September 1987, 11 countries, which together accounted for more than two-thirds of the World's total CFC production, agreed to a protocol regulating the use of CFCs and related halons, known as the Montreal Protocol. In ratifying the Protocol, member states agreed to a freeze on CFC production and consumption at 1986 levels on 1st January 1989 and to reduce this level of production and consumption by 20% by 1993 and by a further 30% by 1998. The Protocol also made provision for amendment of its terms should new scientific data show this to be necessary.

In 1988, Molina and Rowland's hypothesis was largely validated by the British Antarctic Survey team, who discovered a seasonal thinning of the ozone layer above Antarctica during the Antarctic spring. Similar studies since in the Arctic have shown similar seasonal thinning of the ozone layer here, also.

The Montreal Protocol and the gathering scientific data provided the impetus necessary for industry to commence research into alternatives to CFCs and for many other nations to sign the Protocol. More recent data shows that the original measures outlined in the Protocol do not go far enough and the Protocol is currently being revised in light of this. At a meeting in Helsinki in May 1989, member states agreed, in theory, to a 50% reduction in the production and use of CFCs by 1995-6, with a 95% phase-out not later than the turn of the century and a probable total phase-out not later than 2005. In addition, the Protocol may be extended to include other ozone depleting compounds such as carbon tetrachloride and methyl chloroform.

Alternative Refrigerants

In order to give a valid comparison of both existing and possible alternative refrigerants, each compound has been assigned an 'ozone depletion factor' (ODF). R11 is taken as the base and assigned a value of 1.0: all other existing and alternative compounds are rated according to the amount of ozone depletion caused in relation to this. For example, R22 which is now being recommended for many new industrial and commercial installations, has an ODF of only 0.05, or one-twentieth that of R11. Figure 4 shows the ODFs and applications of some of the more widely used refrigerants.

REFRIGERANT	MAJOR APPLICATIONS	OZONE DEPLETION FACTOR, ODF
R11	refrigeration, solvent for degreasing/cleaning, some sterilisation mixtures, blowing agent	1.0
R12	refrigeration, vehicle air conditioning, blowing agent, heat pumps, sterilisation mixtures, propellant	1.0
R22	commercial & industrial refrigeration, air conditioning, refrigerated cargo	0.05
R113	refrigerant, flushing solvent	0.8
R114	large industrial air conditioning, process temperature control, aircraft air conditioning	1.0
R502	commercial & industrial chilling/freezing, air/heat pumps in industrial applications	0.318
13B1	low temperature refrigeration, halon fire extinguishing systems (1301)	11.4

R11 = base = 1.0

Fig. 4

Figure 5 shows a comparison of the ODFs of some existing and proposed alternative refrigerants. It can be seen that the ozone depletion potential of a given CFC or alternative is related to the presence of both chlorine and hydrogen in the molecule. Since it is the chlorine atoms contained within CFCs that are responsible for the interaction with the ozone layer, if no chlorine atoms are present, the compount will have no potential for ozone depletion. In addition, it has been found that the presence of an hydrogen atom destabilises the molecule so that it is broken down in the lower atmosphere, long before it reaches the stratosphere: the very low ODF of R22 relative to that of

R12 reflects the decrease in stability caused by introducing a hydrogen atom into the molecule.

CURRENT REFRIGERANT	ODF	APPLICATION	PROPOSED REPLACEMENT	ODF
R11	1.0	blowing agent, solvent industrial air conditioning	HFA-123	0.02
		blowing agent	HFA-141b	0.10
R12	1.0	refrigerant, sterilisation	HFA-134a	nil
		blowing agent	HFA-142b	0.06
R22	0.05	refrigeration, air conditioning	NONE	
R113	0.8	solvent	HFA-123	0.02
			HFA-141b	0.10
R114	1.0	refrigerant	HFA-124	0.02
R502	0.318	refrigerant, commercial & some ind.	HFA-22	0.05
		refrigerant, industrial	HFA-125	nil

Fig. 5 — A Comparison of the Ozone Depletion Potentials of Current and Proposed Alternative Refrigerants.

In addition to minimal ozone depletion potential, it is also desirable for alternatives to have minimal potential for causing global warming via the greenhouse effect. Although the emission of halocarbons such as CFCs and halons is small compared to emissions of other greenhouse gases such as carbon dioxide and methane, the fact that halocarbons have up to 10,000 times the global warming potential of carbon dioxide, means that their greenhouse potential cannot be ignored. Figure 6 shows the global warming potential (GWP)

CURRENT REFRIGERANT	GWP	APPLICATION	PROPOSED REPLACEMENT	GWP
R11	1.0	blowing agent, solvent industrial air conditioning	HFA-123	0.02
		blowing agent	HFA-141b	0.08
R12	2.9	refrigerant, sterilisation	HFA-134a	0.1
		blowing agent	HFA-142b	0.3
R22	0.3	refrigeration, air conditioning	nil (HFA-22)	
R113	1.4	refrigerant, solvent	HFA-141b	0.08
R114	3.9	refrigerant	HFA-124	0.3
R115	7.5	propellant	HFA-141b	0.08
R502	4.0	commercial & ind. refrigeration	HFA-22	0.3
		refrigerant, industrial	HFA-125	0.2

R11 = base = 1.0

Fig. 6 — A Comparison of the Global Warming Potentials of Current and Proposed Alternative Refrigerants.

of some current refrigerants together with the GWPs of their proposed alternatives, relative to R11, which is taken as the base.

On the basis that alternatives to CFCs should have minimal ozone and greenhouse potentials, the World's CFC manufacturers have set about identifying environmentally benign replacements, the producers have agreed to pool their resources in the environmental and toxicological testing of alternatives: these two testing programmes are known as the Alternative Fluorocarbon Environmental Acceptability Studies, AFEAS, and the Programme for Alternative Fluorocarbon Toxicity Testing, PAFT.

In addition to HFA-22 (R22) which is well proven as a refrigerant, five other HFA (hydrofluoroalkane) alternatives have been identified and are currently undergoing trials. The first two of these, HFA-123 and HFA-134a (replacements for R11 and R12 respectively), should be available commercially by 1993, subject to satisfactory completion of a mandatory two year exposure study. All shorter term studies have already been successfully completed. Three other compounds also undergoing trials are HFA-125 (proposed as a replacement for R502 in industrial and commercial refrigeration) and HFA-141b (a candidate blowing agent).

One factor that initially threatened to delay the introduction of HFA-134a for refrigeration and air-conditioning applications was its compatibility with existing mineral oils. The majority of refrigeration systems require lubricants for the compressor, which is the heart of the refrigeration process. On studying HFA-134a, it was found that, unlike R12, it had a low affinity for existing mineral oils. The major CFC manufacturers declared their intention to cease CFC manufacture by the year 2000 and also set about the development of compatible alternative lubricants: a full range of compatible lubricants will be available by the time the alternative refrigerants are launched commercially.

Alternatives and Sterilisation Mixtures

Returning to sterilisation, we have already seen that R12 is currently used as the diluent for EtO. Once HFA-134a becomes available, it is expected that this will replace R12 in sterilisation mixtures. (Figure 7 shows a comparison of the physical properties of R12 and HFA-134a). It can be seen that the properties of both refrigerants are very similar.

To date, flammability studies involving HFA-134a/EtO mixtures have shown that mixtures up to 16.5% by weight of EtO are non-flammable (cf. 15.9% by weight for R12). Assuming a similar margin of safety as for R12/EtO mixtures, this gives a sterilisation mixture comprising 12.5% by weight of EtO (cf. 12.0% by weight in R12/EtO mixtures).

COMPARISON OF PROPERTIES: HFA-134a & R-12

	HFA-134a	R-12
Chemical Formula	CH_2F-CF_3	CCl_2F_2
Molecular Weight	102.0	120.9
Boiling point (1 bar), °C	-26.5	-29.8
Critical Temperature, °C	100.6	112
Critical Pressure bar	39.45	41.1
Sat. Vapour Density @ BP, kg/m³	5.05	6.33
s.h.c. of liquid @ 25°C, J/kg K	1427	971
s.h.c. of vapour @ 25°C, J/kg K	854	607
Heat of Vap. @ BP, kJ/kg	220*	165
Liquid Thermal Conductivity @ 60°C, W/m K	0.103	0.057
Vapour Thermal Cond. @ 60°C, W/m K	0.018	0.011
Liquid Viscosity @ 25°C, cp	0.205	0.215

* calulated value

Fig. 7

HFA-134a is a somewhat stronger solvent than R12: before introducing HFA-134a/EtO mixtures, more data is required on the compatibility of HFA-134a with plastics and elastomers. In addition to material compatability studies, trials are also underway to determine the rate of desorption of HFA-134a/EtO mixtures from treated materials together with required process times. By the time HFA-134a/EtO sterilisation mixtures are launched commercially, the associated technical data should be readily available.

Alternative Sterilisation Methods

Until HFA-134a and other suitable alternatives do become available in commercial quantities, there are a number of other possibilities for controlling or eliminating discharges of R12 to atmosphere from sterilisation plants.

Firstly, it is possible to use carbon dioxide as the diluent, in place of R12: however, not only does carbon dioxide not form perfect mixtures with EtO, but it is also somewhat more reactive than R12. Consequently, sterilisation chambers using carbon dioxide need to be of stainless steel construction. Sterilisation using carbon dioxide/EtO mixtures may also involve working at higher pressures which ultimately results in additional costs.

Another possible solution, until more HFAs become available, is to make use of refrigerant recovery processes, similar to those used in the refrigeration and air-conditioning industries.

Other possibilities for sterilisation involve the use of irradiation, both gamma and electron beam: there are already a number of facilities in continental Europe using cobalt gamma sources. In addition to the problems of handling radioactive sources and the cost of installations, there are also problems with material compatability.

The Way Ahead

In the interim, until HFA-134a becomes commercially available, it may be possible to substitute sterilisation mixtures containing refrigerants with a lower ozone depletion potential than R12. One such possiblity is HFA-22/EtO mixtures: we have already seen that HFA-22 is widely available today and has only 5% of the ozone depletion potential of R12. In addition, HFA-22 has a vapour pressure of 8 bar at 20°C (cf. 5 bar for R12).

Studies already completed show the limit of flammability of HFA-22/EtO mixtures to be 19.3% EtO by weight. Unlike most other alternative sterilisation mixtures, the HFA-22/EtO mixture should be a drop-in replacement for R12/EtO. Studies in this area are continuing and providing that an HFA-22/EtO mixture can be shown to be both safe and effective, BOC Limited, Special Gases will launch such a product in the near future.

References

(1) Stratospheric Ozone 1988 — UK Stratospheric Ozone Review Group, September 1988.
(2) Technical Progress Report on Protecting The Ozone Layer, Report of The Technology Review Panel, UNEP, 30th June 1989.
(3) Technical Progress Report on Protecting The Ozone Layer, — Refrigeration, Air Conditioning and Heat Pumps: Technical Options Report, UNEP, 30th June 1989.
(4) Report on UNEP Meeting, Nairobi Alliance For Responsible CFC Policy, 15th September 1989.
(5) Freon Fluorocarbons Properties and Applications Bulletin B2 E, C&P Department, Du Pont International SA.
(6) Focus On Ozone — Du Pont de Nemours International SA.
(7) Fluorocarbon/Ozone: Update — September 1989 C&P Department, Du Pont de Nemours International SA.
(8) Environmentally Friendly Chemical Substitutes — P. Glynn, Commission of the European Community, 1989.
(9) The Case For Continued Use of EtO Sterilisation: Pure EtO, EtO/Nitrogen, Carbon Dioxide, CFC Recovery — R. Shaw, C. R. Bard Inc., USA, November 1989.
(10) The Development of Environmentally Acceptable Alternatives To CFCs — A Progress Report — S. W. Kelly, ICI C&P Division, November 1989.
(11) Sur L'oxyde D'ethylene — Wurtz, C. R. Acad Sci (Paris), 48:101, 1859.
(12) Disinfection and Sterilisation — G. Sykes, Pub. E. & F. N. Spon Ltd, London, 1958.
(13) Principles and Methods Of Sterilisation In Health Sciences, 2nd Edition, 2nd Printing — J. J. Perkins, Pub. C. C. Thomas, Illinois, USA, 1970.
(14) Fumigant Composition — Schrader & Bossert, US Pat. No. 2037439, 1936.
(15) The Sterilising Action Of Gaseous Ethylene Oxide (1-4) — Phillips and Kaye, Am. J. Hyg., 50: 280-306, 1949.
(16) BOC Limited, Special Gases, Gas Data and Safety Sheets — 1985: R12 (dichlorodifluoromethane), Ethylene Oxide.

Present and Future UK Legislation Governing Waste Disposal

by
W. K. Townend MPhil, FRSH, FBIM, MInstWM
London Waste Regulation Authority
The County Hall, London SE1 7PB

1. Introduction

1.1 Waste Management legislation in the UK is in the process of being restructured and in the light of experience is being brought up to date to take account of current thinking.

1.2 The Environmental Protection Bill (EP Bill) was introduced into the House of Commons just before Christmas 1989 and received its second reading on 15th January this year and is programmed to be on the statute book by the Summer recess.

1.3 It establishes a new pollution control regime encompassing a number of brand new concepts which will assist regulatory authorities to control pollution of the environment. It builds upon the systems incorporated into the Control of Pollution Act 1974 (COPA) much of which is retained.

Whilst a new regime is proposed nevertheless the total system upon detailed examination proves to be complex with responsibilities shared amongst a number of regulatory bodies with interfaces at different levels and between differing types of organisation.

The Bill takes account of current thinking and the work of The Royal Commission on Environmental Pollution. The House of Lords Select Committee on Science and Technology, The House of Commons Environment Committee and extensive consultation with all interested bodies.

2. Background

2.1 The United Nations Conference on the Human Environment held in Stockholm in 1972 gave the emerging concept of the environment new form and direction.

2.2 It was this concern for the environment that prompted the Conservative Government in 1972 to introduce the Protection of the Environment Bill. During its passage through the House of Lords a number of amendments were made. An attempt too was made to ensure that an envrionmental impact assessment was carried out before embarking on any major projects. The idea stemmed from the USA, where it formed part of their federal National Environmental Policy Act which came into force on 1st January 1970.

2.3 When the Labour Government returned to power in March 1974 they reintroduced the Bill as the Control of Pollution Bill, many of the amendments made in the House of Lords to the original one were incorporated in the new Bill, but the proposals for a general standard and regard being paid to the effects of major projects on the environment were not included, probably causing the change of name of the Bill which accurately described its intentions.

2.4 The Control of Pollution Act 1972 obtained Royal Assent on 31st July 1974. It represented a major development in environmental legislation and with aspects to solid waste management could be regarded as of major significance then. The Act embodied most of the current thinking on waste management and took account of the reorganisation of local government which took place three months previously.

The Act applies to England, Wales and Scotland and a Statutory Order applies similar legislation to Part 1 in Northern Ireland.

3. The Control of Pollution Act 1974

3.1 The Act is divided into four parts. Part I deals with waste on land; Part II pollution of water; Part III noise; Part IV pollution of the atmosphere. It is with Part I that we are concerned. In Section 1 duties of the disposal authority are extended to ensure that adequate arrangements are made by them and other persons for disposing of controlled waste in their area and all waste that is likely to become so situated. This section has never been implemented and it looks now as though it never will be the present Government. Section 2 gives a duty to the disposal authority to investigate what arrangements are needed for disposal in the area and to prepare a plan after consulting with statutory consultees.

3.2 Sections 1 and 2 are of considerable significance as far as waste management is concerned. Section 2 has been in operation since 1st July 1978 requiring disposal authorities to produce a plan, although no time scale is placed on the preparation period.

3.3 Sections 3-11 and 16 introduced a system of licensing for all sites handling controlled wastes. Sections 12-14

LA REGLEMENTATION AU ROYAUME UNI, PRESENTE ET A VENIR DU TRAITEMENT DES DECHETS

Tous les pays développés ont ressenti la necessité d'avoir une politique du traitement des ordures et des déchets, particulierement dans les villes. Cette réglementation variera de pays en pays, sans l'influence de facteurs écononomiques, sociaux, politiques et de la loi qui y rapporte.

Le concepte que le contrôle et la gérance des déchets doit être éffective a l'échele globale commence à se développer à la suite d'événements recents que font paraître que 'les pays développés du nord' tentent de diriger leurs déchets dangereux vers les pays du sud en cours de développement, en particulier l'Afrique et l'Amerique du Sud. Sous l'egide des Nations Unies il se développe un cadre pour la Réglementation de la Gérance des Déchets, qui donnera suite à des accords internationaux. La Communauté Européene est en train de revoir la Directive 75/462/EC qui traite des Déchets et sont en train de considèrer un projet du Directive sur les Déchets Dangereux.

Au Royaume Uni la loi relèvant de la Gérance des Déchets est en revision et doit être mise à jour, les déchets medicaux ont étés definis en 1989 en tent que déchets dangereux, toxiques, ou nuisants la suite des activités des services publics au privés de santé.

Les gaz d'échappement des équipments, d'incinèration sont sous le contrôle de la réglementation nationale, et doivent être conformés aux Directives Globales au Internationales de la Region.

La santé et la securité de personnel de manutention des déchets sont sous le contrôle de la legislation Nationale.

La Réglementation des déchets d'origine des services de santé tant pour les animaux que pour l'homme a, pour objectif, d'assurer dans la mesure du possible et acceptable du point de vue de l'environnement, le contrôle de la separation et de la manutention de ces déchets du point d'origine au point de la destruction finale par un système d'inspections et de rapports formels qui permet un revue à tout stage, pour assurer que ces déchets sont sans danger et que les détritus aprés l'incineration ne presentent aucun danger pour la santé au l'environnement.

tidied up the law with regard to collection and disposal by local authorities.

3.4 Section 17 gives power to the Secretary of State to make regulations with regard to special waste. The Control of Pollution (Special Waste) Regulations 1980 were made under the provisions of this section in 1980. The Regulations provide for the control of difficult waste by requiring consignment notes to be used for waste included on a list in quantities likely to cause danger to health and for medicinal products defined in Section 130 of the Medicines Act 1968. This was in contrast with the method used under the repealed Deposit of Poisonous Wates Act 1972 where all waste not included in a list was subject to the consignment note control.

3.5 Sections 18-30 deal with miscellaneous aspects of public cleansing, implementation and interpretation and contain the authority to recycle materials and sell heat and electricity. Section 30 defines controlled waste as either household, commercial or industrial. There are also provisions with regard to uncontrolled waste.

3.6 The Act has been implemented piecemeal at intervals since 1974 and some sections of Part I have still to be implemented. (See Table 1).

Table 1 Part I

The degree of implementation of Part I of the control of Pollution Act 1974.

Sections	Date of Implementation
1	Not Implemented
2	1st July 1978
3 to 11 inclusive	14th June 1976
12, 13, 14	6th June 1988
15	Not Implemented
16	14th June 1976
17	1st January 1976
18	14th June 1976
19, 29, 21	1st January 1976
22, 23	14th June 1976
24	Sub-section 4 1st april 1977
25, 26	1st January 1976
27	Sub-section 1(9) and 2 — 1st January 1976
28	In its application to Sections 12(6), 21(4) and 26 — 1st January 1976
29 and 30	1st January 1976

Table 1 Part II

Regulations made under the provision of the Act.

Regulations	Date of Implementation
The Control of Pollution (Licensing of Waste Disposal) Regulations 1976 made under the provisions of Sections 3, 5, 6, 10, 11 (England and Wales only)	14th June 1976
The Control of Pollution (Licensing of Waste Disposal) (Amendment) Regulations 1977 (England and Wales only)	16th August 1977
Control of Pollution (Licensing of Waste Disposal) (Scotland) Regulations 1977	16th August 1977
The Control of Pollution (Special Waste) Regulations 1980 made under the provisions of Section 17	17th March 1981
The Collection and Disposal of Waste Regulations 1988 (England and Wales only)	6th June 1988 (Part) 3rd October 1988 (Remainder)

4. The Collection and Disposal of Waste Regulations 1988 (CADOW Regulations)

4.1 In 1988 the Government implemented Sections 12 to 14 of COPA at the same time introducing the CADOW Regulations to apply to England and Wales.

4.2 The Secretary of State for Scotland decided that he has no immediate intention of implementing Sections 12 to 15 or introducing Regulations for Scotland. Legislation with respect to the collection and disposal of waste was updated and consolidated in the Civic Government (Scotland) Act 1982 where Sections 124 and 125 apply.

4.3 In order to illustrate the effects of implementation in England and Wales I will discuss how they relate to the waste produced in hospitals and the philosophy which lies behind their creation and implementation. This should not be looked upon as a legal exercise but a practical way in which they are likely to be interpreted. The final arbiter of course will be the courts.

4.4 All waste from a hospital unless otherwise prescribed falls into the category of household waste. The effect of hospital waste falling into this category means that the local collection authority normally the local District Council or London Borough has a duty to collect the waste free of charge. However, in the case of hospitals this has been defined as a prescribed case and a charge for its collection may be made by the collection authority and the duty to collect does not arise until the collection authority has been requested to collect it.

4.5 If in any part of a hospital there is a factory within the meaning of the Factories Act 1961 then waste from that part will be categorised as industrial waste. The 1988 Regulations also prescribe certain other wastes which arise in a hospital as industrial waste they are:-

(1) Waste from premises where vehicles are maintained.
(2) Laboratory waste.
(3) Waste from a workshop.
(4) Premises occupied by a scientific research association.
(5) Dredging waste.
(6) Construction and demolition waste.
(7) Tunelling waste.
(8) Sewage or sewage sludge.
(9) Clinical Waste.
(10) Waste oil or solvent.
(11) Scrap metal.

This is not a full list but only covers waste likely to be found in hospital. Industrial waste is a category of waste defined in Section 30 of COPA 74. There is no duty for a collection authority to collect this category of waste. They may, however, if requested to do so arrange for its collection but only with the consent of the relevant disposal authority in England.

4.6 It is important for managers to appreciate that they can invoke the duty to collect the waste produced in hospitals except that prescribed as industrial waste.

The complexity and importance of wastes management is not always recognised in hospitals. In the light of the changes in the law it is now vital that a senior manager in each hospital is given the duty to ensure that proper arrangements are made for the collection and disposal of wastes. The Royal Commission on Environmental Pollution in their 11th Report entitled 'Managing Waste: The Duty of Care' were concerned at the standards of waste management in the NHS and recommended that all Regional Health Authorities should prepare and implement waste disposal plans that match the arising and the disposal facilities in health care establishments. The Government in their response pointed out that the Waste Disposal Authorities have a clear duty to prepare plans under the provisions of COPA 74 and should take account of waste produced by the NHS and stressed that the NHS should of course co-operate with disposal authorities in this connection. In the first instance close co-operation with the collection authority is the correct line of communication in England where the two functions of collection and disposal can be separate.

5. Sections 3 to 11 of COPA and the 1988 CADOW Regulations

5.1 These sections deal with the licensing of sites for depositing controlled waste or for the use of plant or equipment for dealing with waste. They apply to England, Wales and Scotland. The Regulations clarify by prescription the cases where plant or equipment is used for dealing with controlled waste or where waste is deposited on land.

Most NHS hospitals cannot be prosecuted for offences under the provisions of Sections 3 to 11 because of the exemptions of Crown land from legal action.

5.2 The penalties for operating a site without a licence being in force include a maximum penalty of two years imprisonment on indictment. The penalties are even more stringent where the waste in question is poisonous noxious or polluting and its presence is likely to give rise to an environmental hazard.

5.3 The Joint Circular 55/76 that accompanied the introduction of COPA 74 made clear that whilst the Act exempted Crown land from prosecution they expected that operating standards meet with the approval of the relevant Waste Disposal Authority.

5.4 In a hospital the plant or equipment that would require a licence include the hospital incinerator if it burns waste. This is clearly stated in Schedule 5 of the 1988 Regulations. The size of incinerator requiring a licence is qualified in Schedule 6 so that an incinerator not burning 'Special Waste' on the premises on which it is produced by means of plant with a disposal capacity of not more than 200 kg per hour should not require a licence. Special waste is defined in The Control of Pollution (Special Wastes) Regulations 1980. If the hospital incinerator burns any of this material and it is unlikely not to if it is being used to dispose of clinical waste and pharmaceuticals then the size qualification does not preclude the incinerator from having a licence.

5.5 A site licence is also required for the storage of special waste on the premises on which it is produced pending its disposal elsewhere. This again is prescribed in Schedule 6 so that a licence is required if over a total of 80 cb m of special waste in containers or a total of over 50 cb m of special waste in a secure place or places is stored. If yellow bagged clinical waste is being accumulated to exceed the amount stated and contains special waste it would be necessary for a licence to be issued.

5.6 Some hospitals in order to meet with the spirit of COPA 74 and the Circular 55/76 have gone through the procedure of obtaining a site licence irrespective of the effects of Crown Immunity in order to satisfy the waste regulation authority that their operational procedures are being carried out to a satisfactory standard. These licences apart from satisfying both the hospitals and the Authority concerning standards, also creates an awareness among the hospital staff of the need for the security of waste streams both inside and outside the hospital, and is of great benefit to the regulation authority in ensuring that satisfactory waste management standards are being practised. It is strongly recommended therefore that hospital management seek from their disposal authority a site licence in all cases where a site licence is necessary under the provisions of COPA 74 and the 1988 Regulations.

6. Clinical Waste

6.1 The derivation of the term 'clinical wastes' is obscure but it first appeared in an official document produced by the UK Health and Safety Commission in 1982 entitled 'The Safe Disposal of Clinical Waste' which defined and categorised clinical waste.

6.2 Waste or refuse is understood in most countries of the world. The adjective, clinical, which is defined in the Concise Oxford Dictionary as meaning 'of or at the sick bed' gives a specific meaning to the waste and more accurately describes the wastes we are dealing with than other definitions which include terms like hospital waste a term which is too imprecise as it covers all wastes from hospitals and does not cover clinical waste from the community.

6.3 The Environmental Protection Agency of the USA use the term infectious waste as it fits into their legislative framework for dealing with Hazardous Waste which they define as 'A solid waste, or a combination of solid wastes, which because of its quality, concentration, or physical, chemical or infectious characteristic may:-

(a) cause or significantly contribute to an increase in mortality or an increase in serious irreversible, or incapacitating reversible illness; or
(b) pose substantial present or potential hazard to human health or the environment when improperly treated, stored, transported, or disposed of, or otherwise managed. Solid wastes are defined in the Statute as solids, liquids, and gas.

and their categories of infectious waste are set out below:

(i) isolation wastes
(ii) cultures and stocks of infectious agents and associated biologicals
(iii) human blood and blood products
(iv) pathological waste
(v) contaminated sharps
(vi) contaminated animal carcasses, body parts, bedding

and the following optional miscellaneous contaminated wastes depending upon decisions taken at the facility:-

(a) wastes from surgery and autopsy
(b) miscellaneous laboratory wastes
(c) dialysis unit wastes
(d) contaminated equipment

6.4 The World Health Organisation in 'Management of Waste for Hospitals' in 1985 classified health care waste into eight main categories:-

(i) general waste
(ii) pathological waste
(iii) radioactive waste
(iv) chemical waste
(v) infectious and potentially infectious waste
(vi) sharps
(vii) pharmaceutical waste
(viii) pressurised containers

6.5 In 1982 the Commission of the European Communities published a Survey of the Collection, Recycling and Safe Disposal of Hospital Wastes in the Member States of the European Communities. An attempt was made to draft a Community Directive in which hospital wastes were categorised as 'Unproblematic' waste that can be disposed of in any way and 'problematic' wastes that must be burned, buried or sterilised.

6.6 The United Kingdom Health and Safety Executive (HSE) Guidance Document 'The Safe Disposal of Clinical Waste' referred to earlier: defines clinical waste as:- 'Waste arising from medical, nursing, dental, veterinary, pharmaceutical, or similar practice, investigation, treatment, care, teaching or research which by nature of its toxic, infectious or dangerous content may prove a hazard or give offence unless previously rendered safe and inoffensive. Such wastes include human or animal tissue or excretions, drugs and medicinal products, swabs and dressings, instruments or similar substances and materials' and categorises them thus:-

Group A

(a) Soiled surgical dressings, swabs and all other contaminated waste from treatment area;

Group A

(b) Material other than linen from cases of infectious disease;

Group A

(c) All human tissues (whether infected or not), animal carcasses and tissues from laboratories, and all related swabs and dressings.

Group B

Discarded syringes, needles, cartridges, broken glass and any other sharp instruments.

Group C

Laboratory and post-mortem room waste other than waste included in Group A.

Group D

Certain pharmaceutical and chemical waste.

Group E

Used disposable bedpan liners, urine containers, incontinence pads and stoma bags.

6.7 With modifications the HSE definition set out in 2.6 has been incorporated into the UK legislation framework. In The Collection and Disposal of Waste Regulations 1988 clinical waste includes:-

(a) any waste which consists wholly or partly of human or animal tissue, blood or other fluids, excretions, drugs or other pharmaceutical products, swabs and dressings, syringes, needles or other sharp instruments, and which may prove a hazard unless previously rendered safe; and

(b) any other waste arising from medical, nursing, dental, blood transfusion, veterinary, pharmaceutical or similar practice, investigation, treatment, care, teaching or research, and which may cause infection.

This definition for all practical purposes is the preferred one as it covers clinical waste produced from health care in the community and of more importance covers activities such as ear piercing, tattooing, and practice of alternative medicines, funeral undertaking as well as animal care.

6.8 Clinical waste can now be dealt with in a number of different ways under the provision of the Regulations. Clinical waste from a private dwelling or residential home is household waste and as such a local collection authority has a duty to collect it if requested to do so. The collection authority because it is so prescribed may make a charge for its collection. The Department of the Environment have stressed that they expect the collection authorities to take account of the social benefits before deciding to make a charge.

All other clinical waste is to be treated as if it were industrial waste. The local collection authority do not have any duty to collect it but may if requested to do so and then only after first obtaining permission from the disposal authority. A disposal authority in England where it is separate from the collection authority may also collect clinical waste where it is prescribed as industrial waste. The authority collecting it has a duty to make a reasonable charge for its collection and disposal.

The disposal of household waste within a private dwelling in normal circumstances does not require a site licence. The Regulations exclude clinical waste from this exemption.

6.9 The storage, transport, transfer, treatment and disposal of clinical waste is continuing to pose major problems particularly in the London area. The London Waste Regulation Authority (LWRA) recognising this established a Member Level Working Party to examine them. They set up an Enquiry so that professional staff of the various interested organisation could identify in detail the problems. The Enquiry began its work in July 1987. On 3rd October 1989 the work of the Enquiry contained in two documents was launched by the Under Secretary of State for the Environment Mrs Virginia Bottomly MP at St Bartholomews Hospital in the City of London.

The documents entitled:-

(a) Guidelines for the Segregation, Handling and Transport of Clinical Waste.

(b) Clinical Waste — An Appraisal
Can be obtained from the LWRA together with a new training video entitled 'Follow the Yellow Bag Code'.

7. Hazardous and Special Wastes

7.1 In order to clarify the terms 'hazardous' and 'special' I have set out below how the terms are defined for the purposes of COPA 74.

'Hazardous Waste'

The presence of waste on land gives rise to an environmental hazard if the waste has been deposited in such a manner or in such a quantity (whether that quality by itself or cumulatively with other deposits of the same or different substances) as to subject persons or animals to a material risk of death, injury or impairment of health or as to threaten the pollution (whether on the surface or underground) of any water supply, and the fact that waste is deposited in containers shall not of itself be taken to exclude any risk which might be expected to arise if the waste were not in containers.

Special waste is defined in the Control of Pollution (Special Waste) Regulations 1980:-

The term 'special waste' shall apply to any controlled waste which — (a) consists of or contains any of the substances listed in Part I of Schedule 1 and by reason of the presence of such substances, (i) is dangerous to life within the meaning of Part II of Schedule 1, or (ii) has a flash point of 21 degrees Celsius or less determined by the methods and with the apparatus laid down by the British Standards Institution in BS 3900: Part A,8: 1976 (EN53), or (b) is a medical product, as defined in section 130 of the Medicines Act 1968(b), which is available only in accordance with a prescription given by an appropriate practitioner as defined in section 58(1) of that Act.

7.2 Special waste is regulated by a 3 day pre-notification consignment note system. This ensures that it is controlled from production through to final disposal and that it is disposed of at a site that holds a relevant disposal licence.

7.3 The definition of hazardous waste appears in COPA 74 to determine the seriousness of the offence of disposing of waste without a licence in contravention of Section 3 of the Act.

7.4 Clinical waste as defined in the previous Chapter could be considered to be hazardous if the consignment did not contain any special waste. If the consignment contained 'special waste' then it would need to follow the consignment note system.

7.5 The yellow coded bag system for clinical waste is now fully and universally accepted. The degree to which it is used varies from hospital to hospital ranging from hospitals that insist that all materials from wards and treatment areas are placed in the bags including eg newspapers, dead flowers, etc following a 'better safe than sorry principle'.

Others arrange for just the clinical waste materials as defined to be placed in the yellow bags. The LWRA have evidence that from samples taken 18% of clinical waste in yellow bags contain special waste mainly in the form of prescription only drugs. There does not appear to be a de minimis qualification for medicinal products that precludes them from being considered 'Special Wastes' and a single pill meets the definition set out in (ii)(b) of the definition of special waste. For example if it was contained in a consignment would need to be dealt with as if it were special waste.

7.6 The regulation authority can direct that where consignments are regularly despatched to the same site, consignment notes need only be furnished to the Authority at regular intervals and not on each occasion.

7.7 The Pharmaceutical Society has issued 'Guide lines for the disposal of Pharmaceutical waste' which should be observed by pharmacists wishing to dispose of unwanted material.
7.8 The London Waste Regulation Authority at the moment operates a collection and safe disposal service for small quantities (less than 50 kg) of hazardous and special wastes. The service is free to the general public and charities and is also available to 'commercial' organisations eg hospitals on a cost recoverable basis. A number of other local authorities also offer this service.
7.9 The LWRA also offer a special collection service on a similar basis to that above for the collection and safe disposal of asbestos wastes.

8. Crown Immunity

8.1 The Royal Commission on Envrionmental Pollution in their 11th Report Managing Waste — The Duty of Care 1985 recommended that Crown Immunity should cease to apply to the NHS with respect to waste management. The Governments response in July 1986 was that whilst they had no immediate plans to remove Crown Immunity they would keep the matter under review.
8.2 The Government quite clearly stated in their response that they expect the NHS to meet and maintain standards required by COPA 74 and supporting regulations. They gave an assurance that evidence that Health Authorities are not complying is thoroughly investigated.
8.3 In the debate in the House of Lords on 14 October 1986, on the National Health Service (Amendment) Bill, an Amendment was carried under a Clause related to health and safety legislation to remove Crown Immunity from the NHS. During the debate, concern was expressed over the storage of materials of a noxious type and the collection and disposal of rubbish, which left much to be desired and often presented a health hazard. Stress was laid upon the dangers of the health of workers and other people which could arise from the disposal of noxious and infected materials, Health and Safety could not be divorced from food hygiene. The question posed as to what the logic was of having one law for private hospital and another for the NHS.
8.4 In the House of Commons on 5th November 1986, the Minister of health, Mr Tony Newton confirmed the removal of Crown Immunity from NHS premises and health authorities in respect of health and safety legislation under the Health and Safety at Work, etc, Act 1974.

With regard to the removal of Crown Immunity under the Control of Pollution Act 1974, the Minister recognised that it might be worthy of consideration in the longer term.
8.5 In reviewing Crown Immunity for catering and the Health and Safety at Work Act the Government took account of a number of incidents that had taken place over the years. The weight of evidence with respect to malpractices in the handling of waste would again have to reach similar proportions before it would be removed from COPA 74. The evidence is available now of malpractices taking place in the handling and disposal of clinical waste from hospitals which is certainly in contravention of COPA 74. At the appropriate time further representations are likely to be made by the industry to see that Crown Immunity is removed.

9. Incineration

9.1 Crown Immunity precludes action being taken against NHS hospitals under the provisions of current 'Clean Air' legislation by local authorities.
9.2 The situation changed with respect to clinical waste incinerators capable of incinerating one tonne or more per hour when the Health and Safety (Emissions into the Atmosphere) Amendment Regulations 1989 came into force on 31st March 1989.
9.3 This required that the incinerators are registered before operation with HMIP. Before registration the Inspector has to clarify that it is fit and that best practicable means are used to prevent emissions and to render such emissions as are emitted harmless.

10. Future Legislation

10.1 The major legislation referred to in the introduction processes some brand new concepts. It is appropriate to discuss them in general terms at this stage in the progress of the EP Bill through Parliament as the detail can and often does change.
10.2 The Bill which when passed will be an enabling Act giving the Secretary of State power to make Regulations which can be changed as circumstances change or new situations arise. Integrated pollution control which will be carried out by a central organisation probably Her Majesty's Inspectorate of Pollution HMIP is a new concept.

Prescribed processes and prescribed substances capable of polluting the environment will be required to be authorised and Regulations may control the substances that will be allowed to be released into anyone or all of the environmental media of air and water or land. Authorisation can include conditions.
10.3 The 'best available techniques not entailing excessive cost' (BATNEEC) will be used to prevent the release of harmful substances and that principle is implied in every authorisation.
10.4 Where processes are designated for central control and substances are likely to be released into more than one environmental medium then as well as the principle of BATNEEC account has to be taken of the 'best practicable environmental option' (BPEO) as respects the substances which may be released to minimise pollution to the environment as a whole.
10.5 The Department of the Environment in its consultation paper 'Air Pollution Control in Great Britain Works Proposed to be Scheduled for prior Authorisation' proposed that for installations incinerating clinical waste at less than one tonne per hour they are to be scheduled for authorisation under the provisions of Schedule B and dealt with by local authorities. In order to provide guidance to manufacturers operations and regulators a set of draft Notes on Best Practicable Means have been issued by HMIP.
10.6 Another new concept is that of 'duty of care' for the producers, importers, holders or carriers of waste or the persons who treat or dispose of waste. Three things will be required:-

(a) They must take care to ensure that the waste is not illegally disposed of or illegally released into the environment.
(b) That a proper description of the waste is prepared by the producer and handed over.
(c) That the waste is only handed over to an authorised person eg a statutorily registered carrier of waste or site holding an appropriate waste management licence.

10.7 The Control of Pollution (Amendment) Act 1989 proposed a regime for the registration of all carriers of waste and will complement the EP Bill in that producers will only be able to hand over their waste to registered carriers.
10.8 The EP Bill at the moment does not have a Clause which refers to Crown Immunity.
10.9 A further new provision in the EP Bill is the power to refuse a waste management licence if the applicant is not a fit and proper person. Apart from legal and financial provisions there is also a requirement that the facility is to be in the hands of a technically competent person.

There are powers for the Secretary of State to prescribe the qualifications of a technically competent person. The Waste Management Industry have co-operated to form the Waste Management Industry Training and Advisory Board. It is working towards having a certificate of technical competence scheme in position by March 1982 for the operators of landfill facilities, treatment plants and the regulators of the waste management industry.

10.10 A consultation paper on Special Waste and the control of its disposal was issued in February 1990. It proposes to redefine special waste to take account of the proposals by the European Commission and the Organisation for Economic Co-operation and Development.

10.11 The major proposals are that to define special waste it must qualify in the following way. For example:-

In Annex A is a list of wastes which are dangerous or difficult to handle. Clinical Waste listed as defined in 6.7 of this paper is one such waste.

In Annex B is a list of substances which if present in waste could make the waste difficult to dispose of.

Viable pathogenic micro-organisms appear in this list.

In Annex C are listed Characteristic Properties which cause waste to be difficult to dispose of one example is 'Infectious' a substance containing viable micro organisms which are known or reliably believed to cause disease in man or other living organisms.

In Annex D is a list of readily identifiable household wastes which are considered to have properties which make them dangerous or difficult to dispose of. 'Clinical Waste' is listed in this Annex.

In order to qualify for the definition of special waste the waste must have at least one of the characteristic properties of either A and C or B and C or AB and C.

10.12 The other major change proposed affects the regulation authorities where it will be the responsibility of the consignees' regulatory authority to monitor the system rather than that of the consignor.

10.13 Consultation on the proposed new system is a two stage exercise phase two will be when the Regulations are framed and are put out for consultation.

11. Conclusion

11.1 In concluding this review of Waste Management Legislation it must be pointed out that it is not complete. It has been carried out in the middle of the process of introducing major new legislation into Parliament so there are as many questions posed as there are answered because the EP Bill is designed as enabling legislation. The regulations prescribing the detail will need to be available before one can complete the jig-saw. However the general direction of the legislation can be determined and it is sufficient for strategic planning to be carried out.

The Control of Pollution: Incinerator Process

by

Mike Bulley
Dip, Chemical Technology, BSc, UED
Auckland Environmental Protection Agency,
PO Box 11-026; Ellerslie, Auckland, New Zealand

Introduction

Over the past 15 years the wastes generated by New Zealand hospitals and particularly clinical wastes have changed significantly. Changes in surgical and clinical procedures as well as the growing use of sterile disposable items has resulted in a large increase of the amount of plastics contained in these wastes. A 1987 survey at Auckland Hospital and the Auckland Blood Transfusion Centre showed that plastics made up 38% and 31% by mass of the wastes being incinerated. Loads containing 50% plastic are not uncommon. The inevitable result of these changes has been a deterioration in the performance of the existing incinerators, smokey chimney stacks, and a poor public image which in the case of at least one incinerator, has led to a legal ban on its use.

In 1985 a new standard for clinical waste incinerators was introduced in New Zealand. Each new incinerator is required to have at least two combustion chambers, the final afterburning chamber to be large enough to maintain the flue gases within it at a minimum temperature of 1,000°C for at least 1.0 seconds in the presence of excess oxygen (> 5%) and in a turbulent condition. These standards were introduced to: (a) adequately destroy any dioxins which it was recognised will be created as products of incomplete combustion in the primary chamber (dioxins being the general term used to describe the 75 congeners of polychlorinated dibenzo-p-dioxins (PCDD's) and the 135 congeners of polychlorinated dibenzofurans (PCDF's)), (b) destroy any cytotoxic drugs which may have been included in the waste and, (c) completely combust the large amounts of carbon black (soot) generated from the combustion of plastics in the primary chamber.

Test Procedures

In March and May 1989 emission tests were carried out on a modern New Zealand designed three chambered incinerator located in Hamilton New Zealand. Samples of the flue gases were extracted immediately downstream of the primary and tertiary chambers.

Test techniques developed for these tests included the following:-

(a) The use of fused silica glass sampling probes to withhstand the high temperatures particularly from the tertiary chamber.
(b) The development of a xenon 127 isotope tracer measurement technique to determine the true tertiary residence time. This method was developed by the Institute of Nuclear Studies DSIR Wellington.
(c) The use of a Nordic modification of the US EPA Method 5 sampling train[1,2] to sample PCDD's and PCDF's.

Standard measuring techniques and methods were used to monitor the other parameters.

Results and Discussion

The carbon monoxide, oxygen and temperature levels recorded at the outlets of the primary and tertiary chambers for the two tests are shown in Fig 1. These readings show the different combustion regimes in the two chambers. Incomplete combustion in the primary chamber characterised by high CO levels (2-5%), and complete combustion in the tertiary chamber characterised by low CO (< 1ppm) and high temperature.

The tertiary chamber carbon monoxide readings were consistently below 1ppm, except for a brief eight minute excursion during Test 1 which resulted from a temporary imbalance caused by an incorrect attempt to change the excess oxygen levels. During this period a maximum reading of 160 ppm. CO was recorded, it also resulted in a visible darkening on the sample train filter and in a visible light smoke emission from the stack for about half a minute.

The hydrogen chloride emission tests showed the stack emission to average 100mg/Nm^3, dry @ 10% oxygen with a range between 62 and 160mg. This average emission level equals the plant licence limit. The control authorities do not at the moment require the installation of a scrubber to control these emissions for the following reasons:-

(a) There is a programme to limit the amount of PVC plastic used by hospitals, as this progresses there is every expectation that stack HC1 levels will reduce.
(d) The installation of a wet scrubber, whilst reducing HC1 levels by around 90%, will give a cold wet plume with no inherent plume rise. This could result in higher ground level concentrations (GLC) of HC1 than if a scrubber had not been present. Fig 2 shows this effect in comparing predicted GLC values for a hot 150mg/m^3 emission versus a cold 20mg/m^3 emission.
(c) The recognition that at this level of emission, the substantial additional cost of a scrubbing system even with a reheat facility, would result in a minimal ground or lung level benefit.

The gas residence times within the tertiary chamber as tested by the xenon 127 isotope method showed the residence times to be 1.7, 1.7 and 1.4 seconds.

The stack particulate emission level was found to be in the range of 50 to 60mg/Nm^3, dry, @ 10% oxygen. This particulate loading was not unexpected as a characteristic of the incinerator is for it to operate with an invisible plume throughout the total burn cycle.

The measured values of the various congeners of PCDD and PCDF at the outlets of the primary and tertiary chambers are shown in the Figure 3 comparison graphs. The values are expressed as ng/Nm^3, dry, and at 12% CO_2. The

CONTROLE DE LA POLLUTION — METHODES D'INCINERATION

L'incinération à hautes températures est devenue, depuis peu, la méthode la plus employée pour les déchets cliniques dans de nombreux pays du monde. Des températures résiduaires après combustion élevées (plus de 1000 degrés Celcius) et persistant à plus d'une seconde après ces mêmes opérations représentent désormais les normes de base. Ces normes sont nécessaires pour pouvoir se débarasser des dioxines et des matières cytotoxiques tout en garantissant que que les incinérateurs opèrent dans une atmosphère sans fumée et stable pendant toute la durée du processus.

Des tests d'émission simultanés ont été effectués á la sortie de chambres de combustion primaires et tertiaires d'un incinérateur moderne fabriqué en Nouvelle-Zélande, à contrôle d'air en trois étapes, traitant des déchets cliniques. Ces tests ont permis d'établir des mesures d'efficacité de l'unité post-combustion concernant la destruction des dioxines. Nous serons en mesure d'établir prochainement une comparaison avec des tests du même ordre faits sur des incinérateurs de déchets cliniques en Californie.

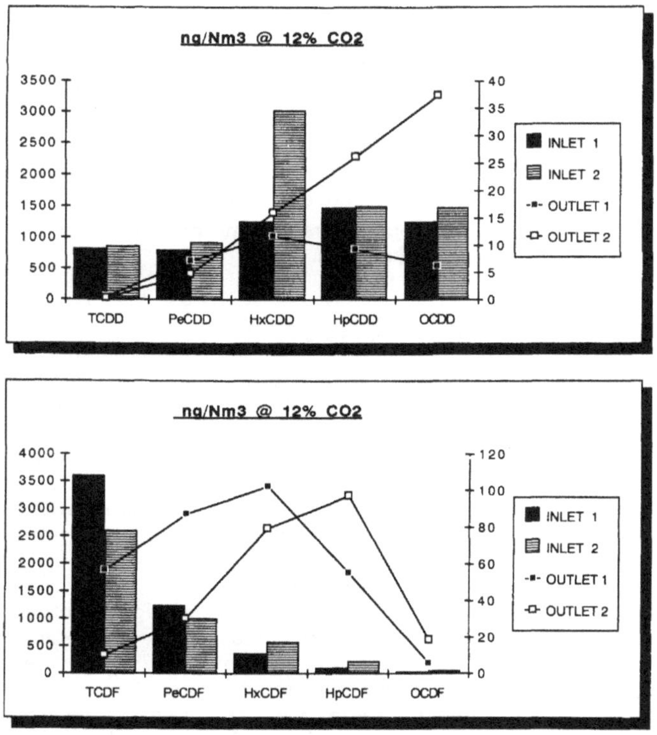

Figure 3.

Comparison with Other Results

No references have been found showing dioxin results before and after an afterburning chamber for an incinerator dedicated to burning clinical wastes. There are some results of dioxin concentrations from hospital waste incinerators at Sutter Hospital, St Agnes Hospital, and Cedar Sinai Medical Centre[3,4,5] published by the California Air Resources Board which could be used for comparative purposes. Figure 4 compares the results from these hospitals with those obtained at Hamilton for the basic groupings of PCDD and PCDF. As can be seen the Hamilton test result is considerably lower. Figure 5 compares those congeners normally used in calculating 2378 TCDD toxic equivalents. Again the Hamilton test results are lower. There is a common pattern in the concentration of individual compounds particularly for the furans. It is possible that residence time and to a lesser extent afterburner temperatures could be responsible for the differences in concentration of the compounds in the emissions from the various hospitals.

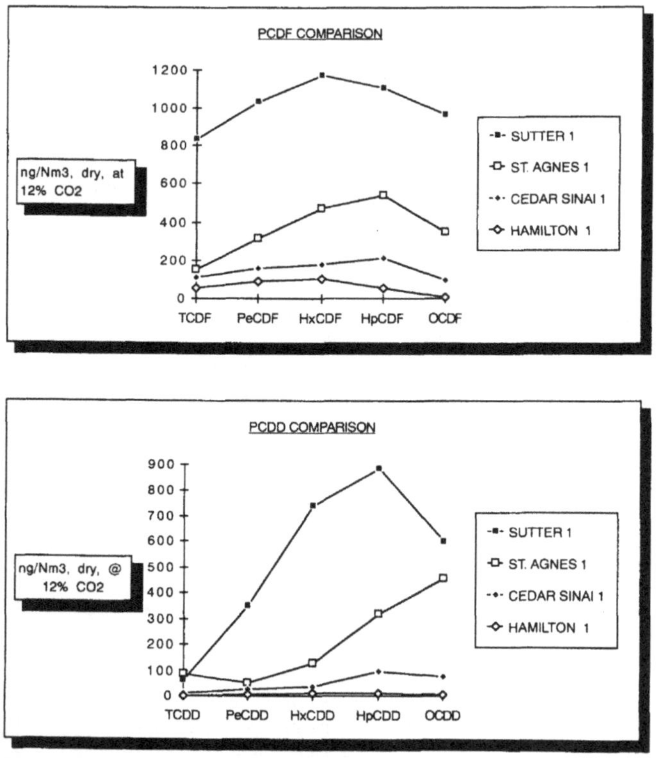

Figure 4.

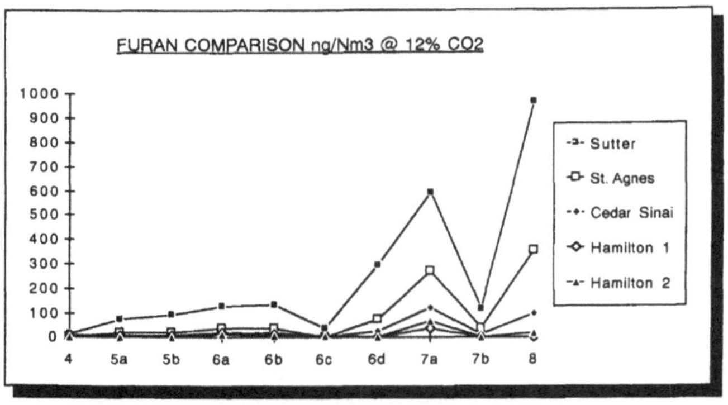

4=2378TCDF; 5a=12378PeCDF; 5b=23478PeCDF; 6a=123478HxCDF; 6b=123678HxCDF; 6c=123789HxCDF; 6d=234678HxCDF; 7a=1234678HpCDF; 7b=1234789HpCDF; 8=OCDF.

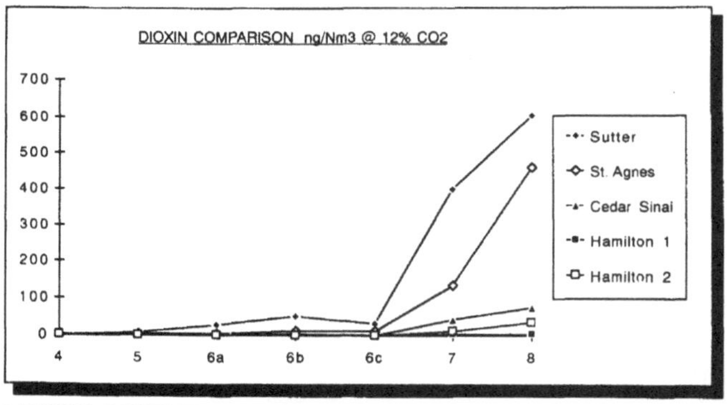

4=2378TCDD; 5=12378PeCDD; 6a=123478HxCDD; 6b=123678HxCDD ; 6c=123789HxCDD; 7=1234678HpCDD; 8=OCDD.

Figure 5.

A considerable amount of work has been done on municipal solid waste (MSW) incinerators with some comparisons being made to the difference in quantity of dioxin emissions between MSW and clinical waste incinerators. A Norwegian paper[6] quotes 2378 TCDD equivalents (Eadon) emissions of 1.3 to 20, and 240ng/Nm^3 for MSW and clinical waste incinerators respectively. Similar comments have been made elsewhere[7]. A probable reason for the higher dioxin levels from clinical waste incinerators is the greater amount of plastics in the clinical waste.

Some published dioxin limits for MSW incinerators are:-

(a) Sweden 0.5 to 2ng/Nm^3 2378 TCDD equiv (Eadon) at 10% oxygen for existing units[8];

(b) Denmark 1ng/Nm^3 @ 10% oxygen 2378 TCDD equiv (Eadon) as from 1991[9]; and

(c) Canada 0.5ng/Rm^3 2378 TCDD equiv (International)[10] R stands for a reference level of 25°C and 1 atmosphere pressure.

In terms of Eadon (86), EPA, and Nordic methods of calculating 2378 TCDD toxic equivalents the emissions of the Hamilton incinerator expressed as ng/Nm^3 at 10% oxygen were as follows:-

	Test 1	*Test 2*
Eadon (86)	6.95	2.49
EPA	2.77	1.42
Nordic	6.95	4.08

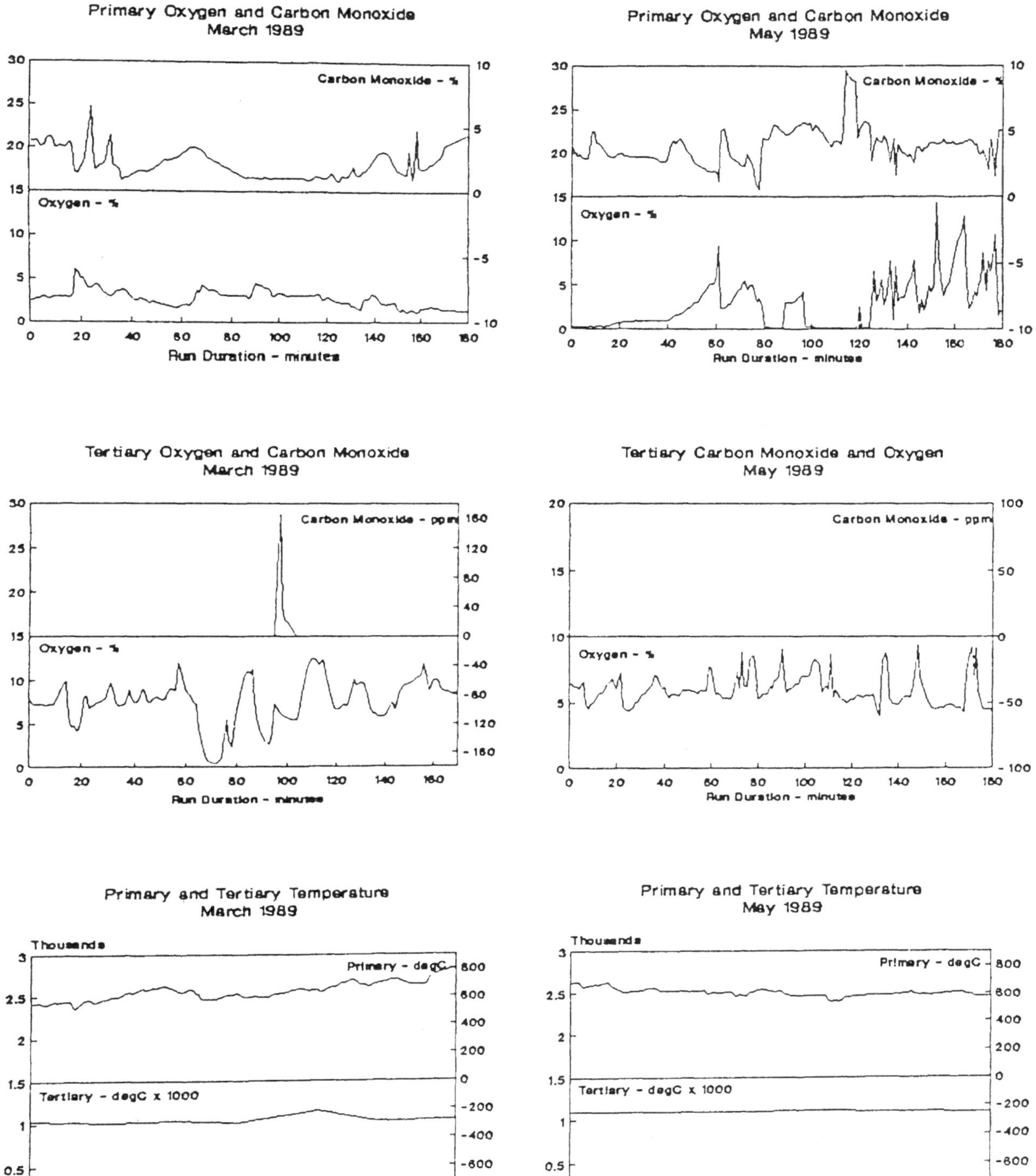

Figure 1.

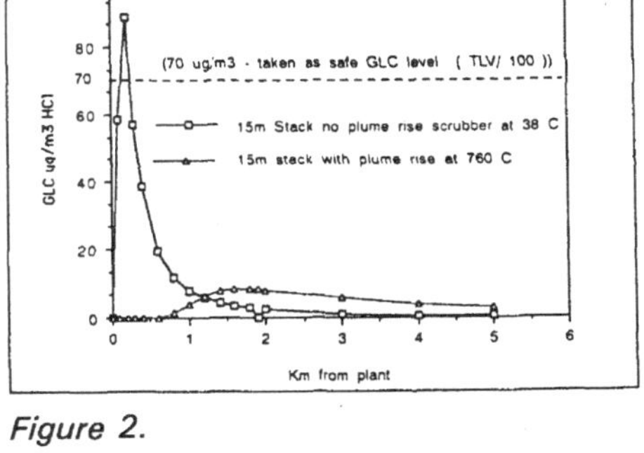

Figure 2.

primary chamber values are shown as columns relating to the values on the left hand axis, and the tertiary chamber values as lines relating to the values on the right hand axis. As can be seen the PCDD and PCDF concentrations are between a hundred to a thousand times more concentrated in the primary chamber. No 2378 TCDD was detected at the exit of the tertiary chamber in either of the two tests.

The graphs show the individual group patterns in each chamber, with the more highly chlorinated congeners tending to predominate in the tertiary chamber. The tests show that PCDD's are more readily destroyed than PCDF's, this may be more apparent than real as the cause could be the additional formation of PCDF's by the breakdown of PCDD's. In assessing the 2378 TCDD equivalent toxicities of the two tests it was found that the PCDF's contributed to more than 80% of the final values.

Conclusion

The work reported in this paper indicates that the Hamilton incinerator operates satisfactorily and that the destruction efficiency for PCDD's and PCDF's is greater than that reported for similar units in overseas studies. Improved destruction efficiencies might be achieved by maintaining oxygen levels in the tertiary chamber between 8 and 9%. (This has been reported as an optimal level in one recent paper[11].)

Acknowledgements

I should like to acknowledge the valuable assistance given to me by Nick Abbott, Alistair Bingham and Chris Edmunds of NECAL/DSIR Auckland for doing the dioxin analyses and helping to set up the sampling trains. I should also like to thank Medical Waste (Waikato) Ltd for permission to publish these results.

References

(1) Hartman, M. et al — National Dioxin Study Tier 4 — combustion sources: sampling procedures. EPA/450/4-84/-041C- Research Triangle Park: United States Environmental Protection Agency 1984.

(2) Joergen, Vikelsloe and Nielsen, Per R — Study of flue gas sampling procedure for the Danish incinerator dioxin program. Paper presented to the 8th International Symposium on Chlorinated Dioxins and Related Compounds, 21st-26th August 1988 Umea, Sweden.

(3) California Air Resources Board Test Report C-87-090; 'Evaluation retest on a hospital refuse incinerator at Sutter Hospital Sacremento Ca', April 1988.

(4) California Air Resources Board Test ARB/SS-87-01; 'Evaluation test on a hospital refuse incinerator at St Agnes Medical Centre, Fresno Ca', January 1987.

(5) California Air Resources Board Test ARB/SS-87-11: 'Evaluation test on a hospital refuse incinerator at Cedar Sinai Medical Centre Los Angeles, Ca' April 1987.

(6) Chemosphere Vol 17, No 11 1988 page N46.

(7) Chemosphere Vol 17, No 11 1988 page N51.

(8) Waste Management Int Bull Vol 25 No 1 Jan-Feb 1988 page 2.

(9) Chemosphere, Vol 17, No 11, 1988 page N28.

(10) Hay, D. J., 'Operating and emission guidelines for Municipal Solid Waste Incinerators. A paper presented at the 10th Canadian Waste Management Conference, October 1988.

(11) Hasselriis, F., 'How control of combustion, emissions and ash residues from municipal solid waste can minimise environmental risk.' AICHE Symposium Services, Vol 84, No 265, 1988 Resource Recovery of Municipal Wastes.

Clinical Waste Disposal: The Private Sector Alternative

by

W. McDonald
Chairman, Waste Technology Ltd,
Interchange House, 6 Cawley Street,
Ellerslie, Auckland, New Zealand

Because of the recently introduced requirements for controlled high temperature incineration of clinical wastes and the necessity for the off gases to be treated at high temperature for long residency times and be released to atmosphere under strict temperature and velocity conditions, the traditional hospital incineration facility has become the subject of considerably more attention than in the past. Ash quality is now a major issue and a high quality ash will also be a necessity, demanding a low carbon content with base metals being measured.

For the purpose of this paper the term Clinical Waste can be regarded as either segregated and classified waste or general hospital waste.

The economic necessity to now consider alternative methods of dealing with the problem includes the alternative of the private sector providing licensed incineration plants together with an approved and licensed handling and transport system.

With Area and District Health Authorities now being encouraged to 'privatise' their operations, other alternatives such as Joint Venture projects and Facility Management contracts have been negotiated or are being negotiated with the private sector on a world wide basis, and are *revenue* driven.

Ancillary services such as laundry services are included where heat recovery and power generation is a necessary component.

Joint Venture agreements may vary depending on local requirements and I detail some alternatives herewith.

Total Private Sector Investment

In this case the private sector are encouraged to provide the total incineration plant and associated services.

A 'Joint Venture' company is formed between the two parties and as a necessary component of the 'JV' agreement the private sector party is required to provide the capital for the total plant to the point of commissioning.

The 'JV' company provides a total waste disposal service including the provision of containers and transport systems to hospitals within the Area or District at a fee set by negotiation for a set contractual term. This is set in place contemporaneously with the 'JV' agreement.

Obviously the availability of a suitable area for the plant is necessary and is usually an existing site. This becomes revenue earning for the hospital as a rental is payable by the company.

Heat recovery and gas treatment equipment is included in the total package where necessary and in the case of heat recovery or power generation (CHP) a supply contract is set on favoured terms.

Equity Joint Venture

A 'Joint Venture' company is formed between the private sector company which must be an experienced operator of similar plants and services and the Health Authority concerned.

The 'JV' shall acquire all plant and equipment and lease all land and premises for its purpose.

In the case of our company we have been providing the plant and equipment at a 'favoured rate', also full training and information in respect of waste segregation, containerisation and transport methods.

The 'JV' company will then contract with neighbouring authorities and Health care interests to collect and dispose of their waste.

Revenue will also be earned from combined heat and power generation from the plant.

Outright Purchase of Plant with Facility Management Contract

This alternative has many variations and as in the previous options is capable of being adjusted to the mutual satisfaction of the parties concerned.

The Health Authority concerned, purchases the total incineration complex to the specifications required, including combined heat and power generation.

A Facilities Management contract is entered into with an experienced operator who will operate and manage the plant and operate the waste collection and associated transport services. Expert in-house training packages are available for the safe handling and segregation of special wastes.

Revenue can be earned from allowing the contractor to bring outside Clinical Waste to the plant from *approved sources* on the payment of a fee or royalty mutually agreed to by the parties.

Again revenue generation from combined heat and power recovery, is an advantage.

There is of course considerable data to collect and many considerations to evaluate prior to embarking on such exercises, some of which I set out below:-

(1) To establish the capacity of the plant required, the waste source area needs to be defined and then likely annual volumes forecast up to 10 or 15 years out ascertained.

(2) Whether segregation is preferred so that only the classified 'Clinical Waste' is separated for incineration (generally about 20% of total waste volume) leaving

EVACUATION DES DECHETS CLINIQUES — SECTEUR PRIVE

Cet article a pour but de souligner les avantages liés à l'utilisation du secteur privé dans des projects à haut niveau de dépenses. Elle permet en effet de faire intervenir une expertise technique, des capitaux et des services de gestion indispensables.

Il existe maintenant des programmes d'amélioration d'efficacité et de productivité. Ceux-ci sont issus de systèmes qui opèrent maintenant de facon rentable depuis cinq ans selon ces nouvelles recommendations.

Un de ces systèmes comprend le code-barre pour tous les récipients et sacs qui indiquent l'identité du contenu aisi que d'autres informations codifiées. Ceux-ci sont identifiés et enregistrés avant de quitter le point de départ ou de ramassage et réidentifiés au moment de l'incinération.

Ainsi des données d'information utiles peuvent apparaitre (volume par rappport à la source par exemple) et les anomalies sont immédiatement repèrables.

Des modèles de sacs et récipinets codés par couleurs sont utilisé en prallèle avec des véhicules spécialement équipés, faisant partie d'un système de transports efficace et rentable.

the remaining waste for disposal at landfill by traditional methods. Economic considerations for heat recovery plant or CHP need to be considered as to whether all waste is needed for incineration or not.

(3) After establishing the volume of waste to be incinerated *daily*, the calorific value of that volume needs to be ascertained together with the average density.

(4) Calculations as to the changes to this data annually up to 10 or 15 years out is essential.

(5) Careful planning of the site which will need to house the plant designed to meet the demands set out above. Full dimensions of building space available including stack requirements are necessary.

It is necessary to design an efficient material handling system to streamline the waste flow from cradle to grave and our company has many options available, with specially designed containers and vehicles.

When selecting plant it is important to anticipate the regulatory requirements governing emissions and ash quality up to 15 years out.

It is difficult to establish this with the goal posts regularly being moved. However, it does seem that we are settling into an area of standardisation for gas residency times of at between one second and two seconds at temperatures between 1,000° and 1,300°C. The presence of excess air and gas turbulence have also become standard requirements. The plant must operate smoke free with total stability on a continuous basis.

It has been necessary to control ash quality. All future plants will almost certainly operate with the ability to efficiently de-ash over 24 hours per day. Some requirements place the maximum carbon content of the ash at as little as one per cent by volume. Accordingly we are designing our plants to meet the low carbon requirements expected.

We have established that the most efficient, safe and productive method of Clinical Waste disposal by high temperature incineration is effected with our mutli chambered solid hearth, controlled air incinerator encompassing automatic loading with container lift, continuous operation, fully automatic and programmed PLC visual screen controls and automatic de-ashing.

Where chlorine levels are excessive in emission tests, gas treatment plants are effectively added at substantial expense.

Chlorine levels have been effectively reduced by a concentrated effort on the part of those responsible for purchasing 'Hospital Supplies' to ensure suppliers eliminate the PVC content of their product. Hospitals and other Health Care areas are giving preference to products which are PVC free. In some cases 'PVC free' products are more expensive but are still given preference.

This policy is market driven and very quickly all manufacturers of medical supplies with PVC content who no longer win tenders or receive orders, seek out alternatives. Tenders and supply contracts should specify very clearly that preference will be given to 'PVC free' products.

Summary

This paper is intended to highlight the potential of involving the private sector in capital intensive projects by providing technical expertise, capital and management skills.

Programmes designed to increase efficiency and productivity are made available. These programmes have evolved from systems which have been efficiently operating for five years within the new guidelines.

One such system involves the bar coding of all containers and bags which have source identification together with other coded information. These are identified and recorded prior to leaving the point of origin or collection point and identified again prior to incineration at the incineration plant.

Valuable information on volume by source and immediate highlighting of missing containers becomes available.

Designs of colour coded bags and containers are all made available together with specially designed vehicles encompassing well organised and efficient transport systems.

Slides of a typical plant will now be shown and should there be time, questions are welcome.

May I at this point congratulate Ray Kensett for having the ability to convince me to attend and present this paper.

The Control of Pollution

by
R. G. Kensett BA, CEng, MIMechE, MCIBSE, MInstE, MBIM, FIHospE

Proposals are now under consideration to review current legislation regarding pollution from all sources. When these proposals are considered in conjunction with the removal of Crown Immunity it is likely to affect all of us concerned with the NHS estate.

Before considering the proposed changes to legislation it is opportune to review both the historical background to pollution control and the current position.

It is important to emphasise however that despite what many of the public appear to think, Crown Immunity does not necessarily imply that lower standards of control are applicable to Government premises.

Many of us are old enough to remember the dreadful fogs and the smog of the late 40s and early 50s which affected our cities. Not only did these conditions virtually bring our cities to a standstill but they contributed in no small measure to high mortality rates from respiratory disease particularly amongst the old and the very young.

Probably the incident which drew the greatest attention and which made legislators realise the need for urgent action was the London smog of 1952 which was reported to have caused some 4,000 excess deaths. Meteorological conditions combined with uncontrolled chimney emissions to bring about appalling conditions which endured for four days throughout the London area.

As a result the public conscience was stirred and a Royal Commission set up under the chairman of Sir Hugh Beaver (the Beaver Committee) to study the problem. The Committee produced two far reaching reports. These reports recognised that the basic problem arose through the uncontrolled gaseous and particulate emissions, laying particular emphasis on sulphur dioxide. As a result and with the support of the late Gerald Nabarro MP (he of the fabulous handlebar moustache) the Clean Air Act of 1956 came into being. No doubt all readers are familiar with the provisions of the Act and have also, as I have, crossed swords with Environmental Health Officers over required chimney heights.

Subsequently people came to appreciate and realise the need to protect our total environment. Greater understanding of the long term effects of environmental pollution was reached by all sections of the population and realisation that, whether we are rich or poor, the conditions under which future generations would live was the inheritance we all leave. As a result pollution became a recognised 'field' of policy and public debate. Environmental legislation had, of course, existed for a long while but generally governments had shown only occasional signs of treating these diverse issues as both politically important and closely related. Since public recognition of the importance of the issues raised, the topic has been a major growth area giving rise to new legislation, new and active pressure groups and a recognition of increasing problems which have arisen, many as the result of new technologies coming into being.

As a result there was the creation of the Department of the Environment in 1970 which included a Central Pollution Unit. This was followed also in 1970 by the appointment of a standing Royal Commission on Environmental Pollution. Subsequently the UK became more closely involved with the EEC and was under pressure to adopt their more positive and rigorous anti pollution measures, with in 1973 the adoption of the European Community Programme of Action on the Environment. In 1974 as we all know virtually everything was reorganised. This included Local Government, River Boards and Water Authorities. The changes included the establishment within Local Authorities of the Environmental Health Inspectorate which replaced the old Public Health Inspectors and the creation of Regional Water Authorities with full responsibility for the complete hydrological cycle including all water pollution and sewerage disposal control.

The control of Pollution Act was introduced in 1974 which was an attempt both to improve and draw together all anti-pollution legislation. The following year saw the passing of the Health and Safety at Work Act which encompassed such separate bodies as the Alkali Inspectorate and the Factory Inspectorate.

This was the position as regards pollution control until in December 1986 when the Department of the Environment published a consultative paper, Air Pollution Control in Great Britain — Review and Proposals. Whilst the reference is specifically to Air Pollution Control the consultative paper also includes other matters of pollution including noise.

The paper was passed to interested bodies for examination and comment. The distribution included the Institute of Hospital Engineering and the Council considered the draft in January/February 1987 and have now made comments to the Department of the Environment.

The summary of the Draft Proposals are (quoting from the Department of Environment accompanying letter)

(i) To retain the principle of control through the use of best practical means but to clarify its breadth of application and allow its use to be adapted to take account of existing and proposed EEC legislation.

(ii) To give Local Authorities powers of control including prior approval over certain processes including some 'offensive' trades.

(iii) To provide a system of 'consents' accessible to the public which will set out the main elements of BPM agreed by the control authorities.

(iv) To improve public access to information about air pollution control.

(v) To make certain changes to the Clean Air Acts 1956 and 1968, the Control of Pollution Act 1974 and the Public Health Acts.

These additional measures when combined with the removal of Crown Immunity may well have considerable effect on the NHS. This is particularly so when it is appreciated that if the changes proposed to present legislation come into being, hospital incinerators will be one of the scheduled processes. In addition it is proposed that revised legislation will include furnaces (ie boilers) which burn waste or waste derived fuels as the alternative to the basic fuel.

The scheduling of NHS incinerators will place both installers and operators under a statutory obligation to meet the required terms of the BPM agreement. The extent to which this duty was carried out would be publicly demonstrated by the terms of consent and by subsequent monitoring of results both of which would be in the public domain.

The Consent System

Best Practical Means would be retained as the basis of air pollution control. Operators of plants included under the proposed two part schedule would be under an obligation to employ (to the satisfaction of the control authority) BPM for

LE CONTRÔLE DE LA POLLUTION

L'auteur presente et decrit les methodes pour le contrôle de la pollution qui s'appliquent aux incinerateurs dans les hôpitaux ainsi qu'aux chaudières.

preventing emission into the atmosphere of any harmful or offensive substances and for rendering harmless and inoffensive any substance that may be emitted. In this connection it should be noted that it is proposed that hospital incinerators will be scheduled processes.

There is the probability of a charge being levied for consents by Local Authorities and the National Inspectorate. The proposals are to apply the new legislation to new plant, existing plant which is substantially modified and existing plant brought back into use following closure for 12 months or longer. It is not expected that retrospective legislation will be applied provided the plant is not already the subject of complaint. However it is expected that the Inspectorate and the plant operator (the DHA) will negotiate and conclude an agreement on the BPM appropriate to the process. It is proposed that this approach will be adopted when introducing the new consent system for existing plants coming within the orbit of the new schedules.

For existing plants which become subject to the new legislation the duty to use BPM would apply and it would be an offence to operate without consent. Owners of processes will be required to notify the controlling authority of each scheduled process within a specified time — three months is suggested, of new legislation coming into force.

The appropriate Authority would then issue a provisional consent which would in effect confirm that the plant had been noted as a scheduled process. Full consent would be given once the required BPM for the process had been agreed. There would also be provision for such consents to be made publicly available.

Other Proposed Changes

Proposals are made to amend existing air pollution legislation when the opportunity arises. This would indicate amending the Clean Air Acts in respect of gaseous emissions. At present the Acts specifically cover grit and dust control with provision to extend the regulations to include fumes. Concern has been expressed that the burning of certain fuels may give rise to harmful gaseous emissions.

It is proposed to include incinerators, large furnaces and those specially designed to burn waste and waste derived fuels in the new schedules with all other combustion processes continuing to be controlled via the Clean Air Acts.

Proposed Schedules and the Application to NHS Premises

Examination of the proposals with regard to revised scheduling shows that no NHS premises will come under the Schedule 'A'; which is in general confined to manufacturing process plants.

It is possible that plants designed for the incineration of toxic and dangerous wastes which are included under Schedule 'A' may be affected but the current proposals are to retain the present Inspectorate's schedule and include all hospital incinerators under Schedule 'B'. No NHS premises would come under the category of 'Offensive Trades'.

Boiler plant unless used with the burning of waste and waste derived fuels appears to remain under the aegis of the Clean Air Act.

Hospital Incinerators are however to be included under Schedule 'B'. This will include incinerators whether or not on NHS premises which dispose of toxic and dangerous wastes.

Other Proposed Changes to Existing Legislation

Clean Air Acts

Consideration is being given to legislation to ease enforcement problems. It would be an offence to burn any material where combustion necessarily gives rise to dark smoke; allowing prosecution not only of the occupier (presumably the DHA in the case of NHS premises) but also of any persons who cause or permit dark smoke to be emitted — this would presumably include incinerator operators. The definition of 'premises' would include open land.

Public Health Act

It is proposed to retain the statutory nuisances provisions of the Act to 'sweep in' all processes which are not scheduled or covered by the requirements of the Clean Air Acts. This will also include domestic nuisance. Subject to Crown Immunity being revoked it is assumed this would include NHS residential accommodation.

It is proposed to amend Part III of the Act to give Local Authorities power — similar to that in the Control of Pollution Act, to deal with noise nuisance — to take action in *anticipation* of a statutory nuisance occurring. It is considered under the proposals that such a power may be appropriate to deal with specific transient nuisances such as demolitions.

It is also proposed to streamline procedures for abatement of nuisance actions similar to that in COPA for noise, which would effectively remove the need for Courts to serve a nuisance order.

It would make the defence of BPM available in all summary proceedings relating to businesses and trades including Water Authorities — although not specifically stated it is assumed this would also apply to the NHS.

It would also oblige Local Authorities to have regard to any relevant Code of Practice that the Secretary of State may issue or approve.

It also makes it clear that the term effluvia will cover odour nuisance.

It will also give Local Authorities default powers to clear accumulation of rubbish and to then reclaim repayment for the clearance.

Finally it will give LAs powers to deal with nuisances from sewerage treatment works.

Comments Arising from the Proposals

The major concern is what will constitute Best Practical Means for pollution control. For example with incinerators, which it appears are likely to be the plant most affected, some EHOs appear satisfied with assurances that the plant complies with the Clean Air Act, is adequate for its purpose and will satisfy the legislation. Others appear to take a far more rigid approach and in one case where local complaints as regards emissions have been raised an EHO suggested in all seriousness that consideration should be given to a gas washer being installed.

The question of BPM is considered further in later sections of the paper but it is obvious that there will be a need for national guidance to ensure common standards are applied.

In addition there is a need for guidance as to who will be responsible for monitoring plant performance. For example will it be the responsibility of the operating authority to prove the plant complies or will the Local Inspectorate have to prove the plants fail to comply? It is doubtful whether any Health Authority has easy access to emission measuring equipment or indeed has the expertise to operate such plant correctly. Similarly it is very doubtful if any Local Authority has the equipment or ability to carry out its own monitoring. It is known from recent experience that the cost of employing a specialist company to carry out such an exercise and to prepare the report would be in the order of £5,000 per test. The question then arises as to who pays? It is surely unfair and unreasonable to expect a Health Authority to fund such an exercise, possibly as the result of a local complaint or even on the whim of an EHO? The obvious answer would seem to be the Health Authority if the plant is shown to be performing badly and the LA if the tests prove satisfactory. This is a further example of many unanswered questions in the proposals.

Similarly reference is made to 'harmful gaseous emissions' without defining what constitutes a harmful emission. For example will such emissions consider health hazards only or will a positive odour which is perfectly safe but perhaps unpleasant constitute a harmful emission?

There is also concern that Part III of the proposed legislation will cover general nuisance which will include noise and transient nuisance such as that occurring with demolitions. Unless common standards are agreed and applied, problems are likely which could have considerable financial implications particularly with regard to building operations and the operation of standby generator plant.

The proposals will also give Local Authorities the power to remove accumulated rubbish and levy a charge for so doing. This could lead to further problems because if a consent to operate an incinerator is withheld it is likely to lead to some accumulation of waste but as we know Local Authorities are very reluctant to handle hospital waste. Again if the waste is transported to an alternative incinerator a far greater hazard would arise from local incineration even if the plant does perhaps leave something to be desired as regards its performance. There are several similar cases where it must be hoped more positive guidance will be given before revised legislation becomes enforceable.

Review of Best Practical Means

Consideration of Best Practical Means must be one of the major points to be debated before the revisions come into force. It is perhaps opportune to review existing methods of limiting both particulate and gaseous emissions and consider also the likely costs involved in applying such means.

Factors Influencing Plant Selection

Apart from the requirement to meet local legislation and the interpretation of what constitutes Best Practical Means other factors influencing the choice of emission control plant are:-

(1) Type and analysis of the auxiliary fuel used.
(2) Constituents of the waste to be incinerated.
(3) Method of firing and type of plant with its likely effect on dust characteristics and particle size distribution.
(4) Required performance relative to local conditions and the application of legislation.
(5) Equipment type and location.
(6) Dust disposal arrangements.

Selection of Emission Control Plant

Until the proposals to review legislation, capital costs of the plant to be used probably received the greatest consideration.

With the higher standards of control proposed it is likely that the following factors will require greater consideration:-

(1) Efficiency of the equipment and its ability to meet local requirements.
(2) Low resistance to gas flow — the resistance to flow will affect fan power and consequently revenue costs.
(3) Small space requirements.
(4) Low operating and maintenance costs.
(5) Low capital costs.

There are, of course, many designs of emission control equipment available, all of which suffer from disadvantages. It is likely that to meet legislation changes it will be necessary, unless national standards are agreed, to compromise between costs and efficiency of control. Common types of equipment available and comment on their performance is as follows:-

Inertia Separators

A typical example is shown on Sketch No. 1A.

The advantages are:-

Low initial cost
Easy installation
Very low resistance to gas flow (not requiring auxiliary fans)
Very limited space requirement
Satisfactory efficiency over the range of larger size particles (generally in the range of 40 microns plus)

The disadvantages are:-

It will not collect smaller particles
It is useless as regards elimination of smoke particles, chemical emissions or odours.
Its efficiency is influenced by particle density and the sail area of particles.
It is unsuitable for use with high stack velocities and thus cannot be used on plant fitted with mechanical draught.
The type of unit shown is normally only suitable for use with steel stacks.

Collectors Operating by Centrifugal Action

These include conventional cyclones, combined fan and cyclone and multi tubular collectors, typical examples are shown on Sketch No. 1B, 2A and B and 3.

The units offer improved efficiency over the inertia separator but again are ineffective as regards smoke, chemical emissions or odours.

They are completely satisfactory as regards collection of solids with multi tubular collectors offering efficiencies in the order of 99.5% on particles of 330 microns plus. There is however a rapid fall off of efficiency with reduction of particle size below 30 microns.

All the plants shown require auxiliary fan power to operate and efficiency depends to a large extent on the operating pressure drop through the unit. Resistance in the order of 75mm WG are typical, giving a fan horse-power in the order of 5Hp on large incinerator installations.

Electrostatic Precipitators

These units will give the ultimate in dust collection efficiency, particularly as regards the collection of solids. It is not proposed to give details on the construction and operation of a precipitator in this paper other than to state the unit operates at high voltage and basically consists of a series of electrodes suspended in either an earthed tube or between earth plates. It is usual to use electrodes negatively charged with the collecting tube or plate positive.

The advantages of a precipitator are:-

(1) high efficiencies maintained over the complete particle size range particularly on smaller particles below 10 microns.
(2) The high efficiencies are maintained irrespective of load variation or changes in the gas volume passed through the unit.
(3) Very low resistance to gas flow (12-15mm WG being typical) which reduces considerably auxiliary fan power compared to mechanical collectors.

The principal disavantages are:-

(1) High capital cost mainly due to the complexity of the electrical auxiliary components necessary.

Diagram No 1
Inertia and Cylone Type Separators

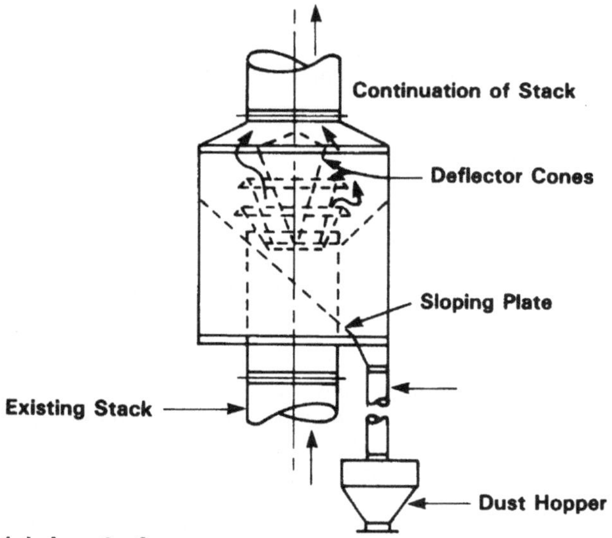

(a) Inertia Separator

Pressure Loss ¼" WG. Suitable for Small Handfired Boilers

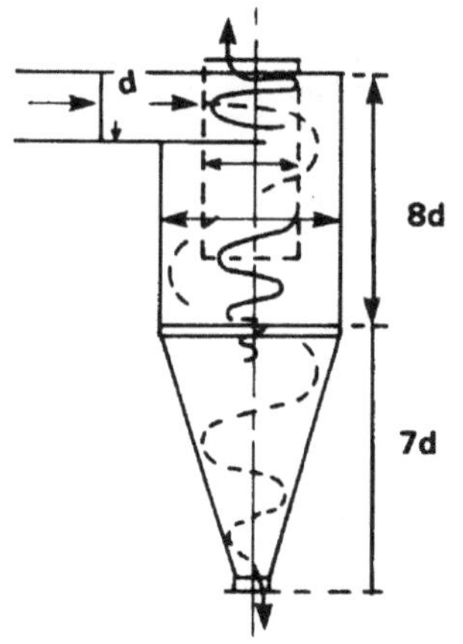

(b) Standard Cyclone. Some Units are fitted with Outlet Scroll for Static Regain. Suitable for small plants as dimensions are large in comparison to gas volume handled. Pressure loss 2" – 3" WG

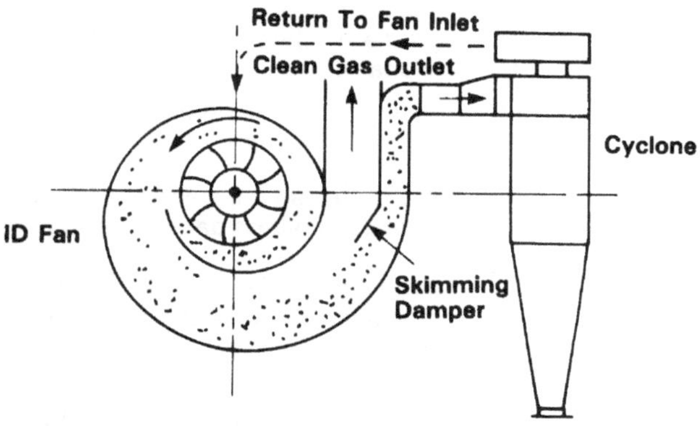

(c) Combined Fan and Grit Arrestor

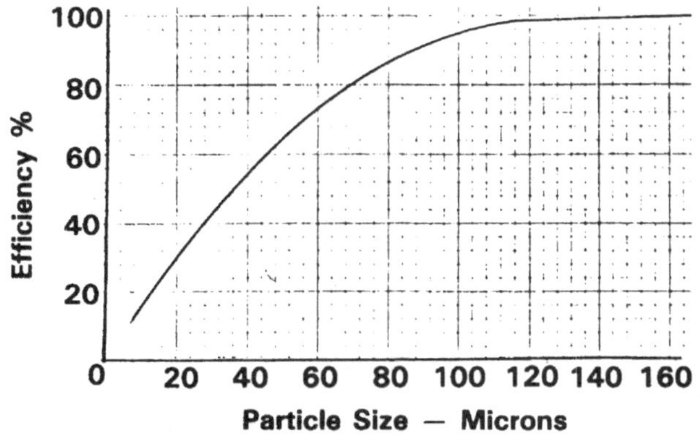

(d) Efficiency Curve for Combined ID Fan and Grit Arrestor

Diagram No 2A/B
Tubular Dust Collector

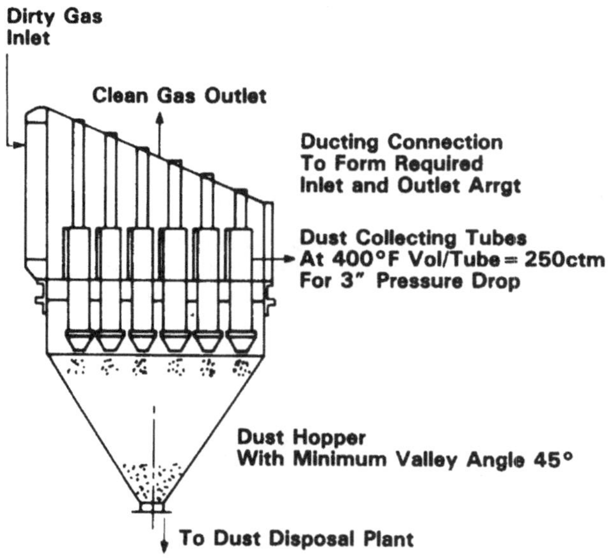

(a) Typical Multitubular Dust Collector Arrgt

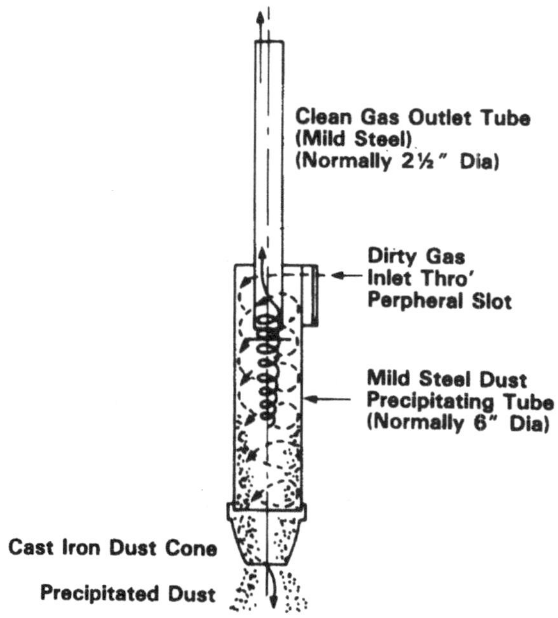

(b) Detail of Single Tube Showing Gas and Dust Paths

Diagram No 3
Special Form of Tubular Collector

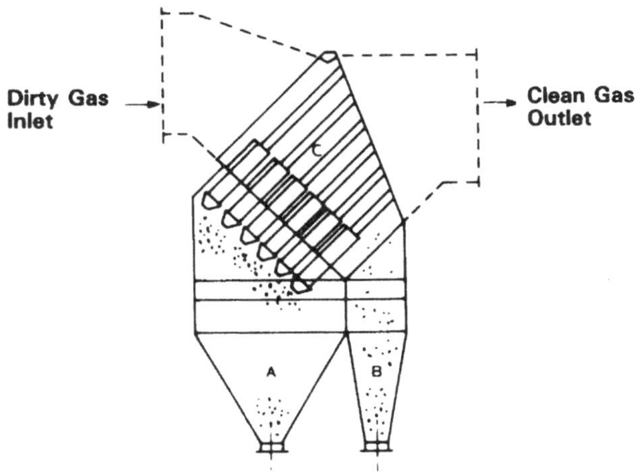

A. Fine dust hopper. Dust being separated via the dust collecting tubes.
B. Coarse dust hopper. Dust is separated by decantation.
C. Standard tube bank.
The simplest method of arranging inlet and outlet ducting is shown in dotted line.

(a) Typical Arrgt of Decantation Type Multitubular Dust Collector.

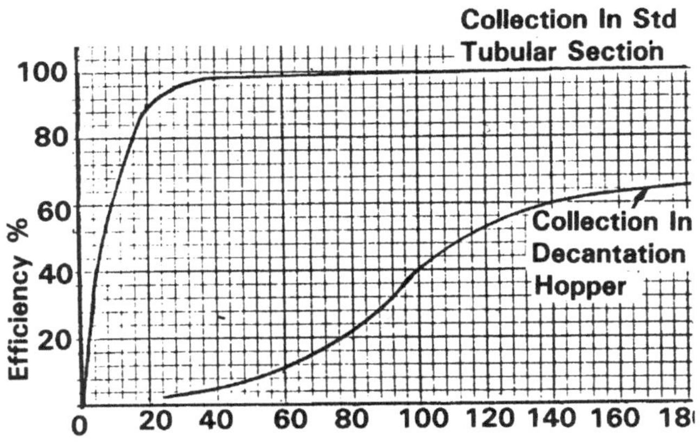

(b) Efficiency Curve for Decantation Collector Showing 'Cut' which can be expected

Simple Precipitator Layout

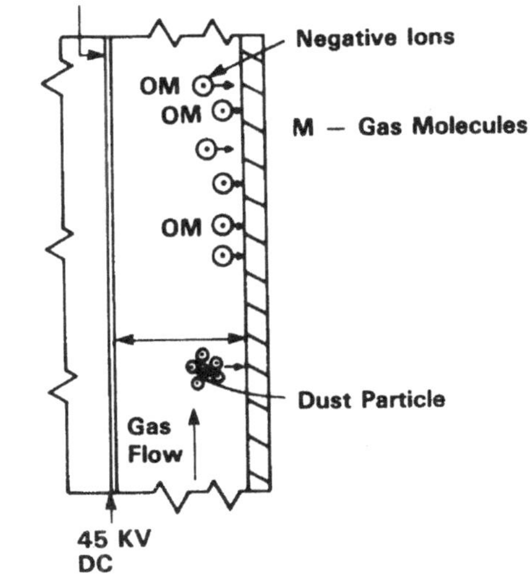

Fp = KQE
Q = Developing Electrical Charge on Each Particle
E = Strength of Electrical Field Between HV and Earthed Electrode
K = Constant
Fp = Developing Precipitating Force

Section On A-A
Showing Particle Charging Phenomena

Diagram No 4
Electrostatic Collector

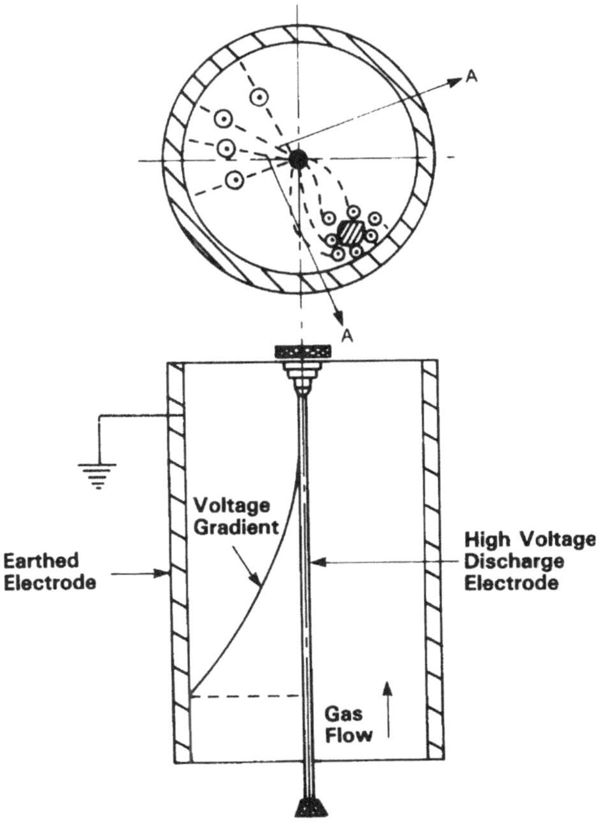

Simple Pipe Precipitator

(2) Large installation space requirements.
(3) Some liability to electrical overloading and therefore flashovers.
(4) Possibility of electrical failure.
(5) High electrical consumption.

It of course suffers from the same disadvantage as all plants so far considered in that it cannot remove chemical emissions nor eliminate odours.

Bag Filters

Whilst these units offer high collection efficiency and can remove some chemical emissions, dependent upon the type of filter material used, there are problems in obtaining a suitable filter cloth which will withstand high gas temperatures without prohibitive costs.

A further disadvantage is a rapid fall off in efficiency as the bags become dirty. There are in situ cleaning methods in use such as reverse jet cleaning but these are costly and difficult to maintain.

Gas Washing

Gas washing plant is probably the only system which will guarantee to remove all stack discharges including chemical emissions and odours. It is known that many Environmental Health Officers consider this is likely to require to be fitted to meet the revised legislation.

The usual form which would be used for limited emission would be the cleaning tower. This usually takes the form of a vertical tower with banks of sprays uniformly distributed across the area to ensure full gas passage coverage. The usual air velocity is in the order of 10 m/s with spray water around 5 litres/min/sq m of cross section.

The factor which makes the major contribution to removal of air impurities is the properly designed scrubber and eliminating surfaces. These must ensure that maximum scrubbing area is available and that moisture is properly removed before final discharge. The principle of operation is to wet the particles as thoroughly as possible thus increasing their density and then removing them from the air stream via the eliminator plates.

The washer requires a settling tank and a filtering system to permit water recirculation.

Commercial systems available are of three main types — the spray type, wet scrubber and combined spray and scrubber.

It is possible to add chemical neutralisers where chemicals or odours are present.

It will be appreciated that corrosion can be a problem especially, for example, where flue gases contain sulphur. In consequence plant protection and treatment can be costly. Resistance to gas flow is also high and in consequence auxiliary fan power is costly. The capital cost of the plant with its auxiliaries such as settling tanks is high. There is of course a continuing maintenance problem as regards cleaning of the plant, in particular of the settlement tanks, unless costly and complex automatic cleaning can be included.

Selection of Plant

Although with the proposed changes to legislation there may well be a requirement to meet a given criteria as regards acceptable emissions, it is likely that the choice of plant will be a compromise between its efficiency, its capital cost and revenue charges. The performance of the collection system is dependent upon the particle sizing and characteristics of the material presented to the collector.

Diagram No. 5 illustrates typical particle sizing curves for various types of incinerator plant. These curves are the result of investigations into plant performance carried out by the author prior to joining the NHS. It is considered that the curve likely to compare most accurately with typical NHS incinerators is that given for a Veterinary Laboratory. The material incinerated was typical of that found in an Acute Hospital analysis and comprised packaging material, animal feeds, bedding (principally straw) and carcases which would be typical of clinical and anatomical wastes. The main characteristic is that some 90% of the ash produced, which would be present in the plant discharge, would be

Diagram No 5
Typical Dust Analysis Curves — Incinerator Plants
Sampling at Incinerator Outlet Flue prior to dust extraction where fitted.
Average dust loading 56 grains/com (4.75 grs/cuft) A & NTP

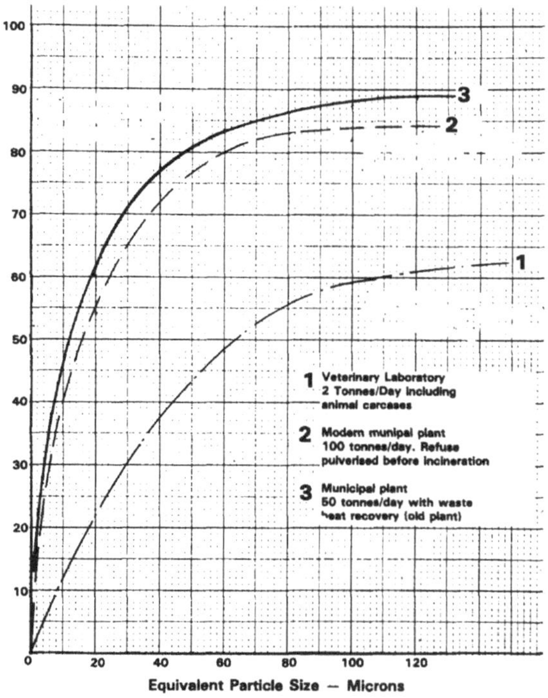

below 120 microns. Diagram No. 6A details the collection efficiency to be expected from the various types of collection equipment discussed in this paper. Based on this data Diagram No. 6B has been prepared which illustrates comparative costs of the various types of dust collection plant. This comparison is based on an assumption of unity cost for a plant giving 50% collection efficiency on the stated dust sizing. It will be appreciated that, with fluctuating costs the general market uncertainty coupled with fluctuating costs and general market uncertainty coupled with individual site peculiarities, it is not possible to quote actual prices but none the less the diagram illustrates typical comparisons for an average site. The comparative cost includes for auxiliary fans, interconnecting ductwork and auxiliary equipment.

Running costs and general revenue charges are difficult to predict because of the large variations in running and operating times and the method of incineration adopted. On all plants, except for the simple inertia separators, there will be an ongoing commitment for regular plant cleaning and for final disposal of the collected material. It will also be understood that it is a complex process to establish chemical emissions which requires specialist knowledge and equipment to complete. Whilst all the systems described and evaluated offer reasonable efficiencies as regards collection of particulate matter, only a gas scrubber will remove chemical emissions. Naturally none can be guaranteed to remove odours as many of these will occur during charging and can persist following plant shutdown. Experience also indicates that odours can emanate from material awaiting incineration.

However, the proposed legislative changes do emphasise that the requirement is to employ Best Practical Means which is likely to lead to protracted discussion on its interpretation.

DIAGRAM NO 6A

Data Including Collection Efficiency on Which Cost v Efficiency Chart (Diagram No 6B) is Based

Dust Grading		Inertia Separator Press Drop 0.3" WG		Combined Fan & Cyclone PD of Cyclone 2.5" WG		Multitubular Coll Press Drop 3" WG		Electrostatic Precip Press Drop 0.5" WG		West Scrubber Press Drop 10" WG	
Size μ	% Present	Effiency %	Catch	Effiency %	Catch	Effiency %	Catch	Effiency %	Catch	Effiency %	Catch
200μ+	29	100	29	100	29	100	29	100	29	100	29
150	4	100	4	100	4	100	4	100	4	100	4
100	11	90	9.9	96	10.6	100	11	100	11	100	11
80	6	85	5.1	88	5.3	100	6	100	6	100	6
70	3.5	75	2.63	80	2.8	100	3.5	100	3.5	100	3.5
60	4.0	58	2.31	75	3.0	100	4.0	100	4.0	100	4.0
50	3.5	42	1.47	64	2.24	100	3.5	100	3.5	100	3.5
40	6.0	32	1.92	55	3.3	99.8	5.98	100	6.0	100	6.0
30	6.0	26	1.56	43	2.59	99.5	5.91	100	6.0	100	6.0
20	7.0	15	1.05	30	2.10	95.0	6.65	100	7.0	100	7.0
10	8.0	4	0.32	16	1.28	70.0	5.62	100	8.0	100	8.0
5	5.0	—	—	5	0.25	42.5	2.13	98	4.9	99	4.95
Below 5	7.0	—	—	—	—	24.5	1.71	91	6.36	97	6.79
Totals	100		59.16		66.46		89.0		99.26		99.74

Diagram No 6B
Cost v Efficiency Based On Units Handling 1000cm/min

Comparison Cost of Plant Supplied and Installed

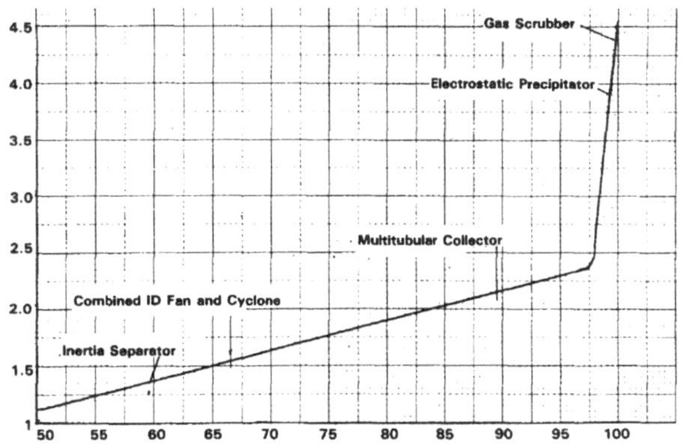

Collection Efficiency based on Data given on Diagram No 6A

In conclusion it is hoped that this paper will have drawn attention to the potential future problems assuming the proposed changes become law, the various factors to be considered in deciding upon the most suitable plant to provide BPM, and will provide some assistance to those of us who will be faced with arguing our corner with the Environmental Health Departments in the future.

Clinical Waste Disposal in the NHS

by

L. W. M. Arrowsmith
Assistant Director and Chief Engineer
Department of Health

Press reportage will have given the impression of far from adequate waste management within the NHS, with incidents of contaminated waste finding its way on to rubbish tips where local children play, of medical records which should have been incinerated turning up in some very unusual places and of complaints about smoke emissions from NHS incinerators. Whilst such incidents are far from commonplace, they are, nevertheless, of considerable concern.

Much of the blame has been laid at the door of NHS Crown immunity, although this was removed from some aspects of the waste handling and disposal process in such legislation as the Health and Safety at Work and NHS (Amendment) Acts. Perhaps the most contentious aspect of Crown immunity relates to incinerator flue — gas emissions; although, under Section 22 of the Clean Air Act 1956, Ministers are required to investigate complaints and this is done and results in action by the health authority concerned.

Until the current proposals, however, the essential legislative requirements which had to be satisfied were the Clean Air Acts 1956 and 1968 and enabling statutory instruments.

Notwithstanding Crown immunity, Ministers have required the health service to comply with the spirit of the Clean Air legislation and current published guidelines such as the Department of Environment's Waste Management Paper 25 'Clinical Wastes', and performance standards given in British Standard 3316. The impending legislation and regulations are likely to bring much change to the policies, processes and management of waste disposal in the NHS.

One of the difficulties in considering current legislative and regulatory developments is the variety of changes taking place and their relative timescales. The major points to examine are the new Environmental Protection Bill, the Best Practicable Means regulations on air pollution, being drawn — up by the Department of the Environment and HMIP, the projected revision of WMP 25 and the loss of Crown Immunity in the NHS.

Currently, the majority of clinical waste is disposed of on-site by incineration, and increasing pressures on existing facilities have led, in some cases, to short term solutions. Contracting out clinical waste for disposal off-site has become more frequent with, in a few cases, some very unsatisfactory results.

A cursory assessment of existing clinical waste disposal facilities in each region and district quickly highlights the scale of the problem facing the NHS, particularly as incineration is to remain the principal means of safe disposal. The Department's data as yet unvalidated, is sufficient to indicate that on age grounds alone the efficiency of some plant is questionable: 63% of reported installations are 10 years old or more and 20% exceed 20 years of age.

Many will not meet the minimum requirements for licencing and others will do so only if operation and maintenance procedures are greatly improved. Some will almost certainly prove impossible to modify to meet the new flue — gas emission regulations. To meet the requirements of new legislation the health service has, therefore, to look at a major incinerator upgrading or replacement programme or alternative means of access to clinical waste incineration or other safe disposal.

Overlying all these considerations is the 'Duty of Care' concept in the Environmental Protection Bill which places a clear 'cradle to the grave' responsibility on generators of waste to ensure its safe, lawful disposal. Ministers in the Department of Health have already indicated, on behalf of NHS managers, acceptance in principle of this duty.

Under the new guidelines health authorities will also be required to obtain licences for incinerator installations, though some have already done so on a solely voluntary basis. This will involve:-

Notification of existing plant to the inspectorate, either HMIP or local authority Environmental Health Officers,
Licensing and authorisation of plant prior to operation,
Designation of a 'Responsible Officer',
Supervision of plant operation and staff training, and
Obtaining planning approval, which will include making environmental impact assessments.

The new emission controls are currently still under the familiar banner 'Best Practicable Means' or 'BPM'. The sixth draft has recently been the subject of consultation with the industry. Clearly a major consideration in any upgrading or replacement proposals will be how quickly the industry can respond and one hopes that HMIP will bear this in mind when setting timescales. When these new regulations are published it is likely that they will rejoice in the European title 'Best Available Technology Not Entailing Excessive Costs' and the latest draft, number 8, indicates this, Mercifully, however, the acronym 'Batneec' should quickly find its way into common usage.

It is difficult to comment on the revision of WMP 25 at this stage as this will take some time — suffice it to say that this too will be a factor which the health service will need to bear very much in mind.

As to Crown immunity, the new NHS Bill seeks to abolish it totally in the NHS although a further provision would empower the Secretary of State for Health by order made by statutory instrument to exclude or modify the appropriate subsection to the extent specified in the order. It is unlikely however, that this power would be used save in the most exceptional of circumstances and, in any case, the Environmental Protection Bill will also seek to remove Crown immunity.

Before considering possible responses, it is worth

EVACUATION DES DECHETS CLINIQUES — PRATIQUES DU NATIONAL HEALTH SERVICE

Cet article prèsente les implications des nouvelles lois prévues sur la gestion et les dispositions générales concernant l'évacuation des déchets cliniques dans les éstablissements de soins de santé.

Ce qui concerne au premier chef la NHS est la ségrégation initiale de ces déchets, puis les options permettant une évacuation sans danger, la gestion et les opérations d'installations sur place, et la formation des personnels techniques et de surveillance. Il s'agira aussi des capacités techniques des éstablissements qui leur permettront le cas échéant d'être mises à niveau selon les nouvelles normes BMP/BATNEEC (Moyens pratiques maximalisés/Rentabilité maximum pour niveau de technologie disponible).

Les avantages issue d'une installation sur place bien gérée, avec recouvrement de chaleur seront examinés dans l'article, ainsi que les occasions de génération de revenus. Ceux-ci seront comparés à ceux qui accompagnent généralement l'évacuation de déchets commerciale.

Une étude systématique des politiques annexes comprendra l'acquisition de matériels à jeter visant à faire diminuer le quantité de matières plastique dans les déchets, les projects d'installations en commun, les capitaux et les dépenses.

considering the question as to whether the NHS has been wrong-footed. To some extent this may be true but since the installation of some of the oldest incinerators there has been a significant change in the procurement of health care devices. For reasons of efficiency and as a result of GMP there has been a move from recycling sterile products to the widespread use of disposable items, for example sharps (syringes and needles), fluid containers etc. Many of these products, with the current focus on environmental issues pose significant problems for incinerator design and operation by the very nature of their materials of construction.

Clearly, NHS General Managers will need to review urgently their waste disposal arrangements. Health authorities are faced with the responsibility for the disposal of waste arising from health care premises, domestic, clinical and community medicine.

Segregation is of critical concern. Regardless of how well managed and careful the waste handling procedure, it is unrealistic to expect correct segregation of waste at all times given the immediate pressures of nursing and other clinical care. Correctly colour coded clinical waste can include a portion of domestic waste and vice versa. Therefore, it may be that in the future all waste arising from medical areas should best be deemed 'clinical'.

The waste arising from dedicated administration blocks, kitchen and industrial areas of hospital premises would continue to be classified as 'domestic'. There remains 'special' clinical waste, the handling and supervision of which is covered by regulations on hazardous waste, for example under the Control of Substances Hazardous to Health Act.

The management of the waste stream, both clinical and domestic, from source to disposal affects policy, procedure, operation and many hospital personnel. Any review of waste disposal policy would need, therefore, to consider:-

Under policy:
Application of 'duty of care',
Method of disposal, and
Procurement of disposable equipment and products.
Under procedure:
Segregation,
On-site collection and transport, and
Training.
Under operations:
On-site incineration and
Transport off-site.
Under the role of personnel, the duties of:
The general manager,
The 'responsible officer',
The medical and nursing staff,
The collection and transport staff, and
The supervisory and operational staff.

Equally, consideration must be given to the need for capital and/or revenue resource allocation. General management have to consider the best use of resources to achieve patient care. Waste arising is a consequence of that care but disposal may be judged to be outwith the hospital remit and a low priority for capital resourcing. Some authorities may therefore consider unconventional financing or private sector disposal.

Two aspects of Government policy have a bearing on the strategic implications and option appraisal.

There is no single solution to waste disposal in the NHS but the current management structures were created precisely to deal with such problems. It will clearly be appropriate for management to hold in mind when considering their strategies, not only the responsibility to meet the new legislation and regulations, but also the Government's concern to see the private sector utilised by the NHS, either directly or in synergy.

Equally, incineration is a large consumer of energy and, in line with the real public and Parliamentary concern for 'green' issues, shared by Ministers in the Department of Health, some thought should be given to on-site heat recovery in addition to generally using processes which combined safe disposal with maximum energy efficiency.

NHS managers will also need to consider appropriate strategic areas. No two Regions are the same, nor any two Districts. In some cases for example, a whole — Region strategy may be appropriate, in others one applying to a group of, or even a single District may be indicated. The Department is aware, for example, of at least one Region which has given preliminary consideration to a Regional waste disposal strategy but concluded that this would present very substantial difficulties and they may be forced to look to other strategic alternatives. In another Region, a joint venture with a private contractor is being considered.

There is no single option, either on method or strategy that the Department of Health favours over any other, however, costs will strongly influence the final decision and local conditions will weigh in the selection process. Each option will have to be examined carefully, taking into account full cost analysis, capital investment, depreciation, revenue costs, energy savings and the potential for income generation. Whatever option is selected the General Manager will retain responsibility under the 'Duty of Care' requirements.

The essential need for proper option appraisal is self evident. Option appraisal exercises should address all aspects of disposal. The assessment of the quantity and type of waste generated within the unit, District or Region may need to be extended to cover potential income generation for example, inter-authority, private health care, local authorities or commercial organisations within the community.

Some of the options presented by a decision to finance the upgrading to full requirements, or replacement of existing plant, within the NHS might be:-

a hospital or District financed incinerator facility with or without heat recovery;
a co-partnership, joint financed incinerator facility with other health authorities;
provision of a site for the Private Sector to develop and manage;
health authority provision and development of a site with a private contract for operation; or
a Regional incinerator facility with or without heat recovery and income generation.

Contracting out similarly presents alternatives, such as letting contracts:-

to another health authority or Regional facility; or
to the private sector for disposal off-site.

If contracting out, Authorities would have to take account of transport; in all cases a 'consignment system' would be operated. Where inter-authority contracts were awarded and hospital transport used, dedicated vehicles would be necessary.

To achieve the levels of performance and emission standards required, incinerator facilities will involve complex combustion and treatment plant possible with heat recovery. Waste burning boilers may prove to be suitable and cost effective alternative provided the requirements of BPM can be met.

A further consideration will be the training which will be essential for supervisory and operation staff of an on-site facility. Indeed, an element of training of supervisory staff should be included in any 'unconventional finance' or private sector option. The extent of training is not yet determined but the objective would be to ensure that best practice procedures, applies to plant performance, will achieve satisfactory combustion, monitoring and recording of test results and emission criteria.

It is clear, therefore, that the NHS faces a substantial but necessary task over the next few years but nevertheless it is one which Parliament and public expect to be carried out.

Printed by Holbrook & Son Ltd., Norway Road, Hilsea, Portsmouth